Dispensing Pharmacy

A Practical Manual

Third Edition

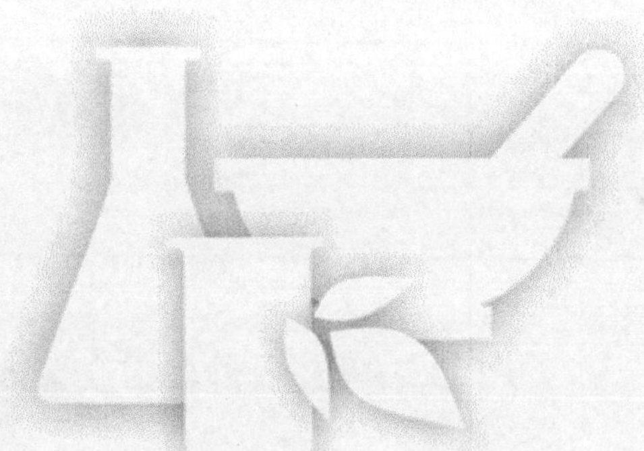

Dispensing Pharmacy

A Practical Manual

Third Edition

Sanmathi. B. S.
M.Pharm.
Assistant Professor
Dept. of Pharmaceutics,
B.S.Anangpuria Institute of Pharmacy
Faridabad, Haryana.
E-Mail ID: sanmathibs@rediffmail.com

Kalpesh K. Mehta
M.Pharm.
Dept. of Pharmaceutics,
S.K. Patel College of Pharmaceutical
Education and Research,
Ganpat University.
Kherva-Mehsana - 382711. Gujarat.
E-Mail ID: kk30180@yahoo.com

Anshu Gupta
Associate Professor and H.O.D,
Dept. of Pharmaceutics,
Swift School of Pharmacy,
Rajpura.
Dist : Patiala
Punjab.

PharmaMed Press
An imprint of BSP Books Pvt. Ltd.
4-4-309/316, Giriraj Lane,
Sultan Bazar, Hyderabad - 500 095.

Dispensing Pharmacy_A Practical Manual *by* **Sanmathi B S, Kalpesh K Mehta and Anshu Gupta**

Seventh Reprint 2025

Published by:

PharmaMed Press
An imprint of BSP Books Pvt. Ltd.
4-4-309/316, Giriraj Lane, Sultan Bazar, Hyderabad - 500 095.
Phone: 040-23445688; Fax: 91+40-23445611
E-mail: info@pharmamedpress.com
www.pharmamedpress.com/pharmamedpress.net

Printed at
Repro India Limited.

Price : Rs. 895.00

ISBN : 978-81-88449-23-1 (Paperback)

Foreword

There are very few books covering most of the practical aspects of Dispensing Pharmacy. A need for such a book written in a simple, direct, lucid and relevant language was appropriately realized. The combined efforts of Mrs. Sanmathi B.S., Mr. Kalpesh K.Mehta, and Anshu Gupta have resulted in publication of this practical book covering the syllabus.

The book gives an overview and insight at the same time. This book has 52 chapters dealing with full of practical illustrations of different dosage forms along with their introduction, Latin term, conversion of Latin term to English, calculation, theory, procedure, dispensing, labeling, category, similar examples, marketed preparation and student exercises.

The subject matter is written with adequate practical and theoretical background and presented in a simple manner for better understanding among the student community.

I hope that, you as a reader, whether you are a student, or a teacher would be pleased, for this book, which should certainly add to your current knowledge, understanding and insights of the practicals.

It is a matter of immense pleasure for me to write a foreward for this book. I wish the authors a great success in this combined venture and hope that their contribution to pharmacy literature will continue endlessly.

N. R. Dave
Ex-Vice Chanceller,
Hemchandracharya North Gujarat University.

Preface to Third Edition

The second edition of this book was well received by the faculty members and the students of various colleges across India and have encourage us to present the third edition with some more experiments, students exercises, figures, marketed products and better readability.

We added aromatic waters, spirits and tinctures in this book and made the book more comprehensive.

We sincerely hope that this new edition will receive appreciations from the academic fraternity.

- Authors

Preface to Second Edition

The immense popularity of the first edition of this book by the faculty members and the students of various colleges across India has encourage us to present the second edition with some more experiments, students exercises, figures, marketed products and better readability.

We are grateful to our colleague and students all over the country for their valuable suggestions and recommendation of the book to their students.

It would be our pleasure for any suggestion and critics in improving the content of the book.

- Authors

Preface to First Edition

Dispensing pharmacy is one of the ancient branch of pharmacy, which deals mainly with the principles of art, science and technology of converting drugs into dosage forms, while dispensing to the patients.

Now-a-days most of the drugs are available in the market as pre-fabricated dosage forms, still students should learn the techniques and skills, which are essential to prepare various pharmaceutical dosage forms.

A number of practical manuals are available for Dispensing pharmacy, but practical aspects like, understanding of Latin terms, conversion and calculation of prescriptions given in Latin, packing (dispensing) techniques, labeling instructions required, for different dosage forms etc., are not found in a single manual. Hence an attempt for the same has been done in this manual.

Certain salient features of this manual are,

- The manual has been mainly divided into four chapters as Liquid, Semisolid, Solid dosage forms and Pharmaceutical incompatibilities.
- Altogether 165 experiments are included in this manual. As per the syllabus, minimum 100 experiments should be covered in the practical of pharmaceutics (Dispensing Pharmacy), which will give the better choice for teachers to select the experiments, depending on the availability of chemical ingredients and time.
- Each chapter begins with a brief introduction to the dosage form followed by the practical examples, which includes,
  - Prescription in Latin,
  - Conversion and calculation of the Latin prescription to English,
  - Theory of the experiment,
  - Procedure,
  - Dispensing,
  - Labelling,
  - Uses with examples of marketed preparations,
  - Student's exercises.

- Pictorial presentation of various types of dosage forms, their method of administration and containers have also been included, whereever essential. (**NOTE:** THE FIGURES ARE INCLUDED IN THIS BOOK ONLY WITH THE INTENSION OF GIVING SUFFICIENT AND ESSENTIAL PRACTICAL KNOWNLEDGE TO THE STUDENTS.)
- Student's exercise is given at the end of each chapter to evaluate the students themselves, about their understanding of the subject.
- Definition, meanings for some important terms and examples of marketed prepration are given at the end of the book.

Certain specific chapters are highlighted in this manual such as, Collodions, Paints, Pessaries, Poultices, Cachets, Tablet triturates, Lozenges and Pastilles which are rarely given in other manuals.

The manual is written in a very simple language, to make both the Diploma and Degree students to understand the topics in better manner. We are presenting a revised edition of the book and hope that, this book will be useful for both the students and teachers of pharmacy.

For further improvement of this book, any suggestions and critics from students and teachers will be greatly appreciated.

- Authors

Acknowledgement

The long cherished dream has come true, today and this is the time to say sincere thanks to all those who have, in some way or the other helped us to sail through.

We take this opportunity to express our sincere gratitude to Shri Ganpatbhai Patel, (Chief Patron, Ganpat University), Shri Anilbhai.T.Patel, (President, Ganpat University, Ex. Ministry of Industry, Gujarat Government), Prof. P.I.Patel, (Director, Ganpat University, Kherva-Mehsana.) for constant support to us to complete this book.

We would like to extend special thanks to Prof. P.D.Bhardia, Principal, (Saffrony college of pharmacy), Dr. M.M.Patel, Principal (Kalol Institute of Pharmacy), Dr. J.K.Patel (Nootan College of Phamacy), Mrs.Jignyasha.A.Raval, Assistant Professor of our college for motivating and sharing their valuable ideas and critical suggestions with us.

We are grateful to other faculty members of the college especially Dr. N.J.Patel, Dr. R.P.Patel, Ritesh B. Patel, Hitesh.R.Patel, Rameshvar.K.Patel, Bhaveshbhai H.Patel, R.M.Patel for their cooperation and critical comments.

We whould like to convey special thanks to T.S.Nagraj, Assistant Prof. S.J.M. College of Pharmacy, Chitradurga and Dr. C.V.S.Subrahmanayam, G.R.R. Pharmacy College Hydrabad for there valuable suggestions and support.

We sincerely thank the non-teaching staff P.I.Patel (Librarian), Mrs. Kiranben Patel, Mrs. Chaulaben Patel, Manish Patel, for their untiring help and support.

We are also very much thankful to our family members Mr. N.T.Venkatesh, Ananya, Mrs. Varsha Mehta, Aditya Mehta, Uday Vyas for their valuable moral support and immense cooperation.

We thank Mr. Amit Patel (Insu4tech), Mr. Hareshbhai M. Purohit & Priteshbhai M. Mehta(Gurudev offset) for the preparation of figures and electronic script.

We also express our thanks to Mr. Anil Shah for bring out this book in a short span of time.

Ganpat University

January 30, 2010

- Authors

Contents

[II] Semisolid Dosage Forms

[III] Solid dosage forms

[IV] Incompatibilities

1 PRESCRIPTION

Prescription is an order written by a physician, dentist or some other registered medical practitioner, to a pharmacist to compound and dispense a specific medicine, for the patient at a particular time.

The prescription (order) contains the directions for the pharmacist, about what type of preparation is to be prepared and how much is to be prepared. It also consists of directions to the patient that, how much medicine is to be taken, how many times is to be taken and how it is to be taken. The prescription provides a common link of mutual understanding between the physician, pharmacist and the patient.

Therefore prescription is a media, through which treatment is provided to the patients by combined skill and services of both the physician and pharmacist.

In olden days, Latin words or abbreviations were frequently used in prescription writing, because medicines were written in Latin language, which was understood all over the world, and such prescriptions remain unknown to the patients, to avoid self medication and it also save the time of the physician.

Now-a-days, prescriptions are written in English language, but still Latin abbreviations are used in prescription writing, specially in dosage instructions.

Parts of prescription:

A typical prescription consists of following parts,

1) Date.
2) Name, age, sex and address of the patient.
3) Superscription.
4) Inscription.
5) Subscription.
6) Signatura.
7) Signature, Address and Registration number of the prescriber.

1) **Date :** Prescriber should write the date on prescription, which helps to the pharmacist to find out the date of prescribing and it avoids the misuse of prescription, number of times for dispensing, specially in case of narcotic drugs and habit forming drugs.

2) **Name, age, sex and address of the patient :** Name, age, sex and address of the patient, must be written on the top of the prescription. This helps to the pharmacist to identify the patient and avoids any chance by giving medicine to another person.
   - Patient's full name should be written instead of surname or nickname.
   - Age and sex of the patient is more important in case of children, to check the dose of the medication.
   - Address of the patient is recorded to contact the patient in the future or to deliver the medicine personally.

3) **Superscription :** The superscription is represented by a symbol "Rx", which is written always at the beginning of the prescription.
   - The symbol "Rx" is considered as a prayer to the God of healing – "Jupiter" for quick recovery of the patient.
   - But now-a-days, this symbol is used as abbreviation of the Latin word "receipe" - means "you take".
4) **Inscription :** This is a main part of the prescription. It consists of the names and quantities of the ingredients.
   - The name of each ingredient is written on a separate line, along with its quantitiy.
   - Last item written is generally the vehicle or solvent.
   - Now-a-days a majority of the drugs are prescribed, which are already prepared in a suitable formulation, so pharmacist is required to dispense the readymade dosage forms of the drug. Therefore compounding (preparation) of the prescription is almost eliminated.
5) **Subscription :** This part consists the direction to the pharmacist, for preparing the particular dosage form and number of doses to be dispensed. But now-a-days, majority of the prescriptions are not compounded (prepared) by the pharmacist. Therefore, the prescribers are not writing the subscription.
6) **Signatura (Signa) :** This part consists of the direction to the patients regarding the administration of the drug. i.e. how, how much and when the dosage form to be administered or applied. It is indicated by a symbol "Signa".
7) **Signature, Address and Registration number of prescriber :**
   - This is the last part of prescription.
   - Prescriber should write his signature, address and registration number, which prevents the danger of dispensing the medicament on a spurious order.
   - The registration number helps to identify the special licence of the prescriber, to prescribe the narcotic and other habit forming drugs.

Handling of prescription : (Dispensing and Compounding of the prescription)

The following procedure should be followed by the pharmacist, during handling the prescription for compounding and dispensing,

1) Receiving the prescription.
2) Reading and checking the prescription.
3) Collecting and weighing the ingredients.
4) Compounding, labelling, packing (dispensing) and delivering to the patients.

Labelling :

After filling the product into a suitable container, it should be labelled properly.

A good quality paper and adhesive should be used, for labelling the containers. The size of the label should be proportional to the size of the container.

The label should bear all necessary informations about the dosage form such as,

- Name of the Dosage form
- Name of the patient, age and sex
- Registration number
- Date of dispensing
- Dose and direction for it's use
- Expiry date
- Storage conditions
- A label should bear certain important warnings or cautions (Auxilliary label) like

  SHAKE WELL BEFORE USE

  STORE IN A COOL PLACE

  KEEP THE CONTAINER LID TIGHTLY CLOSED

  NOT FOR INTERNAL USE

  FOR EXTERNAL USE ONLY

  FOR RECTAL USE

  DO NOT USE AFTER ...... DAYS

  TO BE RUBBED AFTER APPLICATION etc.
- Finally name and address of the pharmacy or manufacturer should be written on the label.

Packing : A properly labeled container is finally packed in neat carton boxes. In case of powders, a good quality of envelope is used for final packing.

An example for a typical prescription:

Sai Hospital
Ashram road, Ahmedabad
Tel.no- 275220301

Date: 12-09-2006

Name: Ramesh kumar Age: 45 Sex-Male
Address: 25, Golden park-II, Sector-2, Gandhinagar.

Rx

Magnessi carbonatis	-	3 i
Magnessi sulphatis	-	3 i
Aquam menthae piperitae..q.s..	-	fl. oz-ii
Fiat: Mistura		Mitte: fl.oz ii

Signa: Cochleare amplum, duo semi hora ante jentaculum sumendum.

(Signature of the prescriber)
Dr.K.K.Mehta
Reg.No.- Guj/125

2 WEIGHTS AND MEASURES

Before dispensing, a pharmacist should understand the various types of calculations, involved in it. Therefore pharmacist should have a thorough knowledge about weights and measures, which are used in the calculations.

Weight : Weight is a measure of the gravitational force, acting on a body and is directly proportional to its mass.

Measure : Measure is the measurement of volume of any substance.

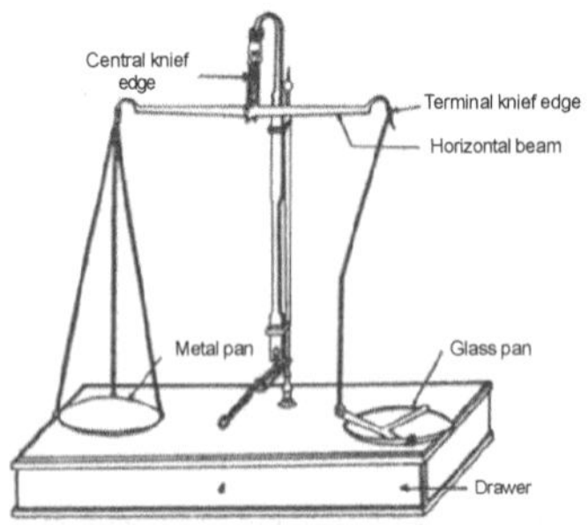

Dispensing balance

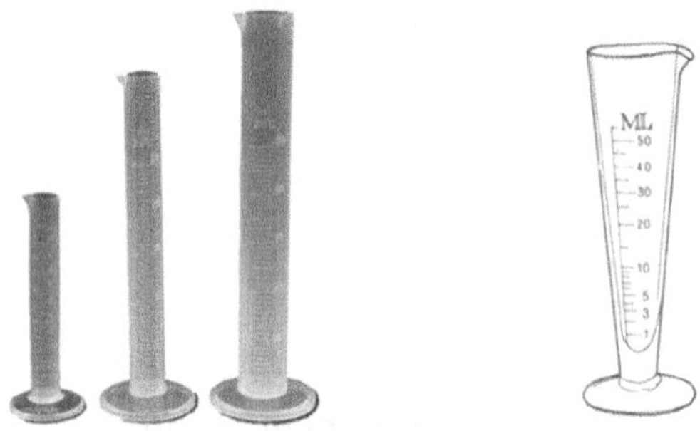

Different measures

There are two systems of weights and measures : 1. The Imperial system
2. The Metric system

1) **IMPERIAL SYSTEM :** It is an old system of weights and measures based on arbitrary and unrelated units like grains, drachms, ounces and gallons.

a) **Measure of weight in imperial system** : Imperial system is divided into two parts for the purpose of measurement of weight as :

i) Avoirdupois system

ii) Apothecaries system

(i) Avoirdupois system : In this system "pound" is the standard unit for weight. Therefore all measures of mass (weight) are derived from the Imperial standard, "pound"(Lb.)

Eg. 1 Lb = 16 oz.
1 Lb = 7000 grains
1 oz. = 7000 / 16 grains
= 437.5 grains.

(ii) Apothecaries system : In this system "grain" is the standard unit for weight. Therefore all the measures of mass (weight) are derived from the "grain".

Eg.	20 grains	=	1 Scruple
	60 grains	=	1 drachm
	480 grains	=	1 ounce
	8 drachms	=	1 ounce
	12 ounce	=	1 pound
	5760 grains	=	1 pound

Abbreviations commonly used in weighing :

Eg.

Latin name	Symbol	English name	Equal to
Granum	gr.	Grain	1 grain
Scrupulus	∋	Scruple	20 grains
Drachma	3	Drachm	60 grains
Uncia oz.	℥	Ounce (Avoir)	437.5 grains
Uncia(Troy)	℥	Ounce (Apothe)	480 grains
Libra	lb	Pound (Avoir)	7000 grains
Libra	lb	Pound (Apothe)	5760 grains

b) **Measurement of Capacity in imperial system :** In both Avoirdupois and Apothecaries system, the standard unit for capacity is "gallon". Therefore all other measures of capacity are derived from gallon.

Eg.	1 gallon	=	160 fluid ounces.		
	1/4 th of a gallon	=	1 quart	=	40 fl.ounce
	1/8 th of a gallon	=	1 pint	=	20 fl.ounce
	1/160 th of a gallon	=	1 fl. ounce		
	1/8 th of one fl.ounce	=	1 fl. drachm		
	1/60th of one fl.drachm	=	1 minim		
	1 fluid ounce	=	480 minims		
	1 fluid drachm	=	60 minims.		

Abbreviations commonly used in measures of capacity :

Latin name	Symbol	English name	Equal to
Minimum	M or m	Minim	1 minim
Fluid drachm	3	fl. drachm	60 minims
Fluid uncia	℥	fl. ounce	480 minims
Octarius	O	Pint	20 fl. ounces
Congius	C	Gallon	160 fl. ounces

2) **METRIC SYSTEM :** The metric system is used in Indian pharmacopoeia,

a) **Measurement of weight in Metric system :** In Metric system "Kilogram" is the standard unit for measurement of weight. Therefore all other measures for weight are derived from kilogram (Kg)

1 Kilogram (Kg)	=	1000 grams (g)
1 Hectogram (hg)	=	100 grams
1 Decagram (dag)	=	10 grams
1 Decigram (dg)	=	0.1 gram
1 Centigram (cg)	=	0.01 gram
1 Milligram (mg)	=	0.001 gram
1 Microgram (mcg)	=	0.000001 gram
1 gram (g)	=	1000 mg
0.1 gram	=	100 mg
0.01 gram	=	10 mg
0.001 gram	=	1 mg

b) **Measurement of capacity in Metric system :** In Metric system, the standard unit for measure is "litre". Therefore all measures of capacity are derived from the litre.

Eg. 1 litre (lt) = 1000 millilitre (ml)

Interconversions of Imperial and Metric units :

Weight measures :

1 grain	= 64.8 mg	= 65 mg (60 mg) (for all practical purposes.)	
1 gram	= 15.43 gr	= 15 gr	"
1 milligram(mg)	= 1/65 gr or 1/60 gr		"
1 kilogram	= 2.2 lb (pounds)		"

Capacity measures :

1 drop	= 1 minim	= 0.06 ml (for all practical purposes)	
1 fl. ounce	= 29.57 ml	= 30 ml	"
1 millilitre (ml)	= 16.23 minims	= 15 minims	"
1 litre	= 33.1 fl. ounce		
1 fl. drachm	= 4 ml		
1 fl. ounce	= 30 ml		
1 ml	= 15 minims		
0.06 ml	= 1 minim		
500 ml	= 1 pint		
1000 ml	= 1 quart		

Domestic measures :

1 drop	= 1 minim	= 0.06 ml
1 teaspoonful	= 1 fl. drachm	= 4 ml (5 ml for all practical purposes)
1 desertspoonful	= 2 fl. drachm	= 8 ml (10 ml for all practical purposes)
1 tablespoonful	= 4 fl. drachm	= 16 ml (15 ml for all practical purposes)
2 tablespoonful	= 8 fl. drachm	= 32 ml (30 ml for all practical purposes)
1 wine glass	= 2 fl. ounce	= 60 ml
1 teacupful	= 4 fl. ounce	= 120 ml
1 tumblerful	= 8 fl. ounce	= 240 ml

Cochleare — Amplum / Magnum / Maximum = One tablespoonful = 16 ml or 15 ml

Cochleare — Medium / Modium / Plenum = One desertspoonful = 8 ml or 10 ml

Cochleare — Minimum / Purvum / Infans = One teaspoonful = 4 ml or 5 ml

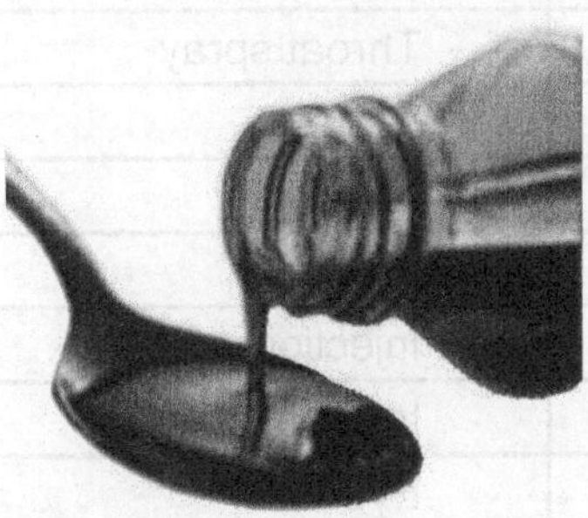

Tablespoonful

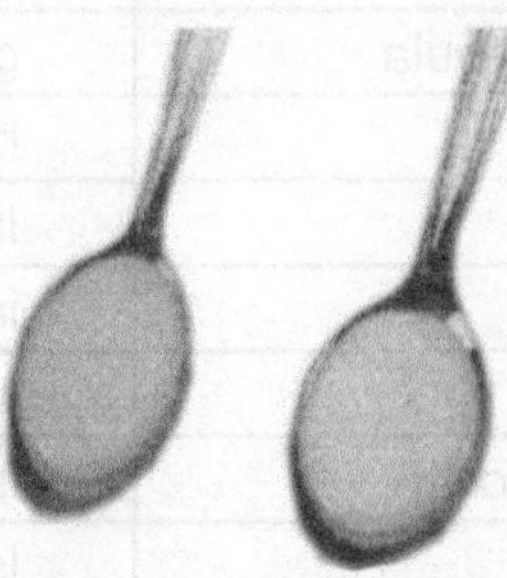

Teaspoonful

3 COMMON LATIN TERMS USED IN PRESCRIPTION WRITING

1. LATIN TERMS FOR DIFFERENT DOSAGE FORMS:

Latin term	Abbreviation	English meaning
Auristillae	Auristill.	Ear drops
Aurinarium	Aurin	Ear cone
Buginarium	Buginar	Nasal bougie
Capsula amylacea	Caps. amylac	Cachet
Capsula	caps.	Capsule
Cataplasma	cataplasm.	Poultice
Cereolus	Cereol	Urethral bougie
Charta	Chart	Powder
Collodium	Coll	Collodion
Collunarium	Collun	Nose wash
Collutorium	collut.	Mouthwash
Collyrium	collyr.	Eye lotion
Cremor	crem.	Cream
Dentifricium	Dentif	Dentrifrice
Emulsio	emul.	Emulsion
Emplastrum	emp.	Plaster
Gargarisma	garg.	Gargle
Gelatina	gelat	Jelly
Guttae	gtt.	Drops
Guttur pigmentum	gtt.pigm	Throat paint
Guttur nebula	gtt.neb	Throat spray
Haustus	ht	Draught
Infusum	Inf.	Infusion
Inhalatio	inhal.	Inhalation
Injectio	inj.	Injection
Insufflatio	insuff	Insufflation
Lamella	lamel	Eye disc.
Linimentum	lin.	Liniment
Linctus	linc.	Linctus
Liquor	liq.	Solution
Lotio	lot.	Lotion

Mistura	mist.	Mixture
Nebula	neb.	Spray solution
Oblatum	oblat	Cachet
Oculus guttae	ocul.gtt	Eye drops
Oculentum	oculent.	Eye ointment
Oleum	ol	Oil
Pasta	past.	Paste
Pastillus	pastill	Pastille
Pessus	pess	Pessary
Pigmentum	pigm.	Paint
Pilula	pil	Pill
Pulvis	pulv.	Powder
Pulvis consperus	pulv. consper	Dusting powder
Sternutamentum	sternut	Snuff
Spiritus	sp	Spirit
Suppositorium	suppos.	Suppository
Syrupus (Syrupi)	syr.	Syrup
Tabletta, Tabella	tab.	Tablet
Trochiscus	troch.	Lozenge
Unguentum	ung.	Ointment
Vapor	vap.	Inhalation

2. LATIN TERMS FOR METHOD OF ADMINISTRATION OR APPLICATION

Latin term	Abbreviation	English meaning
Addendus	addend	To be added
Addatur	add.	Added
Applicandus	applicand.	To be applied
Applicat	—	Let (him) apply
Ad usum externum	Ad. us. enter.	For external use
Agita ante usum	agit. a. us.	Shake before use
Adhibendus	adhib.	To be administered
Capiendus	capiend.	To be taken
Consperge	consper.	Dust, sprinkle
Dolentiparti or Dolentieus partieus or Parti affactae	dolent part p.a.	To the affected part
Da	d	Give

Dandus	dand.	To be given
Detur	d.	To be given
Dolore urgente	dol.urg.	When pain is severe
Deglutiendus	deglut.	To be swallowed
Fiat, Fiant	ft.	Prepared (prepare)
Frequenter	freq	Frequently
Involve	—-	Roll (to be rolled)
Infricandus	infricand	To be rubbed
Instillandus	Instilland.	To be dropped in
Inhaletur	inhal.	Let (it) be inhaled
Mitte	mitt.	Send or supply
Miscendus	miscend.	To be mixed
More solito	mor. so.	In the manner
Quantum libitum	q.lib.	As much as you wish
Quantum sufficiat	q.s.	As much as if sufficient
Quantum vis	—-	As much as you please
Signa	sig.	Label
Sugendus	sugend.	To be sucked
Sumat	sum.	Let be taken
Sumendus	s or sum.	To be taken
Secundum	—-	According to
Sine (s)	—-	Without
Super	—-	Over
Solve	—-	Dissolve
Sicci	—	Dried
Super gossypium	sup. gossyp.	Upon cotton wool.
Super linteum	sup.lint.	Upon lint
Utendus	u or utend.	To be used
Ope penicilli	ope pen	By means of a camel hair brush
Pro usu externo	Pro. us. exter.	For external use
Ut dictum	Ut. dict.	As directed
(Tore) Teratur	—-	Rub
Tere beno	—	Rub Well
Gradation	grad	Gradually

Guttatim	guttatim	Drop by Drop
Lente	—	Slowly
More dicto	m.d.	As directed(As prescribed)
Mode dicto	m.d.	As directed
Prorenata	p.r.n.	Occasionally
Si opus sit	s.o.s.	When required or (When ever necessary)
Statim	stat.	Immediately (At once)
Tussi urgente	tuss. urg.	When the cough is troublesome

3. LATIN TERMS FOR TIME OF ADMINISTRATION:

(A) Times per day

Semel in die	sem in die	Once in a day
Semel die	sem. die	Once a day
Bis in die,	b.i.d.	Twice in a day
Bis die	b.d.	Twice a day
Ter in die	t.i.d.,	Three times in a day
Ter die	t.d.	Three times a day
Quarter in die	q.i.d., q.d.	Four times a day
Sexies in die	sex i.d.	Six times a day
Bis terve in die	b.t.i.d.	Two or three times a day
Ter quaterve die	t.q.d.	Three or four times a day
Vices	vic.	Time or Times
Ter quotidie	ter. quot.	Three timely daily
Ad. tres. vices	Ad. 3 vic.	For three times
Quaque hora	qq.h.	Every hour
Singulis hora	sing. hor.	Every one hour
Cibos (cibum)	c	Meal
Frequentius	freq.	More frequently
Hora decubitus	h. d.	At bed time
Saepe	-	Often
Saepius	-	More often
Saepillime	-	Very often
Quoties opus sit	Quot. o.s.	As often as necessary
Indies or Quotidie	Quot.	Daily

(B) Different times of the day

LATIN TERM	ABBREVIATION	ENGLISH MEANING
Primo mane	prim. m.	Early in the morning
Prima luce	prim. luc.	Early in the morning
Mane	m	In the morning
Omni mane	o.m.	Every morning
Omni nocte	o.n.	Every night
Inter nocte	inter noct.	During the night
Nocte	n	At night
Vespere	vesp.	In the evening
Jentaculum	jentac	Breakfast
Nocte et mane	n.et.m.	Night and morning
Nocte manaque	n.m.	Night and morning

(C) Hour / time

Omni Hora	o.h.	Every hour
Omni quarta hora	o.q.h.	Every four hour
Singulis horis	sing. hora	Every hour
Quaque secunda hora	qq.sec.h.	Every alternate hour
Omni alterna hora	qq.alt.h.	Every alternate hour
Alternis horis	alt. hor.	Every two hours
Tertiis horis	tert. hor.	Every three hours
Quartis horis	quart. hor.	Every four hours
Sextis horis	sext. hor.	Every six hours

(D) Correlated Time

Ante cibos	a.c.	Before meals
Ante (a) (prae)	—-	Before
Post	—-	After
Pro	—-	For or before
Post cibos	p.c.	After meals
Inter cibos	i.c.	Between meals

4. LATIN TERMS FOR VEHICLE USED AND MEANS OF APPLICATION

Latin term	Abbreviation	English meaning
Cochleare – amplum	coch. amp	One tablespoonful
Cochleare – magnum	coch. mag.	One tablespoonful
Cochleare – maximum	coch. max.	One tablespoonful
Cochleare parvum	Coch. parv.	One teaspoonful
Colchleare plenum	Coch. paul	One desertspoonful
Cochleare infans	Coch. inf.	One teaspoonful
Cochleare minimum	coch. min.	One teaspoonful
Cochleare medium	coch. med.	One desertspoonful
Cum	c.	With
Cum duplo	c. dup.	With twice as much
Cum parte aequale	c. pt. aeq.	With an equal quantity
Cum tanto	c. tant.	With as much
Calefac	—-	Warm
Cyathus amplus	cyath. amp.	A tumbler
Cyathus magnus	cyath mag.	A tumbler
Cyathus vinosus	cyath. vin.	A wine glass
Dimidium	Dimid	Half
E. lacte	e. lact.	With milk
Ex. Aqua.	ex. aq.	With water
Ex. Aquae Semicyatho magno	Ex. Aq. Semicyath mag.	With half a tumblerful of water
In	—-	In, into
Misce	m.	Mix
Misce fiat mistura	—-	Mix to make a mixtuer
Poculus	poc	A cup
Partes aequalis	p.aeq.	Equal parts
Semi	ss	Half

5. MISCELLANEOUS

Latin term	Abbreviation	English meaning
Ad	ad.	To. Upto
Ana	aa	Of each (To each)
Ante	a	Before

Aqua	aq	Water
Aqua distillate	aq. dist.	Distilled water
Aquae bullientis or aque ferventis	Aq. Bull Aq. Ferv	Boiling water
Aqua calidae	Aq. cal.	Warm water
Aqua gelidae	Aq. gel	Cold water
Aqua communis	Aq. com	Tap water
Apud	—-	At
Capiti	capiti	To the head
Cibos	cibos	Meals, food
Circa	—-	Around
Contra	—-	Against
Corpori	corp.	To the body
Dexter	dext.	Right
Dosis	dos	A dose
De	—-	Form
Et	—-	And
Hora.	h.	An hour
Infra	—-	Below
Inter	—-	Between
Intra	—-	Within
Ligamentum	liganment	Bandage
Pro dosi	-	As a dose
Pro ratione actatis	Pre.rat. act	According to age
Per	—-	Through
Pone	—-	Behind
Purum	—-	Pure
Simul	—-	Together
Sinister	sinist	Left
Laevo	l.	Left
Mitte	mitt.	Send
Mitte tales	mitt. tal	Send such
More dicto	m. dict.	Prescribed
Omni	omn	Every
Recipe	Rx	Take
Semi	ss	Half
Talis, tales	tal	such

6. LATIN TERMS FOR PARTS OF THE BODY

Latin term		English meaning
Auris		Ear
Auris dexter.		Right ear
Auris laevus		Left ear
Brachis		Arm
Capillis		Hair
Cord		Heart
Corpori		To the body
Cutis		Skin
Digitus		Finger
Dent		Teeth
Gutturi		Throat
Hepar		Liver
Jugulo		Throat
Manus		Hand
Naso		Nose
Naris		Nostril
Oculis		Eye
Oculus dexter		Right eye
Oculus laevus		Left eye
Os, oris		Mouth
Pro oculus		For the eyes
Pectus (Pectori)		Chest (Breast)
Ren		Kidney
Recto		Rectum
Sanguis		Blood
Sterno		To the chest
Talus		Ankle
Tempus (Caput)		Head
Unguis		Nail

7. LATIN TERMS FOR NUMERICALS

Latin term	Abbreviation	English meaning
Unus	I	One
Duo	II	Two
Tres, Tria	III	Three
Quatuor	IV	Four
Quinque	V	Five
Sex	VI	Six
Septem	VII	Seven
Octe	VIII	Eight
Novem	IX	Nine
Decem	X	Ten
Undecim	XI	Eleven
Duodecim	XII	Twelve
Tredecim	XIII	Thirteen
Quatuordecim	XIV	Fourteen
Quindecim	XV	Fifteen
Viginti	XX	Twenty
Viginti Quinque	XXV	Twenty five
Triginta	XXX	Thirty
Quadraginta	XL	Fourty
Quinguaginta	L	Fifty
Sexaginta	LX	Sixty
Septuaginta	LXX	Seventy
Octoginta	LXXX	Eighty
Nonaginta	XC	Ninety
Centum	C	One Hundred
Decenti	CC	Two Hundreds
Trecenti	CCC	Three Hundreds
Quadringenti	CCCC	Four Hundreds
Quingenti	D	Five Hundreds
Mille	M	One Thousand

Note:

s	--	0.25
ss	--	0.5 (Half)
sss	---	0.75

8. LATIN TERMS FOR THE INGREDIENTS:

English term	Latin term
Almond oil	Olei Amygdalae
Aromatic chalk powder	Pulveris cretae aromatici
Aromatic spirit of ammonia	Spiritus ammoniae aromatici
Aspirin (Acetyl salicylic acid)	Acidi acityl salicylici
Antimony potassium tartrate	Antim et potassii tartratis
Amaranth solution	Aquam amaranthi
Ammonium chloride	Ammonii chloride
Boric acid	Acidi borici
Borax	Boracis
Butter	Butyrum
Bitter	Ameri
Benzoic acid solution	Aquam acidi benzoici
Bismuth carbonate	Bismuthi carbonatis
Belladonna green extract	Extracti belladonna viridis
Chalk	Cretae
Calciferol	Calciferolis
Coal	Carbonis
Charcoal	Carbonis ligni
Clove	Caryophylli
Cocoa butter / Theobroma oil	Cacaonis butyri
Cochineal	Coccus
Cherry	Cerasi
Cod liver oil	Morrhuae olei
Coaltar	Picis carbonis
Castor oil	Olei ricini
Cotton	Gossypium
Chloroform water	Aquam chloroformi
Cinnamon water	Aquam cinnamoni
Caffeine	Caffeinae
Calcium lactate	Calcii lactatis
Citrate	Citratis
Compound infusion of gentian	Infusum gentianae compositae
Compound tartrazine solution	Tartrazini liquor compositae
Citric acid	Acidi citrici

Camphor	Camphorae
Dried	Sicci
Dilute Sulphuric acid	Acidi sulphuric diluti
Draught	Haustus
Dilute HCL	Acidi hydrochloridi dilute
Dilute ammonia solution	Diluti liquoris ammoniae
Emulsifying wax	Cerae emulsif
Eucalyptus oil	Olei eucalypti
Ferric citrate	Ferri-et citratis
Ferric iodide syrup	Syrupi ferri iodidi
Ferric perchlorate liquid	Liquoris ferri perchloridi
Ferrous sulphate	Ferri sulphatis
Glycyrrhiza liquid extract	Extracti glycyrrhizae liquidi
Glycerin	Glycerini
Glycerin of tannic acid	Glycerini acidi tannici
Halibut liver oil	Hypoglossi
Hard	Dura
Hyoscine hydrobromide	Hyoscinae hydrobromidi
Infusion of orange peel	Infusum aurantii
Infusion of clove	Infusum caryophylli
Inhalation	Inhalatio
Lobelia ethereal	Lobelia aetheriae
Lemon	Limonis
Lead	Plumbi
Liquid ferric perchloride	Liquoris ferri perchloridi
Lemon syrup	Limonis syrupi
Light kaolin	Lavis kaolin
Liquid extract of glycyrrhiza	Extracti glycyrrhiza liquouris
Liquid phenol	Liquoris phenolis.
Mercurous chloride	Hydragyri sub chloride
Milk	Lactis
Mercurochrome	Merbromini
Magnesium sulphate	Magnesii sulphatis
Magnesium carbonate	Magnesii carbonatis
Magnesium trisilicate	Magnesii trisilicatis
Menthol	Menthilis

Nux-vomica	Nucis vomicae
Orange	Auranti
Oil	Olei
Opium	Opii
Orange syrup	Syrupi aurantii
Orange oil	Olei aurantii
Oleic acid	Acidi oleici
Prepared chalk	Cretae preparatae
Phenol	Carbolici
Potassium	Kalium
Precipitated sulphur	Sulphuris precipitatis
Pure	Purum
Potassium bromide	Potassii bromide
Phenacetin	Phenacetini
Potassium citrate	Potassii citratis
Potassium iodide	Potassii iodidi
Potassium chlorate	Potassii chloratis
Powder	Pulvis
Peppermint water	Aquam manthae piperitae
Piperazine citrate	Piperazinae citratis
Potassium hydroxide solution	Liquoris potassii hydroxidi
Paraffin	Paraffinum
Quinine citrate	Quininae citratis
Quinine sulphate	Quininae sulphatis
Rhubarb	Rhei / Rheum
Raspberry	Rubi idaei
Rose oil	Olei rosae
Starch	Amyli
Silver	Argenti
Spermaceti	Cetaceum
Saffron	Crocus
Sodium	Natrium
Soft paraffin	Paraffinum molle
Sulphurated potash	Potassae sulphuratae
Sugar	Sacchari
Sucrose	Sucrosum

Saccharin	Saccharinum
Salol (Phenyl salicylate)	Salolis
Strong	Fortis / forte
Sweet	Dulcis
Spirit	Spiritus
Soft	Mollis
Syrup	Syrupi
Strychnine HCl solution	Liquoris strychninae hydrochloride
Ferric ammonium citrate	Ferriet ammoni citratis
Sodium salicylate	Sodii salicylatis
Sodium benzoate	Sodii benzoatis
Sodium bicarbonate	Sodii bicarbonatis
Sodium sulphide	Sodii sulphidi
Sodium perborate	Sodii perboratis
Turpentine oil	Terebinthinae olei
Talc	Talcum
Thin	Tanuis
Tincture of nux vomica	Tincturae nucis vomicae
Tincture of catechu	Tincturae catechu
Tincture of hyoscyamus	Tincturae hyoscyami
Tincture of lobelia	Tincturae loberiae aetheriae ethereal
Tincture of stramonium	Tincture stramonii
Tincture of myrrh	Tincturae myrrahae
Tannic acid	Acidi tannicci
Tartaric acid	Acidi tartraci
Wax	Cerae
White wax	Cerae albae
Wool	Lanae
Wood	Lignum
White	Album
Wool Fat	Adipis lanae
Wool alcohol	Lanae alcoholis
Yellow	Flavum
Zinc sulphate	Zinci sulphatis
Zinc oxide	Zinci oxidi

4 DOSAGE FORMS

Drug : A drug is defined as, "a substance which is used in diagnosis, mitigation, treatment, cure or prevention of disease in human beings or animals".

Drugs are rarely administered in their original state. Drugs are formulated into different dosage forms using non-drug components called as "excipients" or "additives".

Dosage forms : Dosage forms are defined as "The suitable preparations containing drug with or without excipients, which are used for convenient and efficacious treatment of the diseases".

Importance of dosage forms (Reasons for converting the pure drug or active ingredients into the dosage forms).

1) To provide safe and convenient delivery of accurate dosage.
2) To protect the drug from oxidation, hydrolysis and reduction process from environmental factors like light, air and moisture.
3) To mask the unpleasant odour and taste of the pure drugs.
   Eg. Tablets, Capsules, Syrups, Coated tablets.
4) To provide maximum (optimum) drug action through inhalation therapy.
5) To protect the drug from decomposition in stomach by acidic pH of gastric juice, after oral administration.
   Eg. Enteric coated tablets.
6) To provide insertion of drug into the body cavities like rectum, vagina, ear or nose.
   Eg. Suppositories, Pessaries, Ear cone, Nasal bougies.
7) To provide maximum drug action from topical administration sites.
   Eg. Ointments, Eye drops, Ear drops, Lotions, Creams.
8) To provide liquid dosage forms of drugs, by dissolving in suitable solvents.
   Eg. Solutions, Mixtures.
9) To provide liquid preparations of drugs, which are insoluble in the vehicles.
   Ex. Suspensions.
10) To provide liquid dosage forms of drugs, which are immiscible with each others.
    Eg. Emulsions.
11) To provide quick onset of action.
    Eg. Injections and I. V. fluids (Parentrals).
12) To provide sustained release action (prolonged action) of drugs by using controlled release mechanism.
    Eg. Microemulsions, Suspensions, Tablets, Sustained release tablets, Capsules.

Dosage forms

Liquid dosage forms

(i) Monophasic liquid dosage forms

A. Solutions

(a) Solutions meant for oral (internal) use

1. mixtures
2. Elixirs
3. Linctuses
4. Syrups

(b) Solutions used only in mouth and throat

1. Mouthwashes
2. Gargles
3. Throat paints
4. Throat sprays

(c) Solutions instilled into body cavities

1. Eye drops
2. Eye lotions
3. Ear drops
4. Nasal drops
5. Nasal wash
6. Nasal sprays
7. Inhalations
8. Douches
9. Enema

(d) Solutions applied to the body surfaces

1. Lotions
2. Liniments
3. Collodions
4. Paints

(ii) Biphasic liquid dosage forms

A. Suspensions
B. Emulsions

Solid dosage forms

1. Tablets
2. Capsules
3. Powders
4. Granules
5. Cachets
6. Lozenges
7. Pastilles
8. Tablet Triturates

Semisolid dosage forms

1. Ointments
2. Creams
3. Pastes
4. Jellies
5. Suppositories
6. Pessaries
7. Nasal bougies
8. Ear Cones
9. Bougies
10. Poultices

5 LIQUID DOSAGE FORMS

Liquid dosage forms are one class of dosage forms, which are meant for either internal, external or parenteral use.

Liquid dosage forms are sub-classified in to,

1) Monophasic liquid dosage forms.
2) Biphasic liquid dosage forms.

Advantages of liquid dosage forms:

1) Liquid dosage forms are easy for administration to children and adults, who are having difficulties in swallowing solid dosage forms like tablets and capsules.
2) The onset of action (bioavailability) is quick, compare to the solid dosage forms, because solids require previous disintegration in the body, before absorption of the drug.
3) Certain substances can be given only in liquid dosage forms, because they are available only in liquid forms and giving such liquids in relatively large dosage in any other forms is not possible. Eg. Castor oil, Liquid paraffin.
4) Certain substances like potassium iodide and potassium bromide cause irritation in stomach, if they are given in solid form (As powder or tablet). Hence, such substances can be given in the form of mixture.
5) Some substances are useful, when they are administered as dispersion (suspension form), because in suspension form, they afford large surface area for maximum adsorption of toxic substances in the alimentary canal.
   Eg. Light kaolin, Bismuth salt.
6) The doses of drug can be easily adjusted accordingly to the need of the patient.
7) Drugs with large doses can be easily administered as liquid dosage forms.
8) Liquid dosage forms are found to be more economical to manufacture compaired to solid and semisolid dosage forms, because they are easy to prepare, require small unit operation, simple machinery and simple procedure..
9) Liquid dosage forms have good appearance due to clear and colourful appearance on visual inspection. This is one more advantage over solid dosage forms to attract the children.

Disadvantages of liquid dosage forms:

1) Liquid dosage forms are less stable compare to the solid dosage forms, because drugs undergoes decomposition by hydrolysis, oxidation or microbial growth. Hence extra preservatives and stabilizers are required to be added.
2) Incompatibility is more in liquid dosage forms, as compared to the solid dosage forms.
3) They are difficult to carry, because of their bulky nature and weight.
4) There are chances of dose variation, if taken either by spoon or measuring cup.
5) Sudden breakage of glass bottle (container), spoils whole amount of the product.

Formulation of Liquid dosage forms

For the preparation of liquid dosage forms along with medicament, following additives are used :

1) VEHICLES :

Sr.no	Type	Examples	Uses
1)	Water	a. Potable water b. Freshly boiled and cooled water c. Purified water d. Distilled water	Used for most of the liquid preparations, where flavouring is not required.
2)	Aromatic waters	a. Chloroform water	Flavouring agent and Preservative.
		b. Cinnamon water	Flavouring agent and Carminative.
		c. Peppermint water	Flavouring agent, Carminative and weak preservative.
		d. Anise water	Flavouring agent and Carminative.
		e. Dill water	Flavouring agent, Carminative (particularly for infants in Gripe water).
3)	Alcohols	a. Ethanol	Solvent, Cosolvent for many liquid preparations like Elixirs, Lotions, Liniments.
		b. Glycerin	Solvent, Cosolvent for many oral preparations and external preparations.
		c. Polyethylene glycol (PEG)	Solvent for liquid prepara tions like Elixirs, Lotions, Liniments and Syrups.
		d. Sorbitol	Solvent, Vehicle for many liquid preparations.
		e. Propylene glycol	Solvent, Cosolvent and Vehicle for many liquid preparations.

4)	Elixirs	Non medicated elixirs a. Low alcoholic elixirs b. High alcoholic elixirs c. Iso-alcoholic elixirs	Aromatics and vehicles for many oral liquid preparations.
5)	Syrups	a. Orange syrup b. Raspberry syrup c. Cherry syrup d. Glycerrhiza syrup e. Cocoa syrup	Most of the syrups are used as sweetening agent, flavouring agent and vehicles in oral liquid preparations .
6)	Infusions	Fresh or concentrated infusions as prescribed, Eg.a. Concentrated infusion of Senna b. Concentrated infusion of Quassia c. Concentrated infusion of Gentian	Used for their corresponding medicinal action.

2) PRESERVATIVES

Benzalkonium chloride	Dichlorophenol
Benzoic acid	Methyl paraben
Cetrimide	Phenol
Chlorbutanol	Phenyl mercuric nitrate
Chloro benzoic acid	Propionic acid
Chloro cresol	Propyl paraben
Dichloro acetic acid	Salicylic acid
Dichloro meta xylenol	Sodium benzoate

3) ANTIOXIDANTS (STABILIZERS)

Ascorbic acid	Maleic acid
Beta-Naphthol	Propyl gallate
Butylated hydroxy anisole (BHA)	Sodium bisulphite
Butylated hydroxy toluene (BHT)	Sodium meta bisulphite
Citric acid	Sodium sulphite
Cysteine	Sodium thiosulphate
Gallic acid	Thioglycerol
Lecithin	Thiourea

4) SWEETENING AGENTS

Cyclamates	Maltose
Dextrose (Glucose)	Malt extract
D-Fructose	Saccharin
Glycyrrihiza glycerin	Sodium saccharin
Glycyrrihiza extract	Sorbitol
Lactose	Sucrose
Tolu Balsam	Liquid Glucose

5) FLAVOURING AGENTS

Flovours	Oils	Spirits
Banana flavour	Anise oil	Aromatic spirit of ammonia
Cardamom flavour	Caraway oil	Chloroform spirit
Ginger flavour	Clove oil	Compound orange spirit
Orange flavour	Lemon oil	Lemon spirit
Pineapple flavour	Orange oil	Peppermint spirit
Vanilla flavour	Peppermint oil	
Chocolate flavour	Rose oil	

6) COLOURING AGENTS

a. Natural colours	Carotene Chlorophill Cochineal Curcumin Red and Yellow ferric oxide Titanium dioxide
b. Artificial colour	Caramel
c. Coal tar colours 1. Blue colour 2. Brown colour 3. Black colour 4. Green colour 5. Red colour 6. Yellow colour 7. Orange colour	 Brilliant blue, Indigo carmine Resorcin brown Naphthol blue (Black) Quinazoline green, Fast green, Brilliant Green Amaranth, Tatrazine (Pink) (Red), Eosin Fast red, Erythrosin Sunset yellow, Quinoline yellow, Tratrazine yellow Orange 'G'

7. Flocculating, Suspending and Wetting agents:

No.	Type	Examples	
1.	Flocculating agents	a. Surfactants	Tweens Spans
		b. Electrolytes	Aluminium chloride Potassium phosphate
		c. Hydrophilic polymers	Hydro-colloids, Bentonite, Alginates, Carbowaxes, Silicates
2.	Suspending and Thickening agents	a. Natural polysaccharides	Gum acacia Gum tragacanth Guar gum Sodium alginate Starch Xantham gum
		b. Semi synthetic Polysaccharides	Methyl cellulose Sodium carboxy methyl cellulose Hydroxy ethyl cellulose Hydroxy propyl cellulose Hydroxy propyl methyl cellulose Micro crystalline cellulose
		c. Inorganic agents	Clays, Bentonite, Kaolin Aluminium hydroxide
		d. Synthetic agents	Colloidal silicon dioxide. Carbomer (Carboxy vinyl polymer)
3.	Wetting agents	——	Alcohol, Glycerin, Polysorbate, Tragacanth mucilage, Sodium alginate, Bentonite dispersion, Surfactants having HLB value between 7 to 9, Sodium lauryl sulphate, Sodium dioctyl sulpho succinate

8. Emulsifying agents

1)	Natural emulsifying agents	a. From vegetable source	Gum acacia, Karaya gum, Tragacanth, Agar, Pectin, Starch, Irish moss, Alginate, Gaur gum, Soyabean.
		b. From animal source	Gelatin, Egg yolk, Casein, Lecithin Wool fat, Serum albumin.

2) Semi-synthetic polysaccharides	—	Methyl cellulose, Carboxy methyl cellulose, Sodium carboxy methyl cellulose, Hydroxy propyl methyl cellulose, Micro crystalline cellulose.
3) Synthetic substances	a. Anionic	Sodium lauryl sulphate, Polypeptide condensates, Trioleyl phosphate, Sarcosinates, Sulfosuccinates, Soaps.
	b. Cationic	Alkoxyalkylamines, Benzalkonium chloride, Cetrimide, Benzethonium chloride.
	c. Non-ionic	Polyoxyethylene, polyoxyethylene alkyl ethers,Polyoxypropylene, Sorbitan esters, Glyceryl esters, Sucrose esters, Polyoxyethylene fatty acid esters, Macrogol esters & ethers.
4) Inorganic substances	—	Magnesium oxide, Milk of magnesia, Magnesium trisilicate, Magnesium aluminium silicate, Bentonite.
5) Alcoholic substances	—	Polyethylene glycols (Carbowaxes), Cholesterol, Lauryl alcohol, Lecithin.

MONOPHASIC LIQUID DOSAGE FORMS:

As the word 'Monophasic' indicates that, this system consists only one (single) phase. It is represented as "True solution" or "Solution".

Solution: Solution is a clear homogeneous mixture, which is prepared by dissolving solid, liquid or gas in another liquid.

In a solution, the component which is present in large amount is known as 'Solvent' and the component present in lesser amount is known as 'Solute'.

Solutions may be used internally, externally or parenterally. Solutions are sub-classified into four types depending on their use as,

i) Solutions meant for internal (oral) use.

ii) Solutions used only in mouth and throat.

iii) Solutions instilled in to body cavities.

iv) Solutions applied to the body surfaces.

Examples for these dosage forms are given in the classification of dosage forms (P.no22).

6 MIXTURES

Latin term: Mistura

Mixtures are liquid (dosage forms) preparations, intended for oral administration, in which drug is dissolved, suspended or dispersed in a suitable vehicle (solvent).

Mixtures generally contain several doses in a bottle. If only one dose of mixture is dispensed (prescribed), then mixture is called as "Draught".

Mixtures are generally used for acute conditions such as cough, diarrhoea, constipation, indigestion. Therefore mixtures are not prepared in large quantity, to keep them for a longer period.

Mixtures should be prepared extemporaneously and supplied only for small number of doses, which can be used up within a short period.

Classification of mixtures: Mixtures are classified as,

1) Simple mixtures containing — Soluble substances only.
2) Mixtures containing — Diffusible solids.
3) Mixtures containing — Indiffusible solids.
4) Mixtures containing — Precipitate forming liquids.
5) Mixtures containing — Slightly soluble liquids.
6) Miscellaneous mixtures.

I. Simple mixture:

Simple mixture is one, which consists of only soluble ingredients. Hence they are also called as 'solutions'.

Eg :- Potassium bromide mixture,
Sodium bicarbonate mixture.

Method:

1) Dissolve the solid substances (drug) in ¾ th of the total volume of the vehicle (The volume of the vehicle initially used is ¾ th in order to keep provision for volume occupied by other ingredients).
2) Examine the solution by holding it against the light. If any foreign particles or undissolved substances are visible, strain the solution through cotton wool.
3) Further, pour a little amount of vehicle over cotton wool to remove (collect) the solution, if it is remaining in it.
4) Add the other ingredients like stabilizers and organoleptic additives.(Volatile liquids/ substances are added at the end, just before adjusting the final volume.)
5) Add the more vehicle, to produce the final volume.
6) Transfer this mixture to a suitable bottle and close thoroughly, polish the bottle to remove finger prints. Fix the label, wrap the bottle and dispense.

II. Mixture containing diffusible solids:

Diffusible solids are those, which do not dissolve in water, but they may be mixed with water upon shaking and evenly diffused throughout the liquid for sufficient time, to ensure uniform distribution in each dose.

In this type of mixtures, upon standing the diffusible solids settle at the bottom of the container, which require re-shaking of the container each time when ever a dose is to be measured.

Hence these mixtures require an auxilliary label "SHAKE WELL BEFORE USE" on their label.

Eg :- The commonly used diffusible solids (drugs) are,

Bismuth carbonate	Magnesium oxide (Heavy or light)
Bismuth subnitrate	Magnesium carbonate (Heavy or light)
	Magnesium Trisilicate

Method:

1) Finely powder the diffusible substances (drug) and other (soluble) substances in a mortar.
2) Measure ¾ th of the total volume of the vehicle. Make a smooth cream by using a small portion of the vehicle by trituration and then add the remaining portion of the measured vehicle. (Reason- Due to the presence of air in the interspace of many powders, they float on the surface of water and do not mix with the vehicle. To prevent this tendency, first a smooth cream is prepared by adding a small amount of vehicle and then it is diluted).
3) Transfer the content to a measure. Rinse the mortar and pestle with little of vehicle and transfer it into the measure.
4) Add any liquid ingredients and make up the final volume by adding more amount of vehicle.
5) Transfer the mixture to a bottle, close throughly, Polish and label. Label should contain auxilliary label like, "SHAKE WELL BEFORE USE".

III. Mixture containing indiffusible solids:

Indiffusible solids are those substances, which do not dissolve in water, and do not remain uniformly distributed (diffused) in the vehicle, for sufficiently longer time. Even after shaking, they immediately settle at the bottom, therefore it is very difficult to measure the accurate dose.

Eg - The commonly used indiffusible solids in mixtures form are,

Phenobarbitone,	Phenacetin,
Quinine salicylate,	Benzoic acid,
Acetyl salicylic acid.	

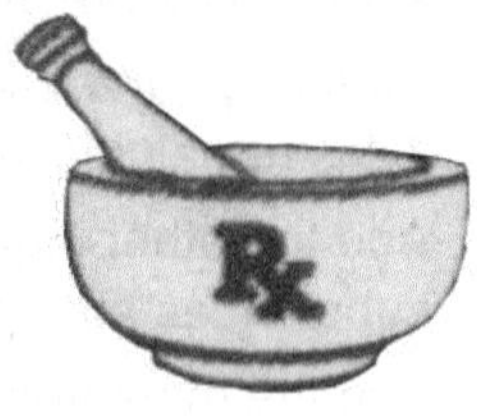

The indiffusible substances are made diffusible by increasing the viscosity of the vehicle by adding suitable suspending agents.

The suspending agent which are used in the mixture containing indiffusible solids are,

1) **Compound powder of tragacanth (C.P.T):** It is a mixture of acacia, starch, sucrose, and tragacanth. It is used in the preparation of mixtures in the proportion of, 2 gm/100 ml of the mixture or 10 grains/ounce of the mixture.

Formula :- Compound tragacanth powder I.P./B.P.

Tragacanth (finely powdered)	15 g
Gum acacia (finely powdered)	20 g
Starch	20 g
Sucrose (finely powdered)	45 g

Procedure: Accurately weigh all the ingredients and mix them uniformly in mortar in the ascending order of their weights and place in a air tight container.

2) **Mucilage of tragacanth (M.T):** It is used in the preparation of mixtures in the proportion of ¼th of the volume of the mixture.

Formula :- Mucilage of tragacanth B.P.C.

Tragacanth, finely powdered	1.25 g
Alcohol (90%)	2.5 ml
Chloroform water ....to....	100 ml

Addition of Tragacanth to water or viceversa, leads to the formation of lumpy product. Therefore alcohol (90%) is used as dispersing agent to disperse tragacanth powder uniformly in water (Chloroform water) for the preparation of Mucilage of Tragacanth.

In this preparation, Chloroform water is used instead of water because on storage, mucilage gets acid nature, due to enzyme action and since its viscosity decreases below pH 4 (at acidic pH). Finally it leads to the rapid deterioration of mucilage. Therefore chloroform water is used as antimicrobial (preservative), to prevent the enzymatic action on Tragacanth.

NOTE : When vehicle used is water or chloroform water or vehicle, which is not medicinally active then either compound powder of tragacanth 2 gm/100 ml of mixture or mucilage of tragacanth (M.T), ¼th of total volume can be used.

But when vehicle is medicinally active, then use only compound powder of tragacanth (CPT), should not use the mucilage of tragacanth because, mucilage of tragacanth is prepared by using alcohol (90%) and chloroform water, which may replace certain amount of medicinally active vehicle and hence decrease it's medicinal and flavouring properties.

Method: [Using compound powder of tragacanth (C.P.T)]

1) Finely powder the indiffusible solid in a mortar, add any diffusible or soluble substances in a mortar. Add the calculated amount of suspending agent and mix thoroughly.
2) Measure ¾ th of the total volume of the vehicle. Triturate the powder with a small quantity of vehicle to form a smooth cream and then add the remaining portion of the measured vehicle.
3) Transfer the content to a measure. Rinse the mortar with little of vehicle and transfer it into the measure.
4) Add if any liquid ingredients present and make up the final volume by adding more of vehicle.
5) Transfer the mixture to a bottle, close throughly, polish, and label. Label should contain auxilliary label like "SHAKE WELL BEFORE USE".

IV. Mixtures containing – Precipitate forming liquids:

These mixtures are prepared by certain liquids, which contain resinous matter. When these liquids are mixed with water, the resin will be precipitated out, this may adhere to the sides of the bottle or form a clotted precipitate, which will not re-diffuse upon shaking. To prevent this problem, compound tragacanth powder or mucilage of tragacanth is used as suspending agent.

Eg : Tincture of Lobelia ether,
Tincture of Stramonium.

Method: [Using compound powder of tragacanth (C.P.T)]

1) Finely powder the indiffusible and diffusible solid in a mortar. Thoroughly mix them with calculated amount of, compound powder of tragacanth.
2) Measure ¾ th of the total volume of the vehicle. Triturate the powder with a small quantity of vehicle, to form a smooth cream and then add the remaining portion of vehicle to make it pourable.
3) Measure the precipitate forming liquid in a dry measure and add it slowly in to the centre of the cream with rapid stirring.
4) Dissolve any soluble ingredients if present, in the sufficient amount of vehicle. Add it slowly with constant stirring to the cream, to avoid local high concentrations, which may neutralize the effect of suspending agent.
5) Transfer the mixture in to a bottle, close throughly, polish and label. Label should contain auxilliary label like "SH AKE WELL BEFORE USE".

V. Mixture containing slightly soluble liquids:

Slightly soluble liquids are not readily diffusible (soluble) and form insoluble portion in the mixture. Hence a suspending agent is needed to dispense such mixtures.

Compound powder of tragacanth (C.P.T) and Muscilage of tragacanth (M.T) are used as suspending agent in the same proportion as discussed in preparation of mixture containing indiffusible solids.

Eg: Liquid extract of glycyrrhiza.

Dispensing: Mixtures are usually dispensed in narrow mouthed, clear bottle and closed throughly with metallic screw cap.

If ingredients are sensitive to the light, they should be dispensed in narrow mouthed, amber coloured (light resistant) glass bottle and should be stored in dark place.

Storage: Mixture should be stored in a cool place. (At temperature not exceding 25° C).

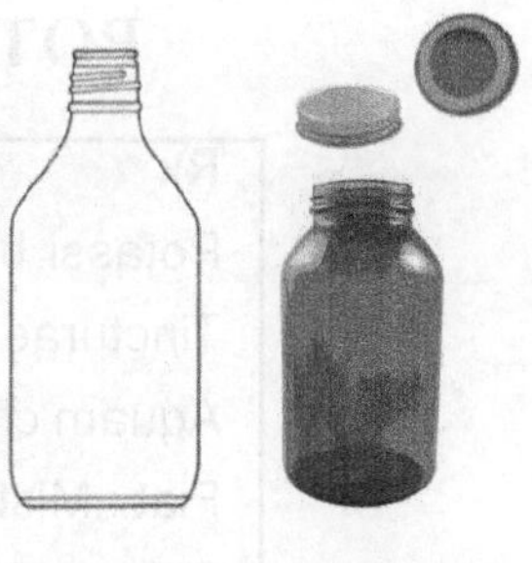

Containers for mixtures

POTASSIUM BROMIDE MIXTURE

Rx	
Potassi bromidi	3 ii
Tincturae nucis vomicae	fl. 3 ii
Aquam chloroformi......q.s.....	fl.oz vi
Fiat : Mistura	Mitte : fl.oz i
Signa : Cochleare magnum ter in die, post cibos sumendum.	

Conversion :

3 ii → 2 drachms	fl.oz vi → 6 fl.oz	fl. 3 ii → 2 fl. drachms
1 drachm = 4 g	1 fl.oz = 30 ml	1 fl. drachm = 4 ml
2 drachms = 8 g	6 fl.oz = 180ml	2 fl. drachms = 8 ml

Calculation : For fl.oz i → 1 fl.oz = 30ml

Potassium bromide $= \frac{8}{180} \times 30 = 1.33\,g$

Tincture of Nux-vomica $= \frac{8}{180} \times 30 = 1.33\ ml$

Chloroform water.... q.s..... ..... = 30 ml

: Label :

POTASSIUM BROMIDE MIXTURE **30 ml**	
Category : Sedative, Bitter tonic.	
Direction : One tablespoonful to be taken, three times a day, after meals.	
Storage : Store in a cool place.	
Mfg. Lic. no. : GU/201 **Batch No.** : XY2	**Mfg. Date :** 12-09-06 **Exp. Date:** 11-09-08
Manufactured By : Roll No - 21 **Name of the college and place:**	

Type	Ingredients	Quantity in imperial	Quantity in metric	Quantity taken
Mixture containing, soluble solid. (Simple mixture)	Potassium bromide	2 dr	8 g	1.33 g
	Tincture of Nux-vomica	2 fl. dr	8 ml	1.33 ml
	Chloroform water...q.s....	6 fl.oz	180 ml	30 ml
	Prepare: Mixture	Send: 30 ml		
	Direction: One tablespoonful to be taken, three times a day, after meals.			

Theory:

This is a mixture containing **soluble solid**, like potassium bromide. Since both potassium bromide and Tincture of nux-vomica are soluble in the vehicle-chloroform water, the mixture can be prepared by the simple solution method.

Potassium bromide acts as sedative and tincture of nux-vomica acts as appetizer. Chloroform water is used as flavoured vehicle and it also acts as preservative.

Procedure:

1) Accurately weigh potassium bromide and dissolve it in about ¾ th of chloroform water, by stirring.
2) Examine the solution for clarity and filter the solution through muslin cloth, if any foreign particles are present.
3) Measure the tincture of nux-vomica and add to the above solution, mix well by stirring and transfer to a measure.
4) Add remaining amount of chloroform water to make up the final volume.

Dispensing: Transfer the mixture to a clear, narrow mouthed glass bottle, close it throughly with metallic screw cap, polish and label.

Direction: One tablespoonful to be taken, three times a day, after meals.

Storage: Store in a cool place.

Uses:

1. Potassium bromide act as sedative. Therefore it is used to induce sleep, when sleeplessness (insomnia) is due to anxiety or overwork or pain.
2. Tincture of nux vomica acts as a bitter tonic, which increases the appetite, in the cases of anorexia due to anxiety. Therefore this mixture is used as a sedative and appetizer.

SODIUM BICARBONATE MIXTURE

Rx	
Sodii bicarbonatis	3 i
Tincturae nucis vomicae	fl. 3 ii
Infusum gentianae comositae...q.s..	fl.oz vi
Fiat : Mistura	Mitte : fl.oz ii
Signa : Cochleare magnum, bis in die, pre cibos sumendum.	

Conversion :

3 i → 1 drachm	fl.oz vi → 6 fl.oz	fl. 3 ii → 2 fl. drachms
1 drachm = 4 g	1 fl.oz = 30 ml	1 fl. drachm = 4 ml
	6 fl.oz = 180 ml	2 fl. drachms = 8 ml

Calculation : For fl .oz ii → 2 fl.oz = 60 ml

Sodium bicarbonate $= \frac{4}{180} \times 60 = 1.33$ g

Tincture of nuxvomica $= \frac{8}{180} \times 60 = 2.66$ ml

Compound infusion of gentian...q.s... = 60 ml

:Label:

SODIUM BICARBONATE MIXTURE **60 ml**	
Category : Appetizer and Antacid.	
Direction : One tablespoonful to be taken, two times a day, before meals.	
Storage : Store in a cool place.	
Mfg. Lic. no. : GU/201 **Batch No.** : XY2	**Mfg. Date :** 12-09-06 **Exp. Date:** 11-09-08
Manufactured By : Roll No - 21 **Name of the college and place:**	

Type	Ingredients	Quantity in imperial	Quantity in metric	Quantity taken
Mixture containing, soluble solid. (Simple mixture)	Sodium bicarbonate	1 dr	4 g	1.33 g
	Tincture of nux-vomica	2 fl. dr	8 ml	2.66 ml
	Compound infusion of gentian.........q.s....	6 fl.oz	180 ml	60 ml
	Prepare: Mixture	Send: 60 ml		
	Direction: One tablespoonful to be taken, two times a day, before meals.			

Theory:

This is a mixture containing **soluble solid like-** Sodium bicarbonate. In this preparation, compound infusion of gentian is used as vehicle, which is used to improve the appetite and to stimulate the gastric secretion. Tincture of nux-vomica contains strychnine, which acts as a bitter tonic and increases the appetite and stimulates the flow of gastric juice.

Sodium bicarbonate is used as an antacid, because when given with bitter tonic like gentian or strychnine before meals, it neutralizes the excessive secretion of hydrochloric acid in the stomach.

All the ingredients are soluble (miscible) in vehicle, therefore this mixture is prepared by simple solution method.

Procedure:

1) Accurately weigh sodium bicarbonate and dissolve in ¾ th of the compound infusion of gentian, by stirring.
2) Filter, if any foreign particles are present.
3) Slowly add tincture of nux-vomica to the above mixture by continuous stirring.
4) Transfer this content to a measure and adjust the final volume by adding more vehicle and mix well.

Dispensing: Transfer the mixture to a clear, narrow mouthed, glass bottle, close it throughly with metallic screw cap, polish and label.

Direction: One tablespoonful to be taken, two times a day, before meals.

Storage: Store in a cool place.

Uses: Sodium bicarbonate mixture is used as appetizer and antacid.

MAGNESIUM SULPHATE AND MAGNESIUM CARBONATE MIXTURE

Rx	
Magnesii sulphatis	3 i
Magnesii carbonatis	3 i
Aquam menthae piperitae..q.s..	fl.oz vi
Fiat : Mistura	Mitte: fl.oz i
Signa : Cochleare amplum semi hora, ante jentaculum sumendum.	

Conversion :

3 i → 1 drachm	fl.oz iv → 6 fl.oz
1 drachm = 4 g	1 fl.oz = 30 ml
	6 fl.oz = 180 ml

Calculation : For fl.oz i →1 fl.oz = 30 ml

Magnesium sulphate $= \frac{4}{180} \times 30 = 0.66$ g

Magnesium carbonate $= \frac{4}{180} \times 30 = 0.66$ g

Peppermint water ...q.s..... = 30 ml

: Label:

MAGNESIUM SULPHATE AND MAGNESIUM CARBONATE MIXTURE	
30 ml	
Category : Antacid.	
Direction : One tablespoonful to be taken, half an hour before Breakfast.	
Storage : Store in a cool place.	
SHAKE WELL BEFORE USE.	
Mfg. Lic. no. : GU/201	**Mfg. Date :** 12-09-06
Batch No. : XY2	**Exp. Date:** 11-09-08
Manufactured By : Roll No - 21	

Name of the college and place:

Type	Ingredients	Quantity in imperial	Quantity in metric	Quantity taken
Mixture containing, diffusible solid.	Magnesium sulphate	1 dr	4 g	0.66 g
	Magnesium carbonate	1 dr	4 g	0.66 g
	Peppermint water.....q.s..	6 fl.oz	180 ml	30 ml
	Prepare: Mixture	Send: 30 ml		
	Direction: One tablespoonful to be taken, half an hour before breakfast.			

Theory:

This is a mixture containing **diffusible solid**. In this mixture magnesium carbonate is diffusible (not soluble) in peppermint water. As per definition, diffusible solids do not dissolve in water, but mix with water upon shaking and evenly diffuse throughout the liquid for sufficient time, to ensure uniform distribution in each dose.

Magnesium sulphate acts as antacid and soluble in peppermint water. Therefore this mixture can be easily prepared, by dispersing magnesium carbonate in peppermint water. Peppermint water is used as flavoured vehicle.

Procedure:

1) Weigh separately and finely powder the magnesium sulphate and magnesium carbonate in a mortar and mix uniformly.
2) Measure ¾th quantity of peppermint water. Triturate the above powder with small portion of peppermint water, until to get a smooth cream. Further dilute this cream with small portion of peppermint water, to make it pourable.
3) Transfer this content in to a measure. Rinse the mortar and pestle with peppermint water and transfer in to the measure.
4) Examine the solution for clarity and filter the solution through muslin cloth, if any foreign particles are present.
5) Adjust the final volume by adding remaining amount of peppermint water.

Dispensing: Transfer the mixture to a clear, narrow mouthed glass bottle, close it throughly with metallic screw cap, polish and label.

Direction: One tablespoonful to be taken, half an hour before breakfast.

Storage: Store in a cool place.

Auxilliary label: SHAKE WELL BEFORE USE.

Uses: Both magnesium sulphate and magnesium carbonate acts as antacid, therefore Compound magnesium sulphate mixture is used as an antacid preparation.

LIGHT MAGNESIUM CARBONATE AND KAOLIN MIXTURE

Rx	
Levis kaolin	gr LX
Levis magnessi carbonatis	gr XV
Sodii bicarbonatis	gr XV
Aquam menthae piperitae...q.s..	fl.oz i
Fiat : Mistura	Mitte : fl.oz i
Signa : Cochleare maximum t.i.d sumendum.	

Conversion :

gr LX → 60 grains
15 grains = 1 g
60 grains = 4 g

gr XV → 15 grains
15 grains = 1 g
fl.oz i → 1 fl.oz = 30 ml

Calculation : For fl.oz i → 1 fl.oz = 30 ml

Light kaolin = $\frac{4}{30} \times 30 = 4$ g

Light magnesium carbonate = $\frac{1}{30} \times 30 = 1$ g

Sodium bicarbonate = $\frac{1}{30} \times 30 = 1$ g

Peppermint water...q.s..... = 30 ml

Type	Ingredients	Quantity in imperial	Quantity in metric	Quantity taken
Mixture containing, diffusible solids.	Light kaolin	60 gr	4 g	4 g
	Light magnesium carbonate	15 gr	1 g	1 g
	Sodium bicarbonate	15 gr	1 g	1 g
	Peppermint water.......q.s...	1 fl.oz	30 ml	30 ml
	Prepare: Mixture	Send: 30 ml		
	Direction: One tablespoonful to be taken, three times a day.			

Theory:

This is a mixture containing **diffusible solids** like, light kaolin and light magnesium carbonate. Light kaolin is purified hydrated aluminium silicate, which acts as antacid and also a good intestinal adsorbent. Light magnesium carbonate acts as antacid. Sodium bicarbonate acts as antacid and is soluble in water. Therefore this mixture is prepared by method, which is used for preparing mixtures containing diffusible solids.

Procedure:

1) Weigh separately the light kaolin, light magnesium carbonate and sodium bicarbonate.
2) Finely powder them in a motor.
3) Measure ¾ th of peppermint water. Out of this, add a small portion to the powder and triturate little thoroughly, until a smooth cream is formed.
4) Then dilute this cream with remaining amount of peppermint water, to make it pourable and strain through a muslin cloth, if any foreign particles present.
5) Transfer this content into a measure and make the final volume with peppermint water.

Dispensing: Transfer the mixture to a clear or amber coloured, narrow mouthed glass bottle, close it throughly with metallic screw cap, polish and label.

Direction: One tablespoonful to be taken, three times a day

Storage: Store in a cool place.

Auxilliary label: SHAKE WELL BEFORE USE.

Uses: Light magnesium carbonate and kaolin mixture is used as antacid.

> **Note:** Light kaolin is a good intestinal adsorbent. Hence it is used in the treatment of food or alkaloid poisoning. It is insoluble in water, it forms a protective coating on mucous membrane of the intestine, hence decreases discomfort. Light kaolin also acts as an antacid. Therefore it is used in symptomatic treatment of intestiinal colitis.
>
> Sodium bicarbonate acts as both antacid and carminative. It expels the gas from the stomach and it potentiates the action of light kaolin.

COMPOUND MAGNESIUM TRISILICATE MIXTURE

Rx	
Magnessi trisilicatis	3 i s
Levis magnessi carbonatis	3 i s
Sodii barcarbonatis	3 i s
Aquam menthae piperitae...q.s..	fl. 3 xxv
Fiat : Mistura	Mitte : fl.oz i
Signa : Cochleare parvum, t.i.d sumendum.	

Conversion :

3 i s → 1.25 drachms	fl. 3 xxv s → 25 fl. drachms
1 drachm = 4 g	1 fl. drachm = 4 ml
1.25 drachms = 5 g	25 fl. drachms = 100 ml

Calculation : For fl.oz i → 1 fl.oz = 30 ml

Magnesium trisilicate = $\frac{5}{100} \times 30 = 1.5$ g

Light magnesium carbonate = $\frac{5}{100} \times 30 = 1.5$ g

Sodium bicarbonate = $\frac{5}{100} \times 30 = 1.5$ g

Peppermint water ...q.s... = 30ml

Type	Ingredients	Quantity in imperial	Quantity in metric	Quantity taken
Mixture containing, diffusible solids.	Magnesium trisilicate	1.25 dr	5 g	1.5 g
	Light magnesium carbonate	1.25 dr	5 g	1.5 g
	Sodium bicarbonate	1.25 dr	5 g	1.5 g
	Peppermint water..q.s...	25 fl. dr	100 ml	30 ml
	Prepare: Mixture Send: 30 ml Direction: One teaspoonful to be taken, three times a day.			

Theory:

This is a mixture containing **diffusible solids,** because both magnesium trisilicate and light magnesium carbonate are diffusible in nature and both are acts as antacids. Sodium bicarbonate is also acts as antacid and is soluble in water. Therefore this mixture is prepared by method, which is used for preparing mixtures containing diffusible solids. Peppermint water is used as flavoured vehicle.

Procedure:

1) Weigh separately, magnesium trisilicate, light magnesium carbonate and sodium bicarbonate.
2) Finely powder them in a motor.
3) Measure $\frac{3}{4}^{th}$ of peppermint water. Add a small amount of peppermint water to the powder and triturate thoroughly, until a smooth cream (paste) is formed.
4) Dilute the cream with small amount of peppermint water to make it pourable and strain through a muslin cloth, to remove if any foreign particles present.
5) Transfer this content into a measure and make the final volume with peppermint water

Dispensing: Transfer the mixture to a clear, narrow mouthed glass bottle, close it throughly with metallic screw cap, polish and label.

Direction: One teaspoonful to be taken, three times a day.

Storage: Store in a cool place.

Auxilliary label: SHAKE WELL BEFORE USE.

Uses: This mixture is used as an adsorbent and antacid. Its action is slow, but continuous for a longer time. It is nontoxic even in large doses. Hence it is widely used in dyspepsia.

Other examples for -- Mixtures containing diffusible solids :

1.

Rx

Light kaolin	20 g
Sodium bicarbonate	5 g
Tincture of hyoscyamus	4 ml
Purified water...q.s....	100 ml

Uses: This mixture is used as antidiarrhoeal and antacid.

2.

Rx

Calcium carbonate	0.1 g
Sodium bicarbonate	0.1 g
Light magnesium carbonate	0.1 ml
Simple syrup	0.1 ml
Aromatic cardamom tincture	0.1 ml
Chloroform water....q.s...	10 ml

Uses: This mixture is used as an antacid and carminative.

3.

Rx

Bismuth carbonate	0.5 g
Sodium bicarbonate	0.4 g
Tincture of Belladonna	0.2 ml
Purified water....q.s....	15 ml

Uses: This mixture is used as antacid.

4.

Rx

Cretae preparatae	gr xxx
Pulveris cretae aromatici	gr xx
Aquam cinnamom...q.s...	fl.oz i

Uses: This mixture is used as antidiarrhoeal.

MIXTURE OF PREPARED CHALK B.P.

Rx	
Cretae preparate	gr xxx
Tincturae catechu	M xv iii
Aquam cinnamoni....q.s...	fl.oz i
Fiat : Mistura	Mitte : fl.oz ii
Signa : Cochleare magnum, quarter in die sumendum.	

Conversion :

gr XXX → 30 grains   M xv iii →18 minims

15 grains = 1 g   15 minims = 1 ml

30 grains = 2 g   18 minims = 1.2 ml

Calculation : For fl.oz ii → 2 fl.oz = 60 ml

Prepared chalk $= \frac{2}{30} \times 60 = 4$ g

Tincture of catechu $= \frac{1.2}{30} \times 60 = 2.4$ ml

Cinnamon water ...q.s.... = 60 ml

Compound powder of tragacanth required is 2 g/ 100 ml of total volume of the mixture

So, Compound powder of tragacanth required for 60 ml = $\frac{2}{100} \times 60 = 1.2$ g

Revised formula:

Prepared chalk	-----	4 g
Tincture of catechu	-----	2.4 ml
Compound powder of tragacanth	-----	1..2 g
Cinnamon water....q.s...	-----	60 ml

Type	Ingredients	Quantity in imperial	Quantity in metric	Quantity taken
Mixture containing, indiffusible solid and volatile liquid.	Prepared chalk	30 gr	2 g	4 g
	Tincture of catechu	18 minims	1.2 ml	2.4 ml
	Cinnamon water....q.s...	1 fl.oz	30 ml	60 ml
	Prepare: Mixture	Send: 60 ml		
	Direction: One tablespoonful to be taken, four times a day.			

Theory:

This is a mixture containing **indiffusible solid-** like prepared chalk. Hence a suspending agent is required, to make prepared chalk as diffusible or distribute evenly in a vehicle for a longer time, so as to ensure that accurate amount of dose can be taken out of the container during measuring of dose. Tincture of catechu acts as astringent and miscible with cinnamon water.

In this mixture, cinnamon water is used as a vehicle, which is medicinally active vehicle, therefore compound tragacanth powder is used as suspending agent, in the concentration of 2 gm/100 ml.

Procedure:

1) Weigh prepared chalk and triturate in a mortar. Add calculated quantity of compound powder of tragacanth (CPT) and mix throughly.
2) Measure ¾ th of cinnamon water, add a little portion of it to the powder mixture gradually and triturate to get a smooth cream. Further dilute this cream with cinnamon water, to make it pourable.
3) Transfer this content to a measure, add tincture of catechu and mix uniformly.
4) Adjust the final volume with cinnamon water.

Dispensing: Transfer the mixture to a clear, narrow mouthed, glass bottle, close it throughly with metallic screw cap, polish and label.

Direction: One tablespoonful to be taken, four times a day.

Storage: Store in a cool place.

Auxilliary label: SHAKE WELL BEFORE USE.

Uses: This mixture is used as astringent, in the treatment of diarrhoea.

PHENACETIN AND CAFFEINE MIXTURE

Rx	
Phenacetini	gr L
Caffeinae	gr xv
Syrupi aurantii	fl. 3 iii
Aquam....q.s......	fl.oz iii
Fiat : Mistura	Mitte : fl.oz i
Signa : Cochleare magnum, dolore urgente capiendus.	

Conversion :

gr L→ 50 grains — fl. 3 iii → 3 fl.drachms

15 grains = 1 g — 1 fl. drachm = 4 ml

50 grains = 3.3 g — 3 fl. drachms = 12 ml

Calculation : For fl.oz i → 1 fl.oz = 30 ml

Phenacetin = $\frac{3.3}{90} \times 30 = 1.1$ g

Caffeine = $\frac{1}{90} \times 30 = 0.33$ g

Orange syrup = $\frac{12}{90} \times 30 = 4$ ml

Water ....q.s.... = 30 ml

Mucilage of tragacanth required is, ¼ th of the total volume of the mixture

So, Mucilage of tragacanth required for 30 ml = $\frac{1}{4} \times 30 = 7.5$ ml

Revised Formula:

Phenacetin	----	1.1 g
Caffeine	----	0.33 g
Orange syrup	----	4 ml
Mucilage of tragacanth	----	7.5 ml
Water...... q.s		30 ml

Type	Ingredients	Quantity in imperial	Quantity in metric	Quantity taken
Mixture containing, Indiffusible solid.	Phenacetin	50 gr	3.3 g	1.1 g
	Caffeine	15 gr	1 g	0.33 g
	Orange syrup	3 fl. dr	12 ml	4 ml
	Water.........q.s...	3 fl.oz	90 ml	30 ml
	Prepare: Mixture	Send: 30 ml		
	Direction: One tablespoonful to be taken, when the pain is severe.			

Theory:

This is a mixture containing **indiffusible solid--** Phenacetin, which acts as analgesic. Due to its indiffusible nature, it does not remain evenly distributed in vehicle for longer time. Hence Phenacetin can be made diffusible in vehicle, by using a suspending agent.

Caffeine acts as analgesic and it is soluble in nature, in the prescribed range. Orange syrup is used as sweetening agent, to mask the bitter (saline) taste of phenacetin.

In this prescription, water is used as a vehicle. Therefore either compound powder of tragacanth or mucilage of tragacanth can be used as suspending agent.

This mixture is prepared by using mucilage of tragacanth, in the concentration of $\frac{1}{4}^{th}$ of the total volume of the mixture.

Procedure:

1) Weigh accurately phenacetin and caffeine separately.
2) Finely powder the phenacetin by triturating in a mortar, add caffeine and mix uniformly.
3) Triturate this powder mixture with mucilage of tragacanth, to form smooth cream.
4) Dilute with water, to make it pourable.
5) Transfer this content to a measure and add orange syrup, mix well.
6) Make up the final volume with remaining amount of water.

Dispensing: Transfer the mixture to a clear, narrow mouthed, glass bottle, close it throughly with metallic screw cap, polish and label.

Direction: One tablespoonful to be taken, when the pain is severe.

Storage: Store in a cool place.

Auxilliary label: SHAKE WELL BEFORE USE.

Uses: This mixture is used as analgesic.

ACETYL SALICYLIC ACID MIXTURE

Rx	
Acidi acityl salicylici	gr x
Potassii citrasis	gr xxx
Aquam chloroformi...q.s...	fl.oz i
Fiat : Mistura	Mitte : fl.oz ii
Signa : Cochleare amplum, apud quartis horis sumendum.	

Conversion :

gr x → 10 grains   fl.oz i → 1 fl.oz = 30 ml

1 grain = 60 mg

10 grains = 600 mg (0.6 g)

gr xxx → 30 grains = 1800 mg (1.8 g)

Calculation : For fl.oz ii → 2 fl.oz = 60 ml

Acetyl salicylic acid = $\frac{0.6}{30} \times 60 = 1.2$ g

Potassium citrate = $\frac{1.8}{30} \times 60 = 3.6$ g

Chloroform water ....q.s...... = 60 ml

Type	Ingredients	Quantity in imperial	Quantity in metric	Quantity taken
Mixture containing Indiffusible solid but due to the presence of alkali citrate. It is Simple mixture.	Acetyl salicylic acid	10 gr	600 mg	1.2 g
	Potassium citrate	30 gr	1800 mg	3.6 g
	Chloroform water ..q.s...	1 fl.oz	30 ml	60 ml
	Prepare: Mixture Send: 60 ml Direction: One tablespoonful to be taken, at every four hours.			

Theory:

This is a mixture containing **indiffusible solid**, because acetyl salicylic acid is insoluble and also indiffusible in water.

If acetyl salicylic acid is prescribed alone, it needs a suspending agent to make it diffusible, but in presence of alkali citrates like, potassium citrate, sodium citrate, and ammonium citrate it is soluble, due to the formation of soluble complexes.

Hence in presence of potassium citrate, acetyl salicylic acid is freely soluble in chloroform water. Therefore this mixture is finally considered as, mixture containing soluble solids(as simple mixture).

Procedure:

1) Dissolve the weighed amount of potassium citrate in $\frac{3}{4}^{th}$ of chloroform water. To this solution, add finely powdered acetyl salicylic acid (aspirin) and dissolve by stirring.
2) Filter the mixture, if any foreign particles are present.
3) Transfer to a measure and make up the final volume with remaining amount of chloroform water.

Dispensing: Transfer the mixture to a clear or amber coloured, narrow mouthed, glass bottle, close it throughly with metallic screw cap, polish and label.

Direction: One tablespoonful to be taken, at every four hours.

Storage: Store in a cool place.

Uses: Acetyl salicylic acid acts as an analgesic and antipyretic, hence this mixture is used as an analgesic and antipyretic.

Note: Potassium citrate is used to dissolve acetyl salicylic acid, because it is insoluble in water. Potassium citrate is mainly used as urine alkaliniser i.e it makes the urine alkaline in the treatment of inflammatory conditions of the urinary bladder and prevents the formation of crystalluria (kidney stones). Therefore, this mixture is also used in the inflammatory and painful condition of the bladder.

SULPHADIMIDINE MIXTURE

Rx	
Sulphadimidine	gr xv
Syrupi aurantii	M xxx
Aquam acidi benzoici	M iii
Aquam amarantii	M iii
Aquam chloroformi...q.s...	fl. 3 ii ss
Fiat : Mistura	Mitte : fl.oz i
Signa : Coch.max., mane et nocte sumendum	

Conversion :

gr xv → 15 grains   M xxx → 30 minims

15 grains = 1 g   15 minims = 1 ml

30 minims = 2 ml

fl. 3 ii ss → 2.5 fl. drachms   3 minims = 0.18 ml ≅ 0.2 ml

1 fl. drachm = 4 ml

2.5 fl. drachms = 10 ml

Calculation : For fl.oz i → 1 fl.oz = 30 ml

Sulphadimidine $= \frac{1}{10} \times 30 = 3$ g

Orange syrup $= \frac{2}{10} \times 30 = 6$ ml

Benzoic acid solution $= \frac{0.2}{10} \times 30 = 0.6$ ml

Amaranth solution $= \frac{0.2}{10} \times 30 = 0.6$ ml

Chloroform water ...q.s...... = 30 ml

Compound powder of tragacanth required is 2 g /100 ml of total volume of the mixture

So, Compound powder of tragacanth required for 30 ml $= \frac{2}{100} \times 30 = 0.6$ g

Revised formula:

Sulphadimidine, in fine powder	3 g
Orange syrup	6 ml
Benzoic acid solution	0.6 ml
Amaranth solution	0.6 ml
Compound powder of tragacanth	0.6 g
Chloroform water…q.s...	30 ml

Type	Ingredients	Quantity in imperial	Quantity in metric	Quantity taken
Mixture containing, indiffusible solid.	Sulphadimidine(fine)	15 gr	1.0 g	3 g
	Orange syrup	30 minims	2.0 ml	6 ml
	Benzoic acid solution	3 minims	0.2 ml	0.6 ml
	Amaranth solution	3 minims	0.2 ml	0.6 ml
	Chloroform water...q.s..	2.5 fl. dr	10.0 ml	30 ml
	Prepare: Mixture Send: 30 ml Direction: One tablespoonful to be taken, at morning and night.			

Theory:

This is a mixture containing **indiffusible solid** like sulphadimidine. Hence suspending agent is required, to make sulphadimidine as diffusible or distribute evenly in a vehicle for a longer time, so as to ensure that, accurate amount of dose can be taken out of the container, each time.

In this prescription chloroform water is used as a vehicle, therefore either compound powder of tragacanth or mucilage of tragacanth can be used as suspending agent. Hence this mixture is prepared by using compound tragacanth powder, in the concentration of 2 gm/100 ml of the total volume of the mixture, as a suspending agent.

Amaranth solution is used to give an attractive colour to the mixture. Benzoic acid solution is used as antimicrobial preservative. Chloroform water is used as flavoured vehicle, which also acts as preservative. Orange syrup is used as sweetening agent and flavouring agent.

Procedure:

1) Accurately weigh sulphadimidine powder and compound tragacanth powder, mix them uniformly in a mortar.
2) To this powder mixture, add chloroform water and triturate so as to form a smooth cream.
3) As the mixture becomes too viscous, it is difficult to strain, therefore remove the foreign particles if present, with the help of glass rod. Dilute the cream with small portion of chloroform water to make it pourable.
4) Transfer this content to a measure. To this, incorporate liquid ingredients like benzoic acid solution, amaranth solution and orange syrup and stir thoroughly with glass rod to get a uniform mixture.
5) Adjust the final volume with chloroform water.

Dispensing: Transfer the mixture to a clear or amber coloured, narrow mouthed glass bottle, close it throughly with metallic screw cap, polish and label.

Direction: One tablespoonful to be taken, at morning and night.

Storage: Store in a cool place.

Auxilliary label: SHAKE WELL BEFORE USE.

Uses: Sulphadimidine acts as a bacteriostatic agent. It is used in the pneumococcal or streptococcal infections and E.coli infections of the urinary tract, hence this mixture is used in the treatment of urinary tract infections (U.T.I.).

BISMUTH CARBONATE MIXTURE

Rx	
Bismuthi carbonatis	gr XV
Cretae preparatae	gr XV
Levis kaolin	gr LX
Tincturae catechu	M XXX
Aquam......q.s.......	fl.oz i
Fiat : Mistura	Mitte : fl.oz i
Signa : Coch.amp.b.i.d, sumendum.	

Conversion :

gr XV → 15 grains
15 grains = 1 g

M XXX → 30 minims
15 minims = 1 ml
30 minims = 2 ml

gr LX → 60 grains
60 grains = 4 g

fl.oz i → 1 fl.oz = 30 ml

Calculation : For fl.oz i → 1 fl.oz = 30 ml

Bismuth carbonate = $\frac{1}{30} \times 30 = 1$ g

Prepared chalk = $\frac{1}{30} \times 30 = 1$ g

Light kaolin = $\frac{4}{30} \times 30 = 4$ g

Tincture of catechu = $\frac{2}{30} \times 30 = 2$ ml

Purified water ...q.s...... = 30 ml

Compound powder of tragacanth required is 2 g /100 ml of total volume of the mixture

So, Compound powder of tragacanth required for 30 ml = $\frac{2}{100} \times 30 = 0.6$ g

Revised formula:

Bismuth carbonate	-----	1 g
Prepared chalk	-----	1 g
Light kaolin	-----	4 g
Tincture of catechu	-----	2 ml
Compound tragacanth powder	-----	0.6 g
Purified water....q.s.....	-----	30 ml

Type	Ingredients	Quantity in imperial	Quantity in metric	Quantity taken
Mixture containing, indiffusible solid.	Bismuth carbonate	15 gr	1 g	1 g
	Prepared chalk	15 gr	1 g	1 g
	Light kaolin	60 gr	4 g	4 g
	Tincture of catechu	30 minims	2 ml	2 ml
	Purified water....q.s...	1 fl.oz	30 ml	30 ml
	Prepare: Mixture Send: 30 ml Direction: One tablespoonful to be taken, two times a day.			

Theory:

This is a mixture containing **indiffusible solid** like prepared chalk, which is indiffusible in nature. Hence to make it diffusible uniformly in the vehicle, suspending agent is required. Prepared chalk is purified native calcium carbonate, which acts as an adsorbent and produces its action by covering the intestinal mucous membrane. It also acts as an antacid.

Bismuth carbonate acts as an antacid. It forms an adhesive coating over intestinal mucosa, hence it also acts as an adsorbent. Light kaolin (kaolin) is purified hydrated aluminium silicate, free from gritty particles, which acts as good intestinal adsorbent. Therefore it is used to stop diarrhoea and dysentery caused by food and alkaloidal poisoning.

Tincture of catechu contains tannic acid, which acts as an astringent. It is liberated slowly from tincture of catechu, therefore its action remains for a longer time. If pure tannic acid is used, its effect is immediate but it has short half life, hence tincture of catechu is preferred than tannic acid. It is used along with other astringent, in the symptomatic treatment of diarrhoea.

The vehicle used is water therefore, either compound tragacanth powder in the ratio of 2 gm/100 ml or mucilage of tragacanth in the ratio of ¼th of total volume of the mixture can be used.

This preparation is prepared by using compound powder of tragacant as suspendind agent.

Procedure:

1) Weigh separately prepared chalk, bismuth carbonate and kaolin powder and mix them in a mortar .
2) To this powder mixture, add calculated quantity of compound tragacanth powder and mix thoroughly.
3) Measure ¾th of final volume of water. From this, add a small portion of water and triturate, so as to form a smooth cream and dilute with remaining portion of water.
4) If foreign particles are present, strain through muslin cloth. If only 2 to 3 particles are present, remove them with glass rod and avoid straining.

5) Add tincture of catechu in to the centre of the cream, with continuous trituration and transfer to a measure and adjust the final volume with purified water.

Dispensing: Transfer the mixture to a clear, narrow mouthed glass bottle, close it throughly with metallic screw cap, polish and label.

Direction: One tablespoonful to be taken, two times a day.

Storage: Store in a cool place.

Auxilliary label: SHAKE WELL BEFORE USE.

Uses: This mixture is used as an antidiarrhoeal preparation.

MIXTURE OF ETHEREAL TINCTURE OF LOBELIA

Rx	
Potassii iodidi	gr xxx
Tincturae lobeliae aetheriae	fl. 3 ii
Aquam........q.s...	fl.oz vi
Fiat : Mistura	Mitte : fl.oz i
Signa : Cochleare magnum, sextis horis sumendum.	

Conversion :

gr xxx → 30 grains
15 grains = 1 g
30 grains = 2 g
fl.oz vi → 6 fl.oz = 180 ml

fl. 3 ii → 2 fl. drachms
1 fl. drachm = 4 ml
2 fl. drachms = 8 ml

Calculation : For fl.oz i → 1 fl.oz = 30 ml

Potassium iodide = $\frac{2}{180} \times 30 = 0.33\text{ g}$

Ethereal tincture of Lobelia = $\frac{8}{180} \times 30 = 1.33\text{ml}$

Purified water...q.s...... = 30 ml

Mucilage of tragacanth required is ¼ th of total volume of mixture

So, Mucilage of tragacanth required for 30 ml = $\frac{1}{4} \times 30 = 7.5\text{ ml}$

Revised formula:

Potassium iodide ---- 0.33 g
Ethereal tincture of lobelia ---- 1.33 ml
Mucilage of tragacanth ---- 7.5 ml
Purified water... q.s ...... 30 ml

Type	Ingredients	Quantity in imperial	Quantity in metric	Quantity taken
Mixture containing, precipitate forming liquid.	Potassium iodide	30 gr	2 g	0.33 g
	Ethereal tincture of Lobelia	2 fl. dr	8 ml	1.33 ml
	Purified water... q.s	6 fl.oz	180 ml	30 ml
	Prepare: Mixture Send: 30 ml			
	Direction: One tablespoonful to be taken, every six hours.			

Theory:

This is a mixture containing **precipitate forming liquid,** like Ethereal tincture of lobelia. Ethereal tincture of lobelia is resinous in nature and precipitated out in the aqueous vehicle. The formed precipitate is indiffusible in nature. Hence this precipitate is made diffusible by using suspending agent. Potassium iodide acts as expectorant and it is soluble in water.

In this prescription purified water is used as a vehicle therefore, either compound powder of tragacanth in the concentration of 2 gm/100 ml or mucilage of tragacanth can be used as suspending agent, in the concentration of ¼th of total volume of the mixture.

This mixture is prepared by using mucilage of tragacanth as a suspending agent.

Procedure:

1) Take calculated quantity of mucilage of tragacanth and mix with equal volume of water in a mortar.
2) Measure Ethereal tincture of lobelia in a dry measure and pour slowly in to the centre of mucilage, with constant stirring.
3) Dissolve separately, potassium iodide in small portion of water. Add this solution to the mixture of mucilage of tragacanth and Ethereal tincture of lobelia and mix uniformly.
4) Transfer the content to a measure and adjust the final volume with water.

Dispensing: Transfer the mixture to a clear, narrow mouthed glass bottle, close it throughly with metallic screw cap, polish and label.

Direction: One tablespoonful to be taken, every six hours.

Storage: Store in a cool place.

Auxillary label: SHAKE WELL BEFORE USE.

Uses: Lobeline is an active ingredient of Ethereal tincture of lobelia, which dilates the bronchioles, relive the bronchial spasm and diminishes the secretion of mucus. Potassium iodide acts as expectorant .

Therefore this mixture is used in the treatment of asthma.

MIXTURE OF TINCTURE OF MYRRH AND POTASSIUM IODIDE

Rx	
Potassii iodidi	gr xxx
Tincturae myrrahae	fl. 3 iii
Tincturae stromonii	fl. 3 iv
Aquam chloroformi...q.s...	fl.oz vi
Fiat : Mistura	Mitte : fl.oz i
Signa : Cochleare amplum q.i.d sumendum.	

Conversion :

gr xxx → 30 grains
15 grains = 1 g
30 grains = 2 g
fl.oz Vi → 6 fl.oz = 180 ml

fl. 3 iii → 3 fl. drachms
1 fl. drachm = 4 ml
3 fl. drachms = 12 ml
fl. 3 iv → 4 fl. drachms = 16 ml

Calculation : For fl.oz i → 1 fl.oz = 30 ml

Potassium iodide $= \frac{2}{180} \times 30 = 0.33$ g

Tincture of Myrrh $= \frac{12}{180} \times 30 = 2$ ml

Tincture of Stramonium $= \frac{16}{180} \times 30 = 2.67$ ml

Chloroform water ...q.s..... = 30 ml

Type	Ingredients	Quantity in imperial	Quantity in metric	Quantity taken
Mixture containing, precipitate forming liquid.	Potassium iodide	30 gr	2 g	0.33 g
	Tincture of Myrrh	3 fl. dr	12 ml	2 ml
	Tincture of Stramonium	4 fl. dr	16 ml	2.67 ml
	Chloroform water...q.s..	6 fl.oz	180 ml	30 ml
	Prepare: Mixture Send: 30 ml Direction: One tablespoonful to be taken, four times a day.			

Theory:

This is a mixture containing **precipitate forming liquid**- like tincture of Myrrh. Tincture of Myrrh is resinous in nature, which yields precipitate in aqueous vehicle. But the resultant precipitate of myrrh is diffusible in nature, therefore no need of using a suspending agent. Tincture of Stramonium and potassium iodide, both are soluble in chloroform water. Therefore this mixture is prepared by simple dispersion method.

Procedure:

1) Divide the chloroform water in to two equal parts.
2) In one part of the chloroform water, add potassium iodide, stir well and add tincture of Stramonium. To this mixture, add tincture of myrrh gradually with continuous stirring.
3) Transfer the content to a measure and adjust the final volume, with remaining half portion of chloroform water.

Dispensing: Transfer the mixture to a clear, narrow mouthed glass bottle, close it throughly with metallic screw cap, polish and label.

Direction: One tablespoonful to be taken four times a day.

Storage: Store in a cool place.

Auxilliary label: SHAKE WELL BEFORE USE.

Uses: Tincture of Myrrh acts as expectorant and astringent to the mucous membrane and Tincture Stramonium contain hyoscyamine, which is used in the treatment of asthma. Potassium iodide acts as expectorant. Therefore this mixture is used as expectorant in the treatment of asthma.

PARALDEHYDE MIXTURE

Rx	
Paraldehyde	M xxx
Syrupi	fl. 3 ii
Extracti glycyrrhiza liquoris	M xxx
Aquam.... q.s....	fl.oz i
Fiat : Mistura (Haustus)	Mitte : fl.oz i
Signa : Utendus more dicto.	

Conversion :

M xxx → 30 minims   fl. 3 ii → 2 fl. drachms

15 minims = 1 ml   1 fl. drachm = 4 ml

30 minims = 2 ml   2 fl. drachms = 8 ml

Calculation : For fl.oz i → 1 fl.oz = 30 ml

Paraldehyde $= \frac{2}{30} \times 30 = 2$ ml

Syrup $= \frac{8}{30} \times 30 = 8$ ml

Liquid extract of Glycerrhiza $= \frac{2}{30} \times 30 = 2$ ml

Water ....q.s...... = 30 ml

Type	Ingredients	Quantity in imperial	Quantity in metric	Quantity taken
Mixture	Paraldehyde	30 minims	2 ml	2 ml
containing,	Syrup	2 fl. dr	8 ml	8 ml
slightly soluble	Liquid extract of glycyrrhiza	30 minims	2 ml	2 ml
liquid.	Water....q.s.......	fl.oz i	30 ml	30 ml
(Simple mixture)	Prepare: Mixture (Draught) Send: 30 ml			
	Direction: To be taken, as directed			

Theory:

This is a mixture containing **slightly soluble liquid** like Paraldehyde, which acts as sedative and hypnotic. Its solubility in water is 1 in 9 parts of water i.e 48 M paraldehyde/ounze. But in this mixture, paraldehyde prescribed is only 30 M/oz. It is in soluble range, hence it forms a simple mixture.

Liquid extract of Glycyrrhiza acts as expectorant and demulcent. It also used as flavouring and sweetening agent. Syrup is used to impart sweetness to the mixture.

Procedure:

1) Take measured quantity of paraldehyde in a previously tared, clear or amber coloured glass bottle and add ¾th quantity of water, close the bottle throughly with metallic screw cap and mix them by vigorous shaking.
2) To this mixture, add syrup and liquid extract of Glycyrrhiza and mix well.
3) Make up the final volume with water, polish and label.

Direction: To be taken as directed.

Storage: Store in a cool place.

Uses: Paraldehyde has both sedative and hypnotic action, but it is most widely used as sedative for inducing the sleep in children. Glycyrrhiza has expectorant and demulcent action, hence it is used in relief of cough. Therefore this mixture is used as a draught as expectorant and sedative.

MIXTURES CONTAINING POTENT MEDICAMENT

A) MIXTURE OF STRYCHNINE HYDROCHLORIDE

Rx	
Strychninae hydrochloridi	1/60 gr
Aquam ...q.s....	fl. 3 ii ss
Fiat : Mistura	Mitte : fl.oz ii
Signa : Cochleare magnum, nocte sumendum.	

Conversion :

1 grain = 60 mg	fl. 3 ii ss → 2.5 fl. drachms
1/60 grains =1 mg	1 fl. drachm = 4 ml
	2.5 fl. drachms = 10 ml

Calculation : For fl.oz ii → 2 fl.oz = 60 ml

Strychinine hydrochloride 1 mg for 10 ml

For 60 ml $= \frac{1}{10} \times 60 = 6$ mg

Water......q.s... = 60 ml

Strychnine hydrochloride is a potent medicament.

∴ its minimum weighable quantity on dispensing balance is, 300 mg.

So for preparation of 60 ml of the mixture, 6 mg of strychnine hydrochloride, is weighed as follows :

Dissolve Strychnine hydrochloride --- 300 mg,

In water --- 100 ml

i.e .100 ml of solution contains = 300 mg of Strychnine hydrochloride

∴ 1 ml of solution contains $= \frac{300}{100} \times 1 = 3$ mg of Strychnine hydrochloride

i.e. 2 ml of solution contains = 6 mg of Strychnine hydrochloride

Revised Formula :

Strychnine hydrochloride solution ----- 2 ml

Water.... q.s....... ----- 60 ml

Type	Ingredients	Quantity in imperial	Quantity in metric	Quantity taken
Mixture containing, potent medicament.	Strychnine hydrochloride	1/60 gr	1 mg	6 mg (2 ml)
	Water ...q.s....	2.5 fl. dr	10 ml	60 ml
	Make : Mixture Send: 60 ml Direction : One tablespoonful to be taken, at night			

Theory :

Strychnine hydrochloride is a alkaloidal salt, obtained from the seeds of Strychnos nuxvomica. It is highly potent medicament used as central stimulant in surgical shock, its maximum dose is 2-8 mg.

Since it is a potent drug, its minimum weighable quantity is 300 mg on dispensing balance. Therefore for preparation of 60 ml of mixture, 6 mg of Strychnine hydrochloride is weighed by dilution method, using water as vehicle.

Procedure :

1) Weigh accurately 300 mg of Strychnine hydrochloride and dissolve in 100 ml of purified water.
2) From the above solution take 2 ml of solution and dilute with 60 ml of purified water and mix uniformly.

Dispensing : Transfer the solution to a amber coloured, narrow mouthed glass bottle. Close it thoroughly with metallic screw cap, polish and label.

Direction : One tablespoonful to be taken, at night.

Storage : Store in a cool and dark place.

Uses : This mixture is used as CNS stimulant, in surgical shock.

B) HYOSCINE HYDROBROMIDE MIXTURE

Rx	
Hyoscine hydrobromidi	0.1 mg
Aquam chloroform...q.s...	fl. 3 ii ss
Fiat : Mistura	Mitte: fl.oz i ss
Signa : Cochleare magnum nocte sumendum.	

Conversion:

fl 3 ii ss $\rightarrow$ 2.5 fl. dr

1 fl. dr = 4 ml

fl. 3 ii ss $\rightarrow$ 2.5 fl. dr =10 ml

Calculation:

For fl.oz i ss $\rightarrow$ 1.5 fl.oz	=	45 ml
Hyoscine hydrobromide	=	0.1 mg for 10 ml
But for 45 ml	=	$\frac{0.1}{10} \times 45 = 0.45\,\text{mg}$
Chloroform water	=	10 ml

Since Hyoscine hydrobromide is a potent medicament, its minimum weighable quantity on dispensing balance is 300 mg. Therefore 0.45 mg of Hyoscine hydrobromide is weighed by double dilution method, using water as a vehicle in two stages, as shown in calculation.

Stage 1 :

Dissolve Hyoscine hydrobromide --- 300 mg,

In water --- 30 ml.

i.e. 30 ml of solution contains 300 mg of Hyoscine hydrobromide

$\therefore$ 1 ml of solution contains = $\frac{300}{30} \times 1 = 10\ \text{mg}$ of Hyoscine hydrobromide.

Stage 2 :

From stage-1, take Hyoscine hydrobromide solution --- 1 ml,

Dilute in water --- 100 ml.

i.e. 100 ml of diluted solution contains = 10 mg of Hyoscine hydrobromide

i.e. 1 ml diluted solution contains = $\frac{10}{100} \times 1 = 0.1\ \text{mg}$ of Hyoscine hydrobromide

$\therefore$ for 0.45 mg of Hyoscine hydrobromide = $\frac{0.45}{0.1} \times 1\,\text{ml} = 4.5\,\text{ml}$ of diluted solution.

Revised formula :

Hyoscine hydrobromide solution, from stage- 2 ----- 4.5 ml

Chloroform water...q.s... ----- 45 ml

Type	Ingredients	Quantity in imperial	Quantity in metric	Quantity taken
Mixture containing, potent medicament.	Hyoscine hydrobromide	0.1 mg	0.1 mg	4.5 ml
	Chloroform water ...q.s...	2.5 fl. dr	10 ml	45 ml
	Make : Mixture Send: 45 ml			
	Direction : One tablespoonful to be taken, at night.			

Theory :

This is a mixture containing potent medicament. Hyoscine hydrobromide is an alkaloidal salt obtained from dried leaves of Atropa belladonna, which acts as parasympatholytic and anti cholinergic, it's maximum dose is 0.6 mg. It is used to reduce the secretions such as sweat, saliva and gastric juice and also used to reduce spasm in cases of intestinal gripping, due to strong purgatives. It is also used as an antidote in opium and chloral hydrate poisoning.

Chloroform water is used as flavoured vehicle, which also acts as a carminative.

Procedure :

1) Accurately weigh 300 mg of Hyoscine hydrobromide and dissolve in 30 ml of purified water (stage 1)
2) From the above solution, pipette out 1 ml of solution into a 100 ml measure and adjust the final volume to 100 ml with purified water and mix well. (Stage 2)
3) From the diluted solution, (Stage 2) pipette out 4.5 ml of solution and transfer to a measure and adjust the final volume upto 45 ml with chloroform water.

Dispensing: Transfer the mixture to a narrow mouthed, amber colored glass bottle. Close the bottle with metallic screw cap and shake well to mix uniformly, polish and label.

Direction : One tablespoon to be taken, at night.

Storage : Store in a cool place.

Uses : This mixture is used as parasympatholytic and anti-cholinergic.

CALCIUM LACTATE MIXTURE

Rx	
Calci lactatis (recentis)	3 ii
Syrupi auranthii	fl. 3 vi
Aquam cinnamoni....q.s.......	fl.oz vi
Fiat : Mistura	Mitte : fl.oz ii
Signa : Cochleare magnum duo b.i.d capiendus.	

Conversion :

3 ii → 2 drachms	fl. 3 vi → 6 fl. drachms
1 drachm = 4 g	1 fl. drachm = 4 ml
2 drachms = 8 g	6 fl. drachms = 24 ml
	fl.oz vi → 6 fl.oz = 180 ml

Calculation : For fl.oz ii → 2 fl.oz = 60 ml

Calcium lactate = $\frac{8}{180} \times 60 = 2.66$ g

Orange syrup = $\frac{24}{180} \times 60 = 8$ ml

Cinnamon water...q.s... = 60 ml

As discussed in theory, i.e.. depending upon the molecular weight of calcium carbonate and lactic acid are required, **for preparation of 8 g of calcium lactate** are found to be,

Precipitated calcium carbonate - 48 grains

Lactic acid BP - 73 minims

But for preparation of 60 ml of mixture 2.66 g of calcium lactate is required, therefore do the calculation for 2.66 g.

i.e. For 8 g of calcium lactate = 48 grains of Precipitated calcium carbonate is required

But for 2.66 g of calcium lactate = $\frac{48}{8} \times 2.66 = 15.96$ grains (1.064 g)

For 8 g of calcium lactate = 73 minims of Lactic acid BP is required,

But for 2.66 g of calcium lactate = $\frac{73}{8} \times 2.66 = 24.27$ minims (1.45 ml)

Type	Ingredients	Quantity in imperial	Quantity in metric	Quantity taken
Mixture for internal use.	Calcium lactate (fresh)	2 dr	8 g	2.66 g
	Orange syrup	6 fl. dr	24 ml	8 ml
	Cinnamon water...q.s..	6 fl. oz	180 ml	60 ml
	Prepare: Mixture	Send: 60 ml		
	Direction: Two tablespoonful to be taken, two times a day.			

Theory:

- Calcium lactate is available as, white granules or powder, which is used as calcium replenisher. Calcium lactate is soluble in water, but freely soluble in hot water. Its solubility also varies and depends upon the method of preparation.
- Calcium lactate is prepared by the reaction between Official lactic acid (Lactic acid B.P.) and calcium carbonate.
- Official lactic acid (Lactic acid B.P.) contains 87.5 % w/w of real lactic acid and lactide. Lactide gets hydrolyses to lactic acid, which has sour taste of milk.
- Freshly prepared calcium lactate has no odour and also has good solubility. Therefore calcium lactate must be prepared in-situ by the reaction between calcium carbonate and lactic acid B.P.
- If the official lactic acid is simply diluted with water, and excess of calcium carbonate is added, only real lactic acid will react to form calcium lactate, but lactide remains unreacted. After filteration, the filtrate consists calcium lactate and lactide. Upon storage of this filtrate, lactide undergoes hydrolysis as lactic acid, which gives sour taste (odour) of milk to the mixture to an undesirable extent.
- Therefore, to avoid this problem, amount of calcium carbonate and lactic acid should be calculated in such a way that complete reaction should takes place between calcium carbonate with both real lactic acid and lactide and there should not be excess of calcium carbonate remains in the mixture.
- This problem is also solved by heating the mixture to boiling for 20 minutes, because lactide hydrolysis to lactic acid. This leads to complete reaction of calcium carbonate to calcium lactate.

$$2(HC_3H_5O_3) + CaCO_3 + 4H_2O \rightarrow Ca(C_3H_5O_3)_2 + 5H_2O + CO_2$$

Lactic acid — Mol.wt. (90x2= 180); Calcium carbonate (100); Calcium lactate (308)

The quantities of calcium carbonate and lactic acid for complete the reaction to form calcium lactate are calculated by considering the above equation and their molecular weights.

Calculation for Lactic acid:

Density of Lactic acid : 1.2 gm / cc, which contains the equivalent of 87.5% w/w of real lactic acid.

To prepare 308 g of calcium lactate: 180 g of lactic acid is required.

But, for 100 g of calcium lactate= $\frac{180}{308} \times 100 = 58.44$ g of lactic acid is required.

But, 100 g of official lactic acid consists only 87.5 g of pure lactic acid.

$$\therefore \quad \frac{100 \times 180}{308 \times 87.5} \times 100 = 66.79\,g \quad \cong 66.8\text{ g}$$

$$\text{Density} = \frac{\text{Mass}}{\text{Volume}}$$

$$\text{or Volume} = \frac{\text{Mass}}{\text{Density}} = \frac{66.8}{1.2} = 55.2\text{ ml}$$

∴ Volume of Lactic acid required is = 55.2 ml

Calculation for Calcium carbonate:

The theoretical amount of calcium carbonate required for 100 g of calcium lactate will be

$$\frac{100}{308} \times 100 = 32.4\text{ g}$$

Therefore, for preparation of calcium lactate,

Calcium carbonate = 32.4 g

Official lactic acid = 55.2 ml are required.

Procedure:

A) Preparation of calcium lactate:

1) Dilute the calculated amount of lactic acid B.P. with ¾th quantity of water.
2) To the dilute lactic acid, add precipitated calcium carbonate and mix well. Boil this mixture for 20 minutes to hasten the reaction.
3) After boiling, allow the mixture to cool to room temperature and filter through a filter paper, to remove excess of calcium carbonate. Wash the filter with small quantity of water.
4) The filtrate contains calcium lactate.

B) Preparation of calcium lactate mixture:

1) For preparation of calcium lactate water is required. This water can be utilised from the cinnamon water. Therefore instead of using cinnamon water a small portion of concentrated cinnamon water is used with major portion of water.

2) Therefore to the above filterate containing calcium lactate, add 1.2 ml of concentrated cinnamon water, orange syrup and mix well.
3) Transfer the content to a measure and adjust the final volume by adding purified water and mix well.

Revised formula :- for preparation of 60 ml of calcium carbonate mixture:

Precipitated calcium carbonate	-----	1.064 g
Lactic acid BP	-----	1.45 ml
To the filtrate (Calcium lactate) add,		
Orange syrup	-----	8 ml
Connecentrated cinnamon water	-----	1.2 ml
Water....q.s...	-----	60 ml

Dispensing: Transfer the mixture to a narrow mouthed, amber coloured, glass bottle, close it thoroughly with metallic screw cap, polish and label.

Direction: Two tablespoonful to be taken, two times a day.

Storage: Store in a cool and dark place.

Uses: This mixture is used as calcium replenisher in the deficiency of calcium.

Student's exercise:

1) Define mixtures and draught. Classify the mixtures.
2) Define diffusible solids, give examples.
3) Define indiffusible solids. How will you prepare them as mixtures?
4) What is C.T.P. or C. P. T.? How it is prepared (What are the ingredients of C.T.P.)?
5) When is the mucilage of tragacanth (M.T.) used in the preparation of mixtures? Give reasons.
6) Define precipitate forming liquids. Give examples.
7) Give the examples for mixtures containing precipitate forming liquids.
8) In what ratio (proportion) compound tragacanth powder and mucilage of tragacanth are used, for preparation of mixtures?
9) Define vehicles, what types of vehicles are used in mixtures.
10) Why chloroform water is used in the preparation of mucilage of tragacanth ?
11) Comment : "Shake well before use' is necessary on the lable of for mixtures containing diffusible and indiffusible solids.
12) Give the examples for soluble substances.
13) List out the mixtures containing diffusible solids.

14) Write the storage conditions for mixtures.
15) Define: antacid, purgative, laxative, expectorant and carminative with examples.
16) Why drugs are formulated as draught ?
17) Which are the various excipients used in preparations of mixtures?
18) Give the examples for slightly soluble liquids.
19) List out the flavouring and colouring agents, used in mixtures.
20) What is Light kaolin and Prepared chalk ? Explain their uses.
21) Comment : Acetyl salicylic acid is a indiffusible solid but it forms a simple mixture (simple solution).

7 ELIXIRS

Elixirs are clear, pleasently flavoured, sweetened, hydroalcoholic liquid preparations meant for oral administration. In elixirs the percentage of alcohol varies form 4 to 40 %.

In Elixirs along with water and alcohol, other substances are also incoprarted such as glycerin, sorbitol, propylene glycol, sweetening agent, flavouring agent and preservatives.

Elixirs are less sweet and less viscous than syrups and may contain less or no sucrose. Elixirs are more stable than syrups and hence preferred over syrups from manufacturing point of view.

Glycerin and syrup are used in elixirs, either for increasing the solubility of medicaments or for sweetening purposes. Propylene glycol may also employed as a substitute for both the solvents, glycerin and alcohol.

Elixirs are classified into two types,

1. **Non medicated elixirs:**

These elixirs do not contain any medicament, but consists some aromatic, pleasantly flavoured substances. These elixirs are used as vehicles, for the preparation of other pharmaceutical liquid formulations.

Eg.
- Simple elixir IP.
- Compound benzaldehyde elixir N.F.
- Isoalcoholic elixir.
- Aromatic elixir.
- Low alcoholic elixir (containing 8 to 10% of alcohol).
- High alcoholic elixir (containing 75 to 78% of alcohol).

2. **Medicated elixirs:**

These elixirs contain some medicinal (therapetically active) substances along with other excipients. These elixirs usally contain potent and nauseous drugs like antibiotics, antihistaminics, antitussives and sedatives.

Eg.
- Phenobarbitone elixir.
- Piperazine citrate elixir.
- Paracetamol elixir.
- Chloral hydrate elixir.
- Chlorpheneramine elixir.
- Terpin hydrate elixir.

The bitter and nauseous taste of the drugs is masked up to a certain limit, due to the presence of flavouring and sweetning agents in hydroalcoholic medium, so that it can be easly taken by children.

The presence of alcohol in elixirs provides following advantages.

1) Alcohol enhances the solubility of drug.
2) Prevents the growth of microorganisums.
3) Does not require extra preservatives, if alcohol quantity is more than 20% in the preparations.

Some elixirs are also available in granules or powder form, because certain active ingredients (drugs) are unstable in solution form.

Eg. • Phenethicillin.

• Phenoxy methyl penicilline.

These types of elixirs are prepared by adding measured amount of water and shake up until a solution is complete. These elixirs should be used with in one week, after their preparation and stored in well closed container in cool place.

Formulation : Generally elixirs contain following ingredients,

Sr.No.	Ingredients	Examples
1	Solvents or Vehicles	Water, Glycerine, Alcohol
2	Preservatives	Propylene glycol, Glycerin, Chloroform, Spirit, Benzoic acid, Methyl paraben and Propyl paraben.
3	Sweetning agent	Sucrose, Saccharin, Syrup, Glycerin, Sorbitol, Invert syrup.
4	Flavouring agents	Aromatic waters, Tincture of lemon, Concentrated raspberry juice, Orange oil.
5	Colouring agents	Amaranth solution, Compound tartrazine - solution.
6	Stabilizers	EDTA, Citric acid.

General method of preparation:

- Elixirs are prepared by simple solution method. Dissolve the alcohol soluble substances in alcohol and water-soluble substances in water.
- In order to maintain the highest possible alcoholic strength at all times and to avoid seperation of alcohol soluble ingredients, always add aqueous solution to the alcoholic solution with continuous stirring. But alcoholic solution should not be added to aqueous solution, because alcohol soluble substance will precipitates out, this precipitate is very difficult to make as diffusible.
- When two solutions are completely mixed, make up the final volume with vehicle. Usually the final mixture obtained will not be clear, but cloudy due to the separation of some of alcohol soluble substances.
- Therefore preparation is allowed to stand for few hours, for complete saturation of hydroalcoholic vehicle and to permit the oil globules of volatile oil to coalesce (aggregate), so as to remove them more easily by filtration using filter aid.
- For removing undissolved oil, purified talc (3 to 5%) is added to the preparation as a filter aid, which has an ability to adsorb excessive amount of oil and removes them from the preparation after final filtration.

- Before filtration, filter paper should be wetted with the hydroalcoholic solution having the same alcoholic strength, so as to avoid any changes in the proportion of water and alcohol in the vehicle, which may develop turbidity.
- For the same reason, collection flask should also be either completely dried or rinsed with same hydroalcoholic vehicle, which is used for the preparation of elixirs.

Dispensing: Elixirs consist alcohol and flavouring agents, which are volatile in nature. Therefore to prevent their volatilisation (evaporation) elixirs should be dispensed in tightly closed, narrow mouthed, screw capped, light resistant bottles.

Medicated elixirs are dispensed in small volume, and non medicated elixirs are dispensed in large volume bottles.

Storage: Elixirs should be stored in a cool place, to prevent the volatilisation at higher temperature.

Label: Label must bear all necessary requirements of liquid dosage forms meant for internal use. In addition, the amount of alcohol content used should be mentioned on the label.

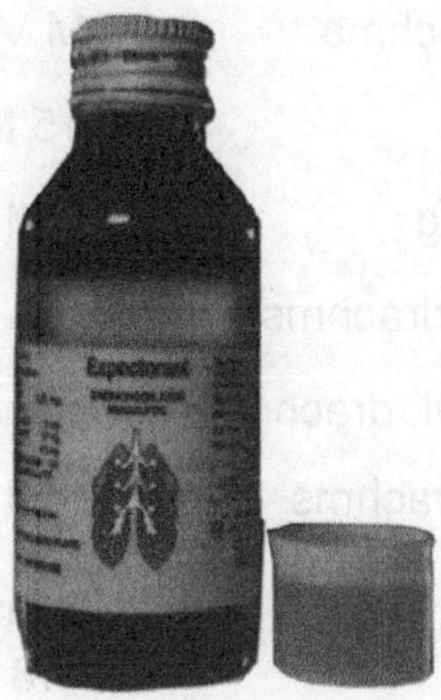

An example for Elixir

PIPERAZINE CITRATE ELIXIR I.P.

Rx	
Piperazinae citratis	3 iv ss
Spiritus chloroformi	M V iii
Glyerini	fl. 3 ii ss
Olei aurantii	q.s
Syrupi	fl. 3 xii ss
Aquam......q.s......	fl. 3 xxv
Fiat : Elixir	Mitte : fl.oz i
Signa :Cochleare minimum duo, nocte sumendum.	

Conversion :

3 iv ss → 4.5 Drachms　　M V iii → 8 minims

1 drachm = 4 g　　15 Minims → 1 ml

4.5 drachms = 18 g　　8 Minims → 0.5 ml

fl. 3 ii ss → 2.5 fl. drachms = 10 ml

fl. 3 xii ss → 12.5 fl. drachms = 50 ml

fl. 3 xxv → 25 fl. drachms = 100 ml

Calculation : For fl.oz i → 1 fl.oz = 30 ml

Piperazine citrate = $\frac{18}{100} \times 30 = 5.4$ g

Chloroform spirit = $\frac{0.5}{100} \times 30 = 0.15$ ml

Glycerin = $\frac{10}{100} \times 30 = 3$ ml

Simple syrup = $\frac{50}{100} \times 30 = 15$ ml

Purified water......q.s.... = 30 ml

Type	Ingredients	Quantity in imperial	Quantity in metric	Quantity taken
Monophasic liquid, for oral use.	Piperazine citrate	4.5 dr	18 g	5.4 g
	Chloroform spirit	8 minims	0.5 ml	0.15 ml
	Glycerin	2.5 fl. dr	10 ml	3 ml
	Orange oil	..q.s..	..q.s..	..q.s..
	Simple syrup	12.5 fl. dr	50 ml	15 ml
	Purified water....q.s..	25 fl. dr	100 ml	30 ml
	Make: Elixir Send: 30 ml. Direction: Two teaspoonful to be taken, at night.			

Theory:

Piperazine citrate acts as anthelmintic. It is in salt form and hence freely soluble in water. Therefore it doesn't requires large amount of alcohol. The alcohol which is present in chloroform spirit is enough, to prepare hydro-alcoholic preparation of piperazine citrate. Chloroform spirit also act as preservative.

Glycerin acts as a co-solvent, to enhance the solubility of drug and also provides soothing effect. Piperazine citrate has unpleasant acid taste, hence sweetening agent like simple syrup and flavouring agent like orange oil are used for masking the unpleasant taste.

Procedure:

1) Accurately weigh the piperazine citrate and dissolve in ¾ th of purified water.
2) Dissolve orange oil in chloroform spirit and add to the piperazine citrate solution, mix well.
3) To the above solution, add simple syrup and glycerin, mix uniformly. Transfer this content to a measure and adjust the final volume with purified water.

Dispensing: Transfer the elixir to a light resistant, narrow mouthed, glass bottle, close it tightly with metallic screw cap, polish and label.

Dose: For treatment of round worms, as a single dose up to 30 ml is given, according to age of the patient.

For children : 9-12 months - 2.5 ml
2 to 3 years - 5 ml
4 to 6 years - 7.5 ml
7 to 12 years - 10 ml

For treatment of Thread worms, 4 to 15 ml daily in divided doses is given.

Direction: Two teaspoonful to be taken, at night.

Storage: Store in a cool place.

Uses: Piperazine citrate expels the round worms and thread worms from the intestine, therefore this elixir is used as anthelmintic.

PARACETAMOL PAEDIATRIC ELIXIR I.P.

Rx	
Paracetamol	gr xxxvi
Ethanol(96%)	fl. 3 ii ss
Propylene glycol	fl. 3 ii ss
Conc. raspberry juice	M xxxvii ss
Chloroform spirit	M xxx
Invert syrup	fl. 3 Vii
Amaranth solution	M iii
Glyerini... q.s. ...	fl. 3 xxv
Fiat : Elixir	Mitte : fl.oz ii
Signa : Cochleare minimum mane et nocte capiendus.	

Conversion :

gr xxxvi → 36 grains

15 grains = 1 g

36 grains = 2.4 g

fl. 3 ii ss → 2.5 fl. drachms = 10 ml.

fl. 3 vii → 7 fl. drachms = 28 ml.

fl. 3 xxv → 25 fl. drachms = 100 ml

M xxxvii ss → 37 minims = 2.5 ml.

M xxx → 30 minims = 2 ml.

M iii → 3 minims = 0.2 ml.

Calculation : For fl.oz ii → 2 fl.oz = 60 ml

Paracetamol = $\frac{2.4}{100} \times 60 = 1.4$ g

Ethanol = $\frac{10}{100} \times 60 = 6$ ml

Propylene glycol = $\frac{10}{100} \times 60 = 6$ ml

Conc. raspberry juice = $\frac{2.5}{100} \times 60 = 1.5$ ml

Chloroform spirit = $\frac{2}{100} \times 60 = 1.2$ ml

Invert syrup = $\frac{28}{100} \times 60 = 17$ ml

Amaranth solution = $\frac{0.2}{100} \times 60 = 0.12$ ml

Glycerin ...q.s....... = 60 ml

Type	Ingredients	Quantity in imperial	Quantity in metric	Quantity taken
Monophasic liquid, for oral use.	Paracetamol	36 gr	2.4 g	1.4 g
	Ethanol	2.5 fl. dr	10 ml	6 ml
	Propylene glycol	2.5 fl. dr	10 ml	6 ml
	Concentrated raspberry juice	37.5 minims	2.5 ml	1.5 ml
	Chloroform spirit	30 minims	2 ml	1.2 ml
	Invert syrup	7 fl. dr	28 ml	17 ml
	Amaranth solution	3 minims	0.2 ml	0.12 ml
	Glycerine..........q.s......	25 fl. dr	100 ml	60 ml
	Make: Elixir	Send: 60 ml		
	Direction: One teaspoonful to be taken, morning and night.			

Theory:

In this preparation, paracetamol is sparingly soluble in water but it is freely soluble in alcohol, therefore alcohol (96%) is used to dissolve paracetamol. Propylene glycol is used as a co-solvent, to increase the solubility of paracetamol.

Paracetamol has an unpleasant taste. Therefore to mask this taste, invert sugar is used as sweetening agent. In this preparation instead of simple syrup, invert sugar is used, because sucrose present in simple syrup is insoluble in alcohol. Along with invert sugar, concentrated raspberry juice is also used, as sweetening and flavouring agent.

Glycerin is used to increase the viscosity of the preparation and also acts as humectant and gives soothing effect.

Procedure:

1) Accurately weigh the paracetamol and dissolve in measured quantity of alcohol (96%) and propylene glycol.
2) To the above mixture, add chloroform spirit and concentrated raspberry juice with stirring.
3) Transfer this content to a measure, add amaranth solution and make up the final volume with glycerin.
4) Filter, if any foreign particles or any undissolved substances are present.

Dispensing: Transfer the elixir to a light resistant, narrow mouthed, glass bottle, close it tightly with metallic screw cap, polish and label.

Dose: 5-10 ml is according to the age of the patient. (**Note** - When dose is less or not a multiple of 5 ml is prescribed, the elixir may be diluted with syrup. The syrup must be freshly prepared.)

Direction: One teaspoonful to be taken, morning and night.

Storage: Store in a cool place.

Label: Label must bear all necessary requirements of liquid dosage forms, meant for internal use. In addition, the amount of alcohol content used in the preparation, should be mentioned on the label.

Uses: Paracetamol paediatric elixir is used as a analgesic and antipyretic for children.

PHENOBARBITONE ELIXIR USP

Synonym : Elixir of luminal

Rx	
Phenobarbitoni	gr vi
Propylene glycol	fl. 3 ii ss
Alcoholis	fl. 3 v
Sorbitol solution	fl. 3 xv
Tartrazini liquor compositae	..q.s..
Olei auranthi	..q.s..
Aquam.......q.s.....	fl. 3 xxv
Fiat : Elixir	Mitte : fl.oz ii
Signa : Cochleare minimum, ter in die sumendum.	

Conversion :

gr vi → 6 grains

15 grains = 1 g

6 grains = 0.4 g

fl. 3 ii ss → 2.5 fl. drachms

1 fl. drachm = 4 ml

2.5 fl. drachms = 10 ml

fl. 3 v → 5 fl. drachms = 20 ml

fl. 3 xxv → 25 fl. drachms = 100 ml

fl. 3 xv → 15 fl. drachms = 60 ml

Calculation : For fl.oz ii → 2 fl.oz = 60 ml.

Phenobarbitone = $\frac{0.4}{100} \times 60 = 0.24$ g

Propylene glycol = $\frac{10}{100} \times 60 = 6$ ml

Alcohol (90%) = $\frac{20}{100} \times 60 = 12$ ml

Sorbitol solution = $\frac{60}{100} \times 60 = 36$ ml

Purified water...q.s..... = 60 ml.

Type	Ingredients	Quantity in imperial	Quantity in metric	Quantity taken
Monophasic liquid, for oral use.	Phenobarbitone	6 gr	0.4 g	0.24 g
	Propylene glycol	2.5 fl. dr	10 ml	6 ml
	Alcohol USP or (90%)	5 fl. dr	20 ml	12 ml
	Sorbitol solution	15 fl. dr	60 ml	36 ml
	Compound tartrazine solution	..q.s..	..q.s..	..q.s..
	Orange oil	..q.s..	..q.s..	..q.s..
	Purified water...... q.s......	25 fl. dr	100 ml	60 ml
	Make: Elixir	Send: 60 ml		
	Direction: One teaspoonful to be taken, three times a day.			

Theory:

This is most popular medicated elixir. It contains 0.4% of phenobarbitone, providing 20 mg of drug in each 5 ml of elixir. Phenobarbitone is slightly soluble in water (1:1000) but freely soluble in alcohol (1:8). Because of its high solubility in alcohol, it is formulated in liquid dosage form as an elixir.

Propylene glycol is used as co-solvent, to increase the solubility of phenobarbitone. Orange oil is used as flavouring agent. Sorbitol solution is used as sweetening agent and it also acts as stabilizer. Compound tartrazine solution is used as colouring agent, to give an attractive colour to the elixir.

After preparation, orange oil remains undissolved, because of low percentage of alcohol (14%)in the elixir. Hence talc is used as a filter aid, to adsorb the undissolved orange oil and then talc can be removed by filteration.

Procedure:

1) Accurately weigh phenobarbitone and dissolve in alcohol (90%), by stirring in a beaker.
2) To the above solution, add propylene glycol, orange oil and sorbitol solution and mix them thoroughly.
3) Add a pinch of purified talc and shake for a few minutes and allow to stand for 1 hour with occasional shaking. Filter the solution. For filteration, soak filterpaper with same strength of alcohol.
4) To the filtrate, add compound tartrazine solution and mix well.
5) Transfer this content to a measure and make up the final volume with purified water.

Dispensing: Phenobarbitone is sensitive to the light, therefore transfer the elixir to a light resistant, narrow mouthed glass bottle, close it tightly with metallic screw cap, polish and label.

Dose: 15 ml daily in divided doses is given, according to age and response of the patient.

(**Note-** When a dose is less than or not a multiple of 5 ml is prescribed, the elixir must be diluted with freshly prepared syrup before administration).

Direction: One teaspoonful to be taken, three times a day.

Storage: Store in a cool and dark place.

Label: Label must bear all necessary requirements of liquid dosage forms meant for internal use. In addition, the amount of alcohol content used in the preparation, should be mentioned on the label.

Uses: Phenobarbitone elixir is used as anticonvulsant and hypnotic.

PAEDIATRIC CHLORAL HYDRATE ELIXIR B.P.

Rx	
Chloral hydrate	ʒ i
Aquam	M xxx
Syrupi aurantii	fl. ʒ V
Syrupi...q.s...	fl. ʒ XXV
Fiat : Elixir	Mitte: fl.oz i
Signa: Coch.min. nocte apud sumendum.	

Conversion :

ʒ i → 1 drachm = 4 g

fl. ʒ V → 5 fl. drachms = 20 ml

fl. ʒ XXV → 25 fl. drachms = 100 ml

M xxx → 30 minims

15 minims = 1 ml

30 minims = 2 ml

Calculation : For fl.oz i → 1 fl.oz = 30 ml.

Chloral hydrate = $\frac{4}{100} \times 30 = 1.2$ g

Purified water = $\frac{2}{100} \times 30 = 0.6$ ml

Orange syrup = $\frac{20}{100} \times 30 = 6$ ml

Simple syrup.....q.s.... = 30 ml

Type	Ingredients	Quantity in imperial	Quantity in metric	Quantity taken
Monophasic	Chloral hydrate	1 dr	4 g	1.2 g
liquid for	Purified water	30 minims	2 ml	0.6 ml
oral use.	Orange syrup	5 fl. dr	20 ml	6 ml
	Simple syrup.....q.s....	25 fl. dr	100 ml	30 ml
	Make: Elixir for a child, six months old. Send: 30 ml Direction: One teaspoonful to be taken, at night.			

Theory:

Chloral hydrate is colorless, transparent or white crystalline powder, soluble in water. Even though it is soluble in water, in this preparation simple syrup is used as a vehicle, because chloral hydrate has slightly acrid odour and bitter taste. To mask this taste, simple syrup is used in higher quantity as a vehicle and also as sweetening agent.

Orange syrup is used as flavouring agent, to mask the acrid odour of chloral hydrate.

Procedure:

1) Accurately weigh the chloral hydrate and dissolve in purified water.
2) To the above solution, add simple syrup and orange syrup with stirring, make up the final volume with simple syrup.

Dispensing: Choral hydrate is volatile in nature and its solution is rapidly deteriorate if exposed to the light, therefore transfer the elixir to a light resistant, narrow mouthed, glass bottle, close it tightly with metallic screw cap, polish and label.

Dose: For child, up to 1 year, 2.5 ml to 5.0 ml is given. (**Note-** When a dose is less than or not a multiple of 5.0 ml is prescribed, the elixir should be diluted with freshly prepared syrup.)

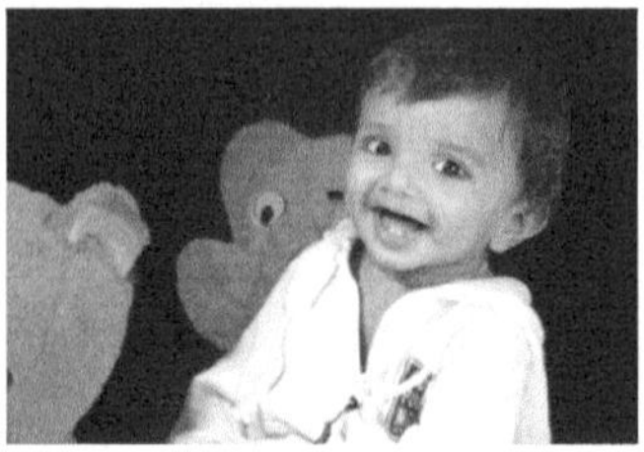

Direction: One teaspoonful to be taken, at night.

Storage: Store in a cool and dark place.

Uses: Chloral hydrate has both sedative and hypnotic action, but it is most widely used as sedative for inducing the sleep in children. Therefore this elixir is used as sedative.

TERPIN HYDRATE ELIXIR I.P.

Rx	
Terpin hydrate	ʒ i s
Glyerini	fl.ʒ x
Alcoholis	fl. ʒ x ss
Syrupi	fl. ʒ ii ss
Oil auranti	0.02 ml (q.s.)
Aquam……q.s…..	fl. ʒ xxv
Fiat : Elixer	Mittle fl.oz.i
Signa: Cochleare magnum, mane et nocte sumendum.	

Conversion :

ʒ i s → 1.25 drachms	fl.ʒ x → 10 fl dr = 40 ml
1 drachm = 4 g	fl.ʒ x ss → 10.5 fl.dr = 42 ml
1.25 drachms = 5 g	fl.ʒ ii ss → 2.5 fl. dr = 10 ml
	fl.ʒ xxv → 25 fl dr = 100 ml

Calculation: For fl.oz.i → 1 fl. oz = 30 ml

Terpin hydrate $= \frac{5}{100} \times 30 = 1.5$ g

Glycerin $= \frac{40}{100} \times 30 = 12$ ml

Alcohol $= \frac{42}{100} \times 30 = 12.6$ ml

Syrup $= \frac{10}{100} \times 30 = 3$ ml

Orange oil $= \frac{0.02}{100} \times 30 = 0.006$ ml (q.s)

Purified water….q.s….. = 30 ml.

Type	Ingredients	Quantity in imperial	Quantity in metric	Quantity taken
Monophasic liquid, for oral use.	Terpin hydrate	1.25 dr	5 g	1.5 g
	Glycerin	10 fl. dr	40 ml	12 ml
	Alcohol	10.5 fl. dr	42 ml	12.6 ml
	Syrup	2.5 fl. dr	10 ml	3 ml
	Orange oil	0.02 ml	0.02 ml	0.006 ml
	Purified water…q.s…	25 fl. dr	100 ml	30 ml
	Prepare: Elixer	Send: 30 ml		
	Direction: One tablespoonful to be taken, morning and night.			

Theory:

Terpin hydrate acts as expectorant. It is slightly soluble in water, but it is highly soluble in alcohol. In this preparation, the content of alcohol is about 42% v/v. Therefore this much amount of alcohol is sufficient, to dissolve terpin hydrate.

Glycerin provides soothing effect and also increases the viscosity of the preparation. Orange oil is used as flavouring agent and syrup is used as sweetening agent. (also acts co-solvent, to increase the solubility of water insoluble compounds).

This elixir is quite viscous in nature, because it is composed of 40% of glycerin and 10% of syrup. It should not be diluted with water, because the alcohol soluble and water insoluble constituents will separate out on dilution.

Due to the presence of high alcohol in this preparation, precipitation or coalescence of terpin hydrate or orange oil does not takes place. Therefore there is no need of adding filter aid, to get a clear solution.

Procedure :

1) Dissolve terpin hydrate in alcohol by stirring.
2) To the above alcoholic solution, add orange oil, glycerin and syrup. Mix uniformly by stirring.
3) Transfer the content to a measure, add sufficient quantity of water to make up the final volume and mix well.

Dispensing: Terpin hydrate, alcohol and orange oil are volatile in nature. Terpin hydrate is sensitive to the light. Therefore transfer the elixir to a narrow mouthed, amber coloured, glass bottle, close it tightly with metallic screw cap, polish and label.

Direction: One tablespoonful to be taken, morning and night.

Storage: Store in a cool and dark place.

Uses: Terpin hydrate elixir is used as, expectorant.

Other examples for Elixirs:

1) **Ephedrine hydrochloride elixir**

Ephedrine hydrochloride	:	0.3 g
Glycerin	:	20 ml
Chloroform spirit	:	4 ml
Lemon spirit	:	0.02 ml
Alcohol	:	10 ml
Invert syrup	:	20 ml
Compound tartrazine solution	:	1 ml
Purified water	:	6 ml
Syrup .....q.s.........	:	100 ml.

Uses: It is used as expectorant and bronchodilator.

2) **Non – medicated elixirs:**

a) **High alcoholic elixir:**

Compound orange spirit	:	4 ml
Saccharin	:	3 g
Glycerin	:	200 ml
Alcohol ....q.s.........	:	1000 ml.

Uses: It is used as flavouring agent and pharmaceutical aid.

b) **Low alcoholic elixir:**

Compound orange spirit	:	10 ml
Alcohol	:	100 ml
Glycerin	:	200 ml
Sucrose	:	320 ml
Purified water .....q.s....	:	1000 ml

Uses: Low alcoholic elixir is used as pharmaceutical aid and flavouring agent.

c) **Aromatic elixir:**

Orange oil	:	0.4 ml
Lemon oil	:	0.2 ml
Syrup	:	40 ml
Alcohol (95%)	:	24 ml
Purified water ....q.s......	:	100 ml

Uses: It is used as flavouring agent and vehicle (flavoured vehicle), for other pharmaceutical liquid preparations.

Student's exercise:

1) Define elixirs.
2) Classify elixirs with examples.
3) Comment : In the preparation of elixers, always aqueous solution should be added to the alcoholic solution.
4) Define filter aid: Why a filter aid is used in the preparation of elixirs ?
5) How will you dispense elixirs? Explain with reasons.
6) Differentiate between elixirs and linctuses.
7) Differentiate between elixirs and syrups.
8) Differentiate between sedatives and hypnotics.
9) What is the use of glycerin in elixirs?
10) Define analgesics and antipyretics with examples.
11) What is the use of high alcoholic elixirs?
12) What is chloral hydrate? (Define chemically)
13) Explain pharmaceutical uses of elixirs.
14) What types of drugs are formulated as elixirs?
15) What are the advantages (roles) of alcohol in elixirs?
16) Define anthalmetics. Give examples.
17) What is the use of propylene glycol in Paracetamol elixir?
18) Mention the colouring and flavouring agents used in elixirs.
19) What is the meaning of paediatric?
20) What is the use of sorbitol in phenobarbitone elixir?
21) What is the difference between invert syrup and simple syrup?
22) Briefly explain the formulation aspects of elixirs.
23) Comment: Elixirs do not require extra preservatives, if concentration of alcohol is high.

8 LINCTUSES

Linctuses are viscous and sweet liquid preparations, containing one or more medicaments used for relief of cough. Linctus contains the medicinal substances, which have expectorant, demulcent or sedative action.

They consists high proportion of syrup and glycerin. Syrup is used as sweetening agent, to mask unpleasant taste of drug and it soothens the sore mucous membrane of the throat. Glycerin makes the preparation viscous and gives the demulcent action, on the mucous membrane of throat.

Linctus should be taken as such, without dilution with water in small dose and must be swallowed slowly, in order to have maximum prolonged action of the drug, on mucous membrane of the throat.

The one dose of linctus is 5 ml and supplied in multi dose container, containing 15-20 doses together.

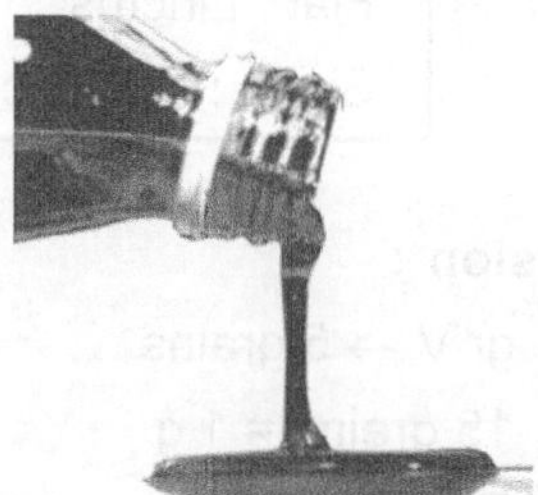

Examples for linctuses :

- Codeine phosphate linctus.
- Nascopine linctus.
- Tolu compound linctus.
- Pholcodine linctus.
- Methadone hydrochloride linctus.

Formulation :

Sr.no	Ingredients	Examples
1	Vehicles/Sweetening agents	Glycerin, Simple syrup, Tolu syrup, Choloform water, Sorbitol solution.
2	Flavouring agents	Lemon syrup, Black current syrup, Tolu syrup
3	Colouring agents	Amaranth solution, Tartrazine.
4	Preservatives	Benzoic acid, Cinnamic acid, Chloroform sprit.
5	Stabilizer	Simple syrup, Invert syrup.

Note: Linctuses are self stabilized, due to the presence of simple syrup or invert syrup, because they acts as preservatives, by exerting high osmotic pressure and kills the microorganisms by dehydration mechanism, due to their high osmotic pressure. Hence there is no need of adding any other stabilizers.

Method of preparation: Linctus is prepared by simple solution method.

1) Dissolve the active ingredients in vehicle, it may be a water or glycerin or syrup.
2) To the above solution, add the other ingredients like colouring, flavouring agents and preservatives. Mix uniformly by stirring.
3) Adjust the final volume with remaining amount of vehicle and dispense in a suitable container.

Dispensing: Linctuses should be dispensed in well filled, well closed air tight, light resistant glass bottle, closed with metallic screw cap.

Directions:
- TO BE SIPPED SLOWLY IN SMALL DOSES.
- DO NOT DILUTE WITH WATER BEFORE USE.

Storage: Linctuses should be stored in a cool place and protected from light.

CODEINE PHOSPHATE LINCTUS

Rx	
Codeine phosphatis	gr V
Syrupi limonis	fl. 3 V
Spiritus chloroformi	M xxx
Aquam	M xxx
Liquoris acidi benzoici	M xxx
Tartrazini liquoris composite	M xv
Syrupi.........q.s.......	fl. 3 xxv
Fiat : Linctus	Mitte : fl.oz ii
Signa : Sip, cochleare minimum et deglutiendus lente t.i.d.	

Conversion :

gr V → 5 grains	fl. 3 V → 5 fl. drachms	M xxx → 30 minims
15 grains = 1 g	1 fl. drachm = 4 ml	15 minims = 1 ml
5 grains = 0.3 g	5 fl. drachms = 20 ml	30 minims = 2 ml
	fl. 3 xxv → 25 fl. drachms = 100 ml	

Calculation : For fl.oz → 2 fl.oz = 60 ml

Codeine phosphate = $\frac{0.3}{100} \times 60 = 0.18$ g

Lemon syrup = $\frac{20}{100} \times 60 = 12$ ml

Chloroform spirit = $\frac{2}{100} \times 60 = 1.2$ ml

Purified water = $\frac{2}{100} \times 60 = 1.2$ ml

Benzoic acid solution = $\frac{2}{100} \times 60 = 1.2$ ml

Coumpound tartrazine solution = $\frac{1}{100} \times 60 = 0.6$ ml

Syrup ....q.s.... = 60 ml.

Type	Ingredients	Quantity in imperial	Quantity in metric	Quantity taken
Monophasic liquid, for oral use.	Codeine phosphate	5 gr	0.3 g	1.8 g
	Lemon syrup	5 fl. dr	20 ml	12 ml
	Chloroform spirit	30 minims	2 ml	1.2 ml
	Purified water	30 minims	2 ml	1.2 ml
	Benzoic acid solution	30 minims	2 ml	1.2 ml
	Compound tartrazine solution	15 minims	1 ml	0.6 ml
	Syrup.... q.s........	25 fl. dr	100 ml	60 ml
	Make: Linctus	Send: 60 ml		
	Direction: Sip, 5 ml spoonful and swallow slowly, three times a day.			

Theory:

Codeine phosphate is an alkloidal salt, hence it is freely soluble in water but its solubility can also be increased by heating. Codeine phosphate has unpleasant bitter taste, therefore to mask this taste, lemon syrup and simple syrup are used as flovouring and sweetening agents respectively.

Simple syrup also acts as vehicle. Benzoic acid and chloroform sprit are used as preservatives. Compound tartrazine solution is used, to give elegant colour to the linctus.

Procedure:

1) Accurately weigh the codeine phosphate and dissolve in water by gentle heating on water bath.
2) To the above solution, add benzoic acid solution, compound tartrazine solution and chloroform sprit. Mix uniformly by continuous stirring.
3) Transfer this content to a measure and add lemon syrup, followed by adjusting the final volume by simple syrup.

Dispensing: Codeine phosphate in solution form is very sensitive to the light, hence it is less stable. Therefore transfer the linctus in to an amber colored, narrow mouthed glass bottle, close it throughly with metallic screw cap, polish and label.

Direction: Sip, 5 ml spoonful and swallow slowly, three times a day.

Storage: Store in a cool and dark place.

Auxilliary label:
- DO NOT DILUTE WITH WATER BEFORE USE.
- STORE IN A COOL AND DARK PLACE.

Uses: Codeine phosphate is an alkloidal salt, it acts as an antitussive and analgesic, in the dose of 10 to 60 mg. Therefore this linctus is used as analgesic and antitussive (cough suppressant).

SIMPLE LINCTUS BPC.

Rx	
Citric acid monohydrate	gr XXXVii ss
Conc. anise water	M XV
Liquor amaranthi	M XXii ss
Chloroformi spiritus	M XC
Syrupi.....q.s......	fl. 3 XXV
Fiat : Linctus	Mitte : fl.oz i
Signa : Sip, cochleare minimum et deglutiendus lente, b.i.d.	

Conversion :

gr XXXVii ss → 37.5 grains
15 grains = 1 g
37.5 grains = 2.5 g
M XV → 15 minims = 1 ml
M XXii ss → 22.5 minims = 1.5 ml
M XC → 90 minims = 6 ml

Calculation : For fl.oz i → 1 fl.oz = 30 ml

Citric acid monohydrate = $\frac{2.5}{100} \times 30 = 0.75$ g

Conc. anise water = $\frac{1}{100} \times 30 = 0.3$ ml

Amaranth solution = $\frac{1.5}{100} \times 30 = 0.45$ ml

Chloroform spirit = $\frac{6}{100} \times 30 = 1.8$ ml

Simple syrup....q.s....... = 30 ml

Type	Ingredients	Quantity in imperial	Quantity in metric	Quantity taken
Monophasic liquid, for oral use.	Citric acid monohydrate	37.5 gr	2.5 g	0.75 ml
	Concentrated anise water	15 minims	1 ml	0.3 ml
	Amaranth solution	22.5 minims	1.5 ml	0.45 ml
	Chloroform spirit	90 minims	6 ml	1.8 ml
	Simple syrup....q.s...	25 fl. dr	100 ml	30 ml
	Make: Linctus	Send: 30 ml.		
	Direction: Sip, 5 ml spoonful and swallow slowly, two times a day.			

Theory :

Citric acid monohydrate and concentrated anise water acts as expectorants and astringents. Both are miscible in water. Even though they are soluble in water, simple syrup is used as vehicle, to mask the unpleasant acid taste (acrid or salty) of citric acid, it also acts as demulcent.

Chloroform spirit and concentrated anise water are used as flavouring agents, chloroform spirit is also acts as preservative and amaranth solution is used as colouring agent.

Procedure:

1) Dissolve accurately weighed citric acid monohydrate, in chloroform spirit.
2) To the above solution, add liquid ingredients like concentrated anise water, simple syrup and amaranth solution. Mix uniformly by continuous stirring.
3) Adjust the final volume by adding sufficient quantity of simple syrup.

Dispensing: Transfer the linctus to a narrow mouthed, light resistant, glass bottle, close thoroughly with metallic screw cap, polish and label.

Direction: Sip, 5 ml spoonful and swallow slowly, two times a day.

Storage: Store in a cool place and protected from light.

Auxilliary label:
- STORE IN A COOL AND DARK PLACE.
- DO NOT DILUTE WITH WATER BEFORE USE.

Uses: Simple linctus is used as demulcent, expectorant in the treatment of cough.

PAEDIATRIC COMPOUND TOLU LINCTUS

Rx	
Benzaldehydi spiritus	M i ss
Citric acid monohydrate	gr vii
Tartrazini liquoris composite	M xv
Glyerini	fl. 3 v
Invert syrup	fl. 3 v
Syrupi tolu...q.s....	fl. 3 xxv
Fiat : Linctus	Mitte : fl.oz i
Signa : Sip, cochleare minimum et deglutiendus lente, b.i.d.	

Conversion :

M i ss → 1.5 minims
15 minims = 1 ml
1.5 minims = 0.1 ml

fl. 3 V → 5 fl. drachms
1 fl. drachm = 4 ml
5 fl. drachms = 20 ml
fl. 3 xxv → 25 fl. drachms = 100 ml

gr vii → 7 grains
1 gr = 60 mg
7 gr = 420 mg

Calculation : For fl.oz i → 1 fl.oz = 30 ml

Benzaldehyde spirit = $\frac{0.1}{100} \times 30 = 0.03$ ml

Citric acid monohydrate = $\frac{0.42}{100} \times 30 = 0.126$ g

Comp. tartrazine solution = $\frac{1}{100} \times 30 = 0.3$ ml

Glycerin = $\frac{20}{100} \times 30 = 6$ ml

Invert syrup = $\frac{20}{100} \times 30 = 6$ ml

Tolu syrup... q.s. ... = 30 ml

Type	Ingredients	Quantity in imperial	Quantity in metric	Quantity taken
Monophasic liquid, for oral use.	Benzaldehyde spirit	1.5 minims	0.1 ml	0.03 ml
	Citric acid monohydrate	7 gr	420 mg	0.126 g
	Compound tartrazine solution	15 minims	1 ml	0.3 ml
	Glycerin	5 fl. dr	20 ml	6 ml
	Invert syrup	5 fl. dr	20 ml	6 ml
	Tolu syrup.....q.s.....	25 fl. dr	100 ml	30 ml
	Make: Linctus Send: 30 ml. Direction: Sip, 5 ml spoonful and swallow slowly, two times a day.			

Theory:

Citric acid monohydrates acts as expectorent and astringent. Tolu syrup is a flavoured syrup, which is prepared from tolu balsam. Tolu balsam acts as expectorant and antitussive. It also acts as demulcent, hence it is used in the treatment of cough and sore throat.

Glycerin is used to increase the viscosity of the linctus and also to give demulcent, soothing effect on mucous memberane of the throat.

Invert syrup is used as sweetening agent. Benzaldehyde spirit is used as preservative.

Procedure:

1) Dissolve citric acid monohydrate, in small portion of tolu syrup by stirring.
2) Add the other liquid ingredients like benzaldehyde spirit, compound tartrazine solution, glycerin and invert syrup and mix uniformly with continous stirring.
3) Adjust the final volume, by adding remainig amount of tolu syrup.

Dispensing: Transfer the linctus to a narrow mouthed, light resistant glass bottle, close thoroughly with metallic screw cap, polish and label.

Direction: Sip, 5 ml spoonful and swallow slowly, two times a day.

Auxilliary label:
- STORE IN A COOL AND DARK PLACE.
- DO NOT DILUTE WITH WATER BEFORE USE.

Storage: Store in a cool place (at temperature not more than 25°C.)

Uses: Tolu linctus is used as demulcent, expectorant in the treatment of cough and sore throat.

Student's exercise:

1) Define Linctuses. What types of medicaments are preferred in linctuses? Give examples.
2) Comment: Linctus should be swallowed slowly, without dilution.
3) Differentiate linctuses and elixirs.
4) What are advantages of glycerin in linctuses?
5) Comment: For preparation of linctuses flavouring and sweetening agents are essential.
6) Mention the general label directions required for linctuses.
7) Define invert syrup. Why it is preferred over simple syrup ?
8) Give minimum 5 examples for linctuses.
9) List out the syrups which are used as sweetening agents in linctuses.
10) Define expectorant and demulcent.
11) Explain in brief - applications of linctuses.
12) How will you dispense linctuses?
13) Define antitussive - give examples.

9 SYRUPS

Syrups are sweet, viscous, concentrated aqueous solutions of sucrose or other sugars in water or any other suitable aqueous vehicle.

Syrups are classified into three types, :

1) **Simple syrup:** When water alone is used for the preparation of solution of sucrose, the preparation is called as simple syrup.

   Eg. Simple syrup I.P. consists 66.7% w/w of sucrose in water.

2) **Medicated syrups:** When syrups contain certain medicinal substances, which are used for therapeutic purpose, are called as medicated syrups.

   Eg.
   - Codeine phosphate syrup
   - Ferrous sulphate syrup
   - Ephedrine sulphate syrup
   - Chlorpheniramine maleate syrup
   - Pseudoephedrine hydrochloride syrup
   - Dextromethorphan hydrobromide syrup.

3) **Flavoured syrups:** When syrups containing only aromatic or flavouring agents, they are called as flavoured syrups. These are used as flavouring agents, for masking the disagreeable, bitter or saline taste of the drugs. They are also used as vehicles, for the preparation of pharmaceutical formulations.

   Eg.
   - Orange syrup,
   - Tolubalsam syrup,
   - Lemon syrup.
   - Cocoa syrup,
   - Raspberry syrup,
   - Cherry syrup,

Formulation of syrups: Syrups consist sucrose as a main ingredient and they also consist other ingredients like,

1)	Vehicles	Purified water, Glycerin.
2)	Chemical stabilizers	a) Poly-hydric alcohols like, Glycerin, Sorbitol and Propylene glycol to prevent the crystallization of sucrose.
		b) Surfactants (eg. Tweens) used to dissolve certain ingredients in the syrup, to make clear solution.
3)	Colouring agents	Amaranth solution, Compound tartrazine solution.
4)	Flavouring agents	Tinctures : Tincture of Lemon Tincture of Ginger
		Fruit Juices : Raspberry juice Wild cherry juice
		Essences : Vanilla flavour Orange flavour
5)	Preservatives	Benzoic acid, Sodium benzoate, Methyl paraben

Methods of preparation : Syrups are prepared by any one of the four following methods, depending upon the physical and chemical properties of the substances, used in the preparation:

1) Simple solution method with the help of heat:

This method is used when the substances are thermostable and non volatile in nature. In this method, sucrose is added to the purified water and heated till it dissolves completely. The solution is allowed to cool and then final volume is adjusted with boiled purified water, to compensate the loss of water during heating.

These syrups do not have any medicinal value.

Eg.
- Simple syrup.
- Tolu syrup N.F
- Cocoa syrup N.F.
- Acacia syrup N.F

Advantages :

1) This method is suitable for thermostable and non-volatile substances.
2) It is less time consuming method.

Disadvantages :

Overheating may causes caramelization of sucrose, which results in the formation of amber or dark coloured syrups, such types of syrups are susceptible to microbial growth.

2) Simple solution method by agitation (without heat):

This method is suitable for thermolabile substances and volatile substances. For small scale, sucrose and other ingredients are dissolved in purified water in a suitable glass stoppered container and allowed to agitate the mixture for longer time until whole amount of sugar and other ingredients get dissolved.

For large scale, syrups are prepared by glass lined tank with mechanical agitators.

Eg.
- Ephedrine sulphate syrup,
- Codiene phosphate syrup.

Advantages:

1) Syrups prepared by this method have maximum stability, because no inversion of sucrose or caramelization takes place..
2) This is most suitable method, for thermolabile and volatile substances.

Disadvantages:

This is a more time consuming process.

3) Percolation (extraction) method:

In this method, sucrose is percolated with purified water as a menstrum. The menstrum (it may be purified water or flavoured liquid), is allowed to pass through a column of crystaline sucrose to dissolve it. The percolate is collected and repassed repeatedly, until whole amount of sucrose has been dissolved. Finally sufficient purified water is added to make up the final volume.

Eg.
- Tolu syrup.
- Squill syrup.

4) Addition of sucrose to a prepared medicated liquid or flavoured liquid:

This method is used when the medicaments are available in the form of tinctures, fluid extracts and other liquid forms to medicate the syrup. The alcohol present in these liquids helps to dissolve resinous or oleoresinous substances. Alcohol also acts as preservative.

Addition of this type of liquids to syrup causes the precipitation of alcohol soluble substances, due to presence of water. This precipitate is removed by allowing the mixture to stand for some hours, for the separation of insoluble constituents and then filtered. But this method cannot be employed, if the insoluble constituents are having some medicinal properties. Eg. Aromatic eriodictyon syrup NF.

Medicaments commonly used in syrups are :

Medicaments	Examples
Antipyretics	Paracetamol
Antibiotics	Lincomycin hydrochloride
Antiemetics	Chlorpromazine hydrochloride
Antihistaminics	Chlorpheniramine meleate
Antitussives	Dextromethorphan hydrobromide
Analgesics	Meperidine hydrochloride
Adrenergics	Pseudoephedrine hydrochloride
Sedatives	Chloral hydrate
Iron supplement	Ferrous sulphate
Electrolytes	Sodium (Na+), Potassium (K+), Calcium(Ca++).

Advantages of syrups:

1) Syrup retards (prevents) oxidation reaction, because it is partialy hydrolysed into reducing sugars, as dextrose and laevulose, which acts as anti-oxidants and prevent the oxidation of the medicament.
2) Syrup prevents the growth of micro-organisms, which are chief causes of decomposition, because strong solution of sucrose (66.7% w/w) has great osmotic pressure due to which, it withdraws water from the microorganisms.

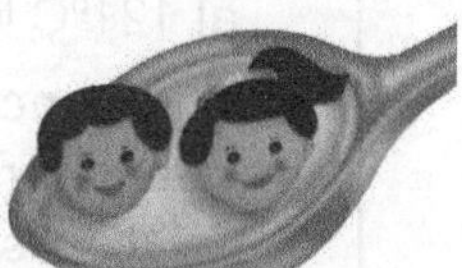

3) Because of its palatable sweet taste, it is used as a sweetening agent for masking of bitter, saline and nauseous taste of the drugs.
4) Syrups are very much liked by youngsters and children, due to their sweet taste.
5) Syrup is also used as vehicle, in many pharmaceutical preparations.

Disadvantages of syrups:

1) If syrups are not concentrated (diluted syrup) or containing less than 66.7% w/w, it leads to microbial growth, hence it requires addition of extra preservatives.

2) If syrup is highly concentrated, it leads to crystallization of sucrose. Hence to prevent crystallization, polyhydric alcohols (polyols) like glycerin, sorbitol or propylene glycol are required.
3) Syrups are not suitable for diabetic patients.
4) Syrups are not suitable for patients who are on a restricted calorie intake.
5) Pleasant taste of syrups will attract the children, to take more than required dose. This may leads to 'dental carries' and 'gingivitis'.

Note:

1) Only small quantities of syrup should be prepared and which should be used within few months. If large quantities are to be prepared then they should be well preserved by adding suitable preservatives, to prevent microbial contamination.
2) Now-a-days, syrups are prepared using artificial sweetening agents. They have the advantage over syrups, which are prepared by natural sugars (sucrose), because they do not contain any carbohydrate (glucose, sucrose, dextrose) and hence they can be given to diabetic patients. Synthetic syrups are more stable than sugar based syrups.

   Eg.- For synthetic sugar - Saccharin
3) In the syrups, sugars or sugar substitutes provides viscosity (viscous nature) to the preparation. But synthetic sugars do not provide (exert) viscosity. Hence to improve the viscosity of such preparation, viscosity imparting (thickening) agents like methyl cellulose, Hydroxy ethyl cellulose are used.
4) **Caramelization:** When syrup is heated, inversion of sucrose occurs as dextrose and levulose, but over heating degrade the levulose into caramel. Hence solution converts into colourless to yellowish brown. This process is called as "caramelization".
5) Syrups cannot be sterilized by autoclave, because autoclaving of syrup at 121°C leads to caramelization.
6) The concentration of the syrup is measured using an apparatus **"Saccharometer"** at warm condition, if the specific gravity of the sugar solution is known.

Dispensing of syrups: Simple flavoured syrups are dispensed in bulk volumes, but medicated syrups should be dispensed in small volumes.

Syrups should be dispensed in well dried, completely filled and well stoppered bottles because, moisture present in the wet bottles and atmospheric moisture causes fermentation of the sucrose. Therefore they should be dispensed in narrow mouthed, amber coloured (light resistant) bottles, fitted with white, poly propylene moulded or black thermosetting plastic screw cap.

Storage: Syrups are very sensitive to light, moisture and temperature. Cold place induces the crystallization of sucrose and warm place (higher temp) favours fermentation and also caramelization. Therefore syrups should be stored at fairly cool temperature, not exceeding 25 ºC, in dark place.

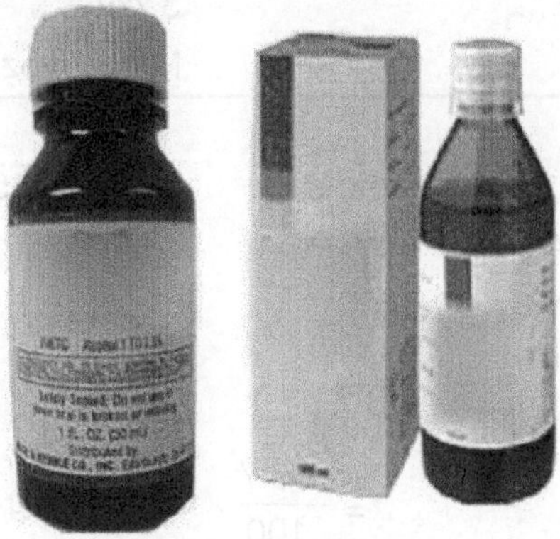

Containers for syrup

Label: The label must bear all necessary requirements of liquid dosage forms. In addition it should contain auxilliary label like '**Store at fairly cool temperature, not exceeding 25°C in dark place**'.

Invert syrup : It is prepared by acid hydrolysis of sucrose present in syrup. It is more sweeter then simple syrup because furctose is sweeter than sucrose. (if sweetness of sucrose is 100, fructore is 173).

Fructore is releatively less stable to heat and hence syrup darkarns, if not stored at cool conditions.

SIMPLE SYRUP I.P

Rx	
Sacchari	3 xvi sss
Aquam....q.s.....	3 xxv
Fiat : Syrupi	Mitte : fl.oz ii

Conversion :

3 xvi sss → 16.75 drachms   3 xxv → 25 fl. drachms = 100 ml

1 drachm = 4 g

16.75 drachms = 66.7 g

Calculation : For fl.oz ii → 2 fl.oz = 60 ml

Sucrose $= \frac{66.7}{100} \times 60 = 40$ g

Purified water...q.s.. = 60 ml

Type	Ingredients	Quantity in imperial	Quantity in metric	Quantity taken
Monophasic liquid, for pharmaceutical aid.	Sucrose	16.75 dr	66.7 g	40 g
	Purified water ....q.s....	25 fl. dr	100 ml	60 ml
	Make: Syrup Send: 60 ml			

Theory:

Simple syrup is a concentrated or nearly saturated solution of sucrose in purified water. It contains 66.7% w/w of sucrose. Hence the solubility of sucrose in water, at such a high concentration is slow. Therefore to increase the solubility of sucrose, syrup is prepared by heating.

Sucrose is a disaccharide, which partially hydrolyzed into monosaccharides as dextrose (glucose) and laevulose (fructose). These monosaccharides are called as "invert sugars" and reaction is called as "Inversion".

$$\underset{\text{Sucrose}}{C_{12}H_{22}O_{11}} + H_2O \xrightarrow{\text{Partial hydrolysation}} \underset{\text{Dextrose}}{C_6H_{12}O_6} + \underset{\text{Laevulose}}{C_6H_{12}O_6}$$

The inversion of sucrose is confirmed by measuring its optical rotation. After inversion, if the solution of sucrose rotates the polarized light to the right side, then it is considered as dextro-rotatory. If same solution rotates the polarized light to the left side, then it is considered as levo-rotatory.

Procedure:

1) Accurately weigh sucrose and dissolve in ¾th of total volume of purified water in a beaker.
2) Heat this solution on a water bath with occasional stirring, until whole amount of sugar completely dissolves (Do not do overheating).
3) Allow the solution to cool. After cooling, filter through the muslin cloth, to remove foreign particles, if present.

Dispensing: Syrup should be always dispensed in dry bottles, because moisture content present in the wet bottle is sufficient to cause fermentation.

After preparation of syrup it should be cooled to room temperature, before filling into the bottle or if syrup is filled in to the bottle, it should be occasionally shaked until, that attains room temperature. Because moisture will condense on the inner side of upper part of the bottle. These water molecules after running down, dilute the upper layers of the syrup, which leads to fermentation of sucrose.

Therefore transfer the syrup to a well dried, narrow mouthed, amber coloured , well filled glass bottle, close it thoroughly with plastic screw cap, polish and label.

Storage: If syrup is prepared in large quantity, then it should be always stored in loosely stoppered bottle, because if fermentation takes place carbon dioxide will liberate, which increases the pressure inside the bottle and may leads to bursting of container (bottle).

Warm place favours the fermentation and cool place induces crystallization, therefore syrup should be stored at fairly cool temperature not exceeding 25 °C, in dark place.

Auxilliary label: STORE AT FAIRLY COOL TEMPERATURE, NOT EXCEEDING 25°C IN DARK PLACE.

Uses: Simple syrup is used as a pharmaceutical aid, in the preparation of many pharmaceutical products for the following reasons.

1) It has palatable (pleasant) sweet taste. Hence it is used as a sweetening agent in the preparations, containing bitter and nauseous substances.
2) It is also used as vehicle for many liquid preparations like linctuses, elixirs.
3) In syrups, sucrose undergo hydrolysis into reducing sugars, as dextrose and levulose, which acts as anti-oxidants. Hence syrup reduces the oxidation of the preparations.
4) Simple syrup consists 66.7% w/w of sucrose, which is sufficient to exert osmotic pressure. Due to its high osmotic pressure, it withdraws water from the microorganisms and leads to dehydration and finally death of microorganisms. Hence it acts a "self preservative".

Note: If we prepare simple syrup with all precautions, it does not require any preservatives, to prevent the growth of microorganisms, because of its concentrated nature and the scarcity of required water, to promote the growth of microbes. This fact is understood by following points:

1) Syrup I. P. has density at 20 °C = 1.313.
2) It means that 1000 ml syrup weighs= 1313 g.
3) But Simple syrup I. P. contains, 667 g sucrose in 1000 g syrup.
4) When 1000 g syrup contains 667 g sucrose :

   1313 g syrup will contain $= \frac{667 \times 1313}{1000 \times 1} = 875.5$ g sucrose.
5) Therefore, the quantity of water present in the syrup,

   1313 – 875.7 = 437.3 ml.
6) It means, 437.3 ml water is used to dissolve 875.7g sucrose.
7) Since the solubility of sucrose in water is 1 in 0.5 ml, hence, to dissolve 875.7 g sucrose: 875.7 x 0.5 = 437.85 ml water is required, which is more or less equal to the water present in the syrup to form the solution.

   Thus, there is practically no additional water is available, for the growth of micro-organisms. Hence it acts as self preservative.

FERROUS SULPHATE SYRUP U.S.P

Rx	
Ferri sulphatis	3 X
Acidi citrici	gr XXX
Spiritus menthae piperitae	M XXX
Sacchari	3 CCVi
Aquam....q.s....	fl. 3 CCL
Fiat : Syrupi	Mitte : fl.oz iii
Signa : Cochleare magnum, omni nocte post sibos sumendum.	

Conversion :

3 X → 10 drachms	gr XXX → 30 grains
1 drachm = 4 g	15 grains = 1 g
10 drachms = 40 g	30 grains = 2 g
3 CCVi → 206 drachms	M xxx → 30 minims
1 drachm = 4 g	15 minims = 1 ml
206 drachms = 825 g	30 minims = 2 ml
	fl. 3 CCL → 250 fl.dr = 1000 ml

Calculation : For fl.oz iii → 3 fl.oz = 90 ml

Ferrous sulphate $= \frac{40}{1000} \times 90 = 3.6$ g

Citric acid $= \frac{2}{1000} \times 90 = 0.18$ g

Peppermint spirit $= \frac{2}{1000} \times 90 = 0.18$ ml

Sucrose $= \frac{825}{1000} \times 90 = 74$ g

Water ....q.s.... = 90 ml

Type	Ingredients	Quantity in imperial	Quantity in metric	Quantity taken
Monophasic liquid, for oral use.	Ferrous sulphate	10 dr	40 g	3.6 g
	Citric acid	30 gr	2 g	0.18 g
	Peppermint spirit	30 minims	2 ml	0.18 ml
	Sucrose	206 dr	825 g	74 g
	Purified water...q.s.....	250 fl. dr	1000 ml	90 ml
	Make: Syrup	Send: 90 ml		
	Direction:One tablespoonful to be taken, every night after meals.			

Theory:

Ferrous sulphate is a salt, hence it is freely soluble in water. But ferrous (Fe++) form of the ferrous sulphate is readily oxidized by reacting with dissolved oxygen of water into ferric (Fe+++) form, which will precipitate as basic ferric salt. This results in discoloration of the solution from green to reddish brown colour.

Therefore to overcome this problem, ferrous sulphate is added to the purified water, containing some amount of sucrose (which provides a reducing environment) because sucrose partially hydrolysis into reducing sugars as dextrose and laevulose, which acts as antioxidants and prevents the oxidation of ferrous form into ferric form.

To dissolve ferrous sulphate in water, only a small amount (portion) of sucrose should be used, otherwise if whole amount of sucrose is used, it gives high viscosity to the solution and which causes difficulties in filtration. The remaining major portion of sucrose is dissolved, at the end of the preparation.

Citric acid is used as stabilizer, to prevent the discoloration of syrup from green to reddish brown by chelating, if any ferric ions formed as a result of auto-oxidation (during storage). Peppermint spirit is used as flavouring agent to mask the unpleasant taste of ferrous ion (specific iron taste) of the preparation.

Procedure:

1) Dissolve $\frac{1}{4}^{th}$ of sucrose in $\frac{3}{4}^{th}$ of total volume of purified water.
2) To the dilute sucrose solution, add ferrous sulphate with stirring until, it completely dissolves.
3) To the above solution add citric acid, peppermint spirit, mix well and filter.
4) To the filtrate, add remaining amount of sucrose and dissolve by continuous stirring, then add purified water to make up the final volume. Mix well and (if necessary) filter through muslin cloth.

Dispensing: Transfer the syrup to a well dried, narrow mouthed, amber coloured glass bottle, close it thoroughly with plastic screw cap, polish and label.

Direction: One tablespoonful to be taken, every night after meals.

Auxilliary label: Store at fairly cool temperature, not exceeding 25°C, in dark place.

Uses: Ferrous sulphate syrup is used as iron supplement, in anemic patients.

CODEINE PHOSPHATE SYRUP I.P. / B.P.C.

Rx	
Codeine phosphate	3 i s
Chloroformi spiritus	fl. 3 vi s
Aquam	fl. 3 iii sss
Syrupi....q.s.......	fl. 3 CCL
Fiat : Syrupi	Mitte : fl.oz ii
Signa : Cochleare maximum, bis in die sumendum	

Conversion :

3 i s → 1.25 drachms = 5 g

fl. 3 Vi s → 6.25 fl. drachms = 25 ml

fl. 3 iii sss → 3.75 fl. drachms = 15 ml

fl. 3 CCL → 250 fl. drachms = 1000 ml

Calculation : For fl.oz ii → 2 fl.oz = 60 ml

Codeine phosphate $= \frac{5}{1000} \times 60 = 0.3$ g

Chloroform spirit $= \frac{25}{1000} \times 60 = 1.5$ ml

Purified water $= \frac{15}{1000} \times 60 = 0.9$ ml

Syrup ....q.s...... = 60 ml

Type	Ingredients	Quantity in imperial	Quantity in metric	Quantity taken
Monophasic liquid, for oral use.	Codeine phosphate	1.25 dr	5 g	0.3 g
	Chloroform spirit	6.25 fl. dr	25 ml	1.5 ml
	Purified water	3.75 fl. dr	15 ml	0.9 ml
	Syrup......q.s.....	250 fl. dr	1000 ml	60 ml
	Make: Syrup	Send: 60 ml		
	Direction: One tablespoonful to be taken, two times a day.			

Theory:

This preparation consists 0.46 to 0.54% of Codeine phosphate. Codeine phosphate acts as analgesic and antitussive (expectorant). It is freely soluble in water. Chloroform spirit is used as flavouring agent and also as a preservative. Syrup is used as sweetening agent and also as vehicle.

All the ingredients are miscible (soluble) in water, hence it is prepared by simple solution method by agitation, without aid of heat. Codeine phosphate in solution form is very sensitive to the light, hence it should be protected from light.

Procedure:

1) Accurately weigh codeine phosphate and dissolve in ¾ th quantity of purified water.
2) To the above solution, add chloroform spirit, mix well and adjust the final volume with syrup.

Dispensing: Transfer the syrup to a well dried, narrow mouthed, amber coloured glass bottle, close it thoroughly with plastic screw cap, polish and label.

Direction: One tablespoonful, to be taken two times a day.

Storage: Codeine phosphate is sensitive to the light and chloroform spirit contains volatile oil and alcohol. Sucrose will crystallize at lower temperature and higher temperature favours the fermentation. Therefore it should be stored in dark place at temperature, not exceeding 25ºC.

Auxilliary label: STORE AT FAIRLY COOL TEMPERATURE, NOT EXCEEDING 25°C IN DARK PLACE.

Uses: Codeine phosphate syrup is used as analgesic and antitussive (expectorant).

COMPOUND FERROUS PHOSPHATE SYRUP B.P.C.

Synonym: Parrish's food

Rx	
Iron wire	gr vi sss
Phosphoric acid	fl. 3 i s
Calcium carbonate	gr xx ss
Potassium bicarbonate	gr i ss
Sodium phosphate	gr i ss
Cochineal	gr v s
Sucrose	3 xvii ss
Orange flower water	fl. 3 i s
Purified water.... q.s....	fl. 3 xxv
Fiat: Syrupi	Mitte : fl.oz i
Signa: Cochleare amplum post jentaculum capiendus.	

Conversion :

gr vi sss → 6.75 grains	3 xvii ss → 17.5 drachms
15 grains = 1 g	1 drachm = 4 g
6.75 grains = 0.45 g	17.5 drachms = 70 g
gr xx ss → 20.5 grains = 1.37 g	
gr v s → 5.25 grains = 0.35 g	fl. 3 i s → 1.25 fl. drachms = 5 ml
gr i ss → 1.5 grains = 0.1 g	fl. 3 xxv → 25 fl. drachms = 100 ml

Calculation : For fl.oz i → 1 fl.oz = 30 ml

Iron wire = $\frac{0.45}{100} \times 30 = 0.135$ g

Phosphoric acid = $\frac{5}{100} \times 30 = 1.5$ ml

Calcium carbonate = $\frac{1.37}{100} \times 30 = 0.411$ g

Potassium bicarbonate = $\frac{0.1}{100} \times 30 = 0.03$ g

Sodium phosphate = $\frac{0.1}{100} \times 30 = 0.03$ g

Cochineal = $\frac{0.35}{100} \times 30 = 0.105$ g

Sucrose = $\frac{70}{100} \times 30 = 21$ g

Orange flower water = $\frac{5}{100} \times 30 = 1.5$ ml

Purified water.....q.s...... = 30 ml

Type	Ingredients	Quantity in imperial	Quantity in metric	Quantity taken
Monophasic liquid, for oral use.	Iron wire (Filings)	6.75 gr	0.45 g	0.135 g
	Phosphoric acid	1.25 fl. dr	5 ml	1.5 ml
	Calcium carbonate	20.5 gr	1.37 g	0.411 g
	Potassium bicarbonate	1.5 gr	0.1 g	0.03 g
	Sodium phosphate	1.5 gr	0.1 g	0.03 g
	Cochineal	5.25 gr	0.35 g	0.105 g
	Sucrose	17.5 dr	70 g	21 g
	Orange flower water	1.25 fl. dr	5 ml	1.5 ml
	Purified water.... q.s....	25 fl. dr	100 ml	30 ml
	Make: Syrup	Send: 30 ml		
	Direction:One tablespoonful to be taken, after breakfast.			

Theory:

Ferrous phosphate syrup is prepared by chemical reaction between iron and phosphoric acid and other electrolyte supplements like calcium carbonate, potassium bicarbonate and sodium phosphate.

The electrolytes such as calcium (Ca++), sodium (Na+) and potassium (K+) are also supplied in phosphate form.

In this preparation, half of the portion of phosphoric acid reacts with iron and forms ferrous acid phosphate. Remaining half of the portion of phosphoric acid reacts with calcium carbonate, potassium bicarbonate and sodium phosphate and forms corresponding phosphates.

But the amount of phosphoric acid is insufficient to complete this reaction. Hence the excess of acid phosphate present in ferrous acid phosphate {$Fe(H_2Po_4)_2$} is used to complete the reaction.

The following reactions takes place, during the preparation of ferrous phosphate syrup.

Fe + $2H_3PO_4$ → $Fe(H_2PO_4)_2$ + H_2O
Iron Phosphoric acid (Ferrous acid phosphate)

$CaCO_3$ + $2H_3PO_4$ → $Ca(H_2PO_4)_2$ + CO_2 + H_2O
Calcium carbonate Calcium dihydrogen phosphate

$KHCO_3$ + $2H_3PO_4$ → KH_2PO_4 + CO_2 + H_2O
Potassium carbonate Potassium dihydrogen phosphate

Na_2HPO_4 + $2H_3PO_4$ → $2NaH_2PO_4$ + CO_2 + H_2O
Sodium phosphate Sodium dihydrogen phosphate

Cochineal is used as colouring agent, which is obtained by aqueous extraction of cochineal. In this preparation it is used as masking agent to mask, if any colour change of the preparation occurs, due to oxidation of constituents during storage.

Orange flower water is used as flavouring agent. Sucrose is used to prepare syrup, which is used as sweetening agent to mask the specific iron taste of the preparation. It also helps in giving viscous nature to the preparation and also acts as preservative, because of its higher concentration.

Procedure:

1) Cut the iron wire into small pieces.
2) Dilute phosphoric acid with water and divide it into two equal portions.
3) In a small flask, take iron pieces and half of the portion of diluted phosphoric acid and gently heat on a water bath until a whole amount of iron dissolves. (Note: Heating should not be done at higher temperature because if water evaporates, a solid mass will be formed, which will not dissolve in water).
4) In a separate beaker, take second portion of diluted phosphoric acid and dissolve calcium carbonate, potassium bicarbonate and sodium phosphate one by one with continuous stirring.
5) When phosphoric acid reacts with calcium carbonate and potassium bicarbonate, there is effervescence due to release of CO_2. Allow this CO_2 to evolve completely.
6) Mix the above both solutions (contents) with stirring and allow it to stand for a while, to complete the reaction.
7) After completion of reaction, the resulting solution contains the impurities like iron-carbide and carbon, which are derived from the iron solution. To remove these impurities, filter the solution.
8) In a conical flask, boil cochineal with water for about 15 minutes. To this solution, add sucrose and again boil for 15 minutes. Cool, strain and add sufficient purified water to produce required volume.
9) Mix this coloured syrup with mixture containing ferrous acid phosphate, calcium acid phosphate, potassium phosphate and sodium phosphate.
10) Add the orange flower water and then add sufficient purified water to make final volume.

Dispensing: Transfer the syrup to a well dried, narrow mouthed, amber coloured glass bottle, close it thoroughly with plastic screw cap, polish and label.

Direction: One tablespoonful to be taken after breakfast.

Auxilliary label: STORE AT FAIRLY COOL TEMPERATURE, NOT EXCEEDING 25 °C IN DARK PLACE.

Uses: Ferrous phosphate syrup is used as iron and electrolyte supplement to the patients, who are suffering from anaemia.

TOLU SYRUP

Synonym: Balsam of tolu syrup

Rx	
Tolu balsam	gr x ix
Sacchuri	3 xvi ss
Aquam....q.s......	fl. 3 xxv
Fiat : Syrupi	Mitte : fl.oz i
Signa : Cochleare minimum, bis in die sumendum.	

Conversion :

gr xi x → 19 grains — 3 xvi ss → 16.5 drachms

15 grains = 1 g — 1 drachm = 4 g

19 grains = 1.25 g — 16.5 drachms = 66 g

fl. 3 xxv → 25 fl. drachms = 100 ml

Calculation : For fl.oz i → 1 fl.oz = 30 ml

$$\text{Tolu balsam} = \frac{1.25}{100} \times 30 = 0.375 \text{ g}$$

$$\text{Sucrose} = \frac{66}{100} \times 30 = 19.8 \text{ g}$$

Purified water ....q.s...... = 30 ml

Type	Ingredients	Quantity in imperial	Quantity in metric	Quantity taken
Monophasic liquid, for internal use.	Tolu balsam	19 gr	1.25 g	0.375 g
	Sucrose	16.5 dr	66 g	19.8 g
	Purified water......q.s.......	25 fl.dr	100 ml	30 ml
	Make: Syrup Send: 30 ml Direction: One teaspoonful to be taken, two times a day.			

Theory:

Tolu balsam is a solid or semisolid balsam, obtained by incisions from the trunk of Myroxylon balsumum. It contains about 80% of resin, 20% of aromatic principles and balsamic acids. The resin consists free cinnamic acid (12-15%) and free benzoic acid (8%).

Cinnamic acid and benzoic acid are highly soluble in hot water than cold water. Hence extraction of these acids is done by decoction method. Melting of balsam at elevated temperature in water facilitates greater surface area for balsam and hence fast solubilization of active constituents.

To prevent the loss of volatile constituents during boiling, vessel should be covered by covering dish. On cooling, undesirable acid crystallizes out, which are removed by filtration. Sucrose is used to prepare syrup, which acts as sweetening agent to mask resinous taste of balsam.

The percentage of sucrose is 66% w/w, hence it also acts as preservative, due to its higher osmotic pressure.

Procedure:

1) Take accurately weighed tolu balsam in a tarred vessel.
2) Add boiled purified water, and cover the vessel lightly and boil the contents on water bath gently for half an hour with occasional stirring.
3) After boiling, add more purified water to adjust the specified volume to compensate the loss of water due to evaporation during heating. Then cool to room temperature and filter the solution, to remove foreign particles or any undissolved substance if present.
4) To the filtrate, add remaining portion of sucrose and dissolve by warming on a water bath.
5) Finally add sufficient purified water to adjust the final volume.

Dispensing: Transfer the syrup to a well dried, narrow mouthed, amber coloured glass bottle, close it thoroughly with plastic screw cap, polish and label.

Direction: One teaspoonful to be taken, two times a day.

Storage: Store in a dark place at temperature, not exceeding 25 ºC.

Auxilliary label: STORE AT FAIRLY COOL TEMPERATURE, NOT EXCEEDING 25 °C IN DARK PLACE.

Uses: Tolu balsam has expectorant action. Hence this syrup is used as common ingredient of cough mixtures. This syrup is also used as flavouring agent, due to the presence of volatile principles.

ORANGE SYRUP

Rx	
Tincturae aurantii	M XC
Syrupi...q.s....	fl. 3 XXV
Fiat : Syrupi	Mitte : fl.oz ii

Conversion:

M XC → 90 minims — fl. 3 XXV → 25 fl. drachms

15 minims = 1 ml — 1 fl. drachm = 4 ml

90 minims = 6 ml — 25 fl. drachms = 100 ml

Calculation: For fl.oz ii → 2 fl.oz = 60 ml

Orange tincture = $\frac{6}{100} \times 60 = 3.6$ ml

Syrup ....q.s...... = 60 ml

Type	Ingredients	Quantity in imperial	Quantity in metric	Quantity taken
Monophasic liquid, for pharmaceutical aid.	Orange tincture	90 minims	6 ml	3.6 ml
	Syrup....q.s...	25 fl. dr	100 ml	60 ml
	Make: Syrup	Send:60 ml		

Theory:

Orange syrup is a flavored syrup, prepared by using orange tincture. Orange tincture is obtained by the maceration of fresh orange peel with alcohol (90%), for 7 days. Orange peel is the fresh outer part of pericarp of fruit Citrus aurantium. Fresh orange peel consists more volatile oil, compare to dried peel, hence fresh orange peel is used for extraction. Orange peel is sliced into small pieces, to expose more surface area for the solvent action.

Orange syrup is prepared by dissolving freshly prepared orange tincture in the syrup, which is used as flavouring and sweetening agent (flavoured syrup) in the preparation of many pharmaceutical liquid dosage forms like linctuses, elixirs, etc..

Procedure:

1) Mix freshly prepared orange tincture in small portion of the syrup, then add sufficient syrup to produce final volume.
2) Transfer to an amber coloured, narrow mouthed, glass bottle, tightly close with a plastic screw cap, polish and label.

Dispensing: Transfer the orange syrup to a well dried, narrow mouthed, amber coloured glass bottle, close it thoroughly with plastic screw cap, polish and label.

Storage: Store in a dark place at temperature, not exceeding 25 ºC.

Auxilliary label: STORE AT FAIRLY COOL TEMPERATURE, NOT EXCEEDING 25 °C IN DARK PLACE.

Uses: Orange syrup is used as flavoured syrup (both flavouring and sweetening agent) for masking the unpleasant bitter and nauseous taste of the drugs, in many pharmaceutical liquid dosage forms.

Note:

Formula for orange tincture:

Ingredients	**Quantity**
Fresh orange peel in thin slices	25 g
Ethanol (90%).... q.s...	100 ml

LEMON SYRUP

Synonym: Citric acid syrup

Rx	
Tincturae limonis	fl. 3 i
Acidi citrici	3 vi
Aquam	fl. 3 xxv
Syrupi....q.s.....	fl. 3 CCL
Fiat : Syrupi	Mitte : fl.oz iii

Conversion :

fl. 3 i → 1 fl. drachm = 4 ml

3 vi → 6 drachms = 24 g

fl. 3 XXV → 25 fl. drachms = 100 ml

fl. 3 CCL → 250 fl.dr = 1000 ml

Calculation : For fl.oz iii → 3 fl.oz = 90 ml

Lemon tincture = $\frac{4}{1000} \times 90 = 0.4$ ml

Citric acid = $\frac{24}{1000} \times 90 = 2.16$ g

Purified water = $\frac{100}{1000} \times 90 = 9$ ml

Syrup ...q.s...... = 90 ml

Type	Ingredients	Quantity in imperial	Quantity in metric	Quantity taken
Monophasic liquid, for pharmaceutical aid.	Lemon tincture	1 fl. dr	4 ml	0.4 ml
	Citric acid	6 dr	24 g	2.16 g
	Purified water	25 fl. dr	100 ml	9 ml
	Syrup.....q.s...	250 fl. dr	1000 ml	90 ml
	Make: Syrup	Send: 90 ml.		

Theory:

Lemon syrup is a flavoured syrup prepared by using lemon tincture, which is obtained by the maceration of fresh lemon peel with alcohol 96%, for seven days.

Lemon syrup is prepared by dissolving citric acid in purified water and adding the syrup to this solution. To this solution, lemon tincture is added and final volume is adjusted with syrup.

In this preparation syrup is used as vehicle, hence to prevent the discolouration of syrup, citric acid is used as a stabilizer.

Procedure:

1) Dissolve accurately weighed citric acid in purified water by stirring.
2) To this solution, add syrup and mix well.
3) Add freshly prepared lemon tincture and adjust the final volume by adding sufficient amount of syrup.

Dispensing: Transfer the syrup to a well dried, narrow mouthed, amber coloured glass bottle, close it thoroughly with plastic screw cap, polish and label.

Storage: Store in a dark place, at temperature not exceeding 25 ºC.

Auxilliary label: STORE AT FAIRLY COOL TEMPERATURE, NOT EXCEEDING 25 °C IN DARK PLACE.

Uses: Lemon syrup is used as a flavoured vehicle.

Note:

1) The syrup should not be dispensed, if it has terbinthine odour and taste or shows other indications of deterioration.
2) Being acidic in nature, this syrup is not suitable as a vehicle for preparations containing alkaline ingredients, because it leads to the precipitation of such substances.
   Eg. phenobarbitone sodium.

Other examples of syrups:

1) Vasaka syrup

Vasaka liquid extract	—	500 ml
Glycerin	—	100 ml
Syrup....q.s....	—	1000 ml

Uses: It is used as expectorant and bronchodilator.

2) Piperazine citrate syrup U.S.P.

Piperazine citrate	—	18 g
Syrup... q.s.....	—	100 ml

Uses: It is used as anthelmintic in the treatment of tape worms and round worms.

3) Chlorpheniramine maleate syrup

Chlorpheniramine maleate	—	0.4 g
Syrup ....q.s ...	—	1000 ml

Uses: It is used as antihistaminic and antiallergic.

4) Chloral hydrate syrup

Chloral hydrate	—	4 g
Water	—	2 ml
Simple syrup... q.s....	—	100 ml

Uses: It is used as hypnotic, particularly in children to induce sleep.

Student's exercise:

1) Define syrups. Classify the syrups with examples.
2) What are the advantages and disadvantages of syrups, prepared by the aid of heat?
3) Give the examples for stabilizers, used for preparation of syrups.
4) Mention the type of medicaments used in syrups with examples.
5) Explain advantages and dis-advantages of syrups.
6) Define caramalization. How it can be avoided?
7) What is the storage conditions required for syrups?
8) What is saccharin? why it is preferred in the preparation of syrups?
9) How will you dispense syrups?
10) How syrup acts as self preservative?
11) How citric acid acts as stabilizer, in ferrous sulphate syrup?
12) What is cochineal?
13) Explain in brief the principle involved in the preparation of parrish's food.
14) What is Tolu balsam? what for it is used?
15) Explain how Orange tincture is prepared.
16) What is the concentration of simple syrup. I.P.?

10 MOUTHWASHES

Latin terms: Collutoria --- Mouthwashes,

Collutorium --- Mouthwash

Mouthwashes are aqueous solutions in concentrated form with pleasant taste, flavor and odour, which are used for rinsing, deodorizing, cleansing, refreshing or antiseptic action in mouth or buccal cavity. Mouthwashes generally contain medicaments like,

Astringents : Zinc sulphate, Zinc chloride

Antiseptic and antibacterial agents : Phenol, Hydrogen peroxide, Thymol and Sodium perborate

Deodorants : Sodium bicarbonate and Sodium chloride.

Sodium chloride and sodium bicarbonate are incorporated as hypertonic solutions, to remove the debris from the mouth and leaving the deodorant effect in mouth cavity.

Along with the medicaments, mouthwashes also contain other additives like flavouring agents, colouring agents and sweetening agents, glycerin, alcohol and surfactants. They have pH between 5.0 to 9.5. Mouthwashes are supplied in concentrated form, therefore they should be used, after suitable dilution with warm water.

Examples for Mouthwashes:

- Hydrogen peroxide mouthwash
- Compound sodium chloride mouthwash
- Compound thymol glycerin mouthwash
- Glycerin tannic and Zinc chloride mouthwash
- Phenol mouthwash

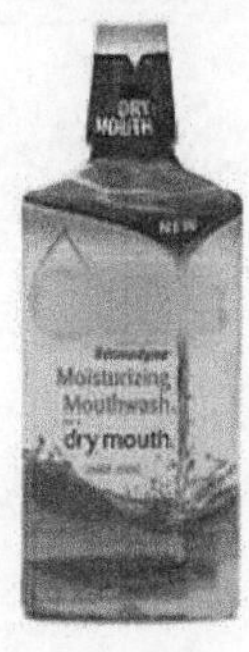

An example for Mouthwash

Formulation:

Sr. No.	Ingredients type	Examples
1	Vehicles	Chloroform water, Peppermint water
2	Sweetening agents	Simple syrup
3	Flavoring agents	Aromatic water, Chloroform water, Peppermint water
4	Colouring agents	Amaranth solution.
5	Surfactants	Tween 20, Tween 80, Sodium lauryl sulphate , Spans
6	Humectants	Glycerin, Sorbitol

Method of preparation: Mouthwashes usually consists soluble ingredients. Hence they are prepared by simple solution method.

Dispensing: Mouthwashes should be dispensed in a clear, fluted, narrow mouthed, glass or plastic bottles with colored plastic screw cap, in order to distinguish them from the preparations meant for internal use.

Label: Label should bear all necessary requirements of liquid dosage forms except dose. In addition, it should also contain auxiliary labels like:

- FOR EXTERNAL USE ONLY.
- DILUTION RATIO WITH WARM WATER.
- NOT TO BE SWALLOWED IN LARGE QUANTITIES.

Direction: Dilute with equal volume of warm water before use.

Storage: Mouthwashes should be stored in a cool place (or at room temperature).

COMPOUND SODIUM CHLORIDE MOUTHWASH B.P.C

Rx

Sodii chloridi	gr LXXX
Sodii bicarbonatis	gr XL
Liquor amarantis	M L
Aquam menthae piperitae...q.s..	fl.oz X
Fiat : Collutorium	Mitte : fl.oz ii

Signa : Cum duplo aqua calidae aequales, pro utendum et rinse oris omni mane.

Conversion :

gr LXXX → 80 grains	M L → 50 minims
15 grains = 1 g	15 minims = 1 ml
80 grains = 5.3 g	50 minims = 3.3 ml
gr XL → 40 grains = 2.7 g	fl.oz X → 10 fl.oz = 300 ml

Calculation : For fl.oz ii → 2 fl.oz = 60 ml

Sodium chloride $= \frac{5.3}{300} \times 60 = 1.06$ g

Sodium bicarbonate $= \frac{2.7}{300} \times 60 = 0.54$ g

Amaranth solution $= \frac{3.3}{300} \times 60 = 0.66$ g

Peppermint water ....q.s... = 60 ml

Type	Ingredients	Quantity in imperial	Quantity in metric	Quantity taken
Monophasic liquid, used only in mouth or buccal cavity.	Sodium chloride	80 gr	5.3 g	1.06 g
	Sodium bicarbonate	40 gr	2.7 g	0.54 g
	Amaranth solution	50 minims	3.3 ml	0.66 ml
	Peppermint water....q.s..	10 fl.oz.	300 ml	60 ml
	Make: Mouthwash Send: 60 ml			
	Direction: Dilute with an equal volume of warm water, before use and rinse the mouth every morning.			

Theory:

It is a mouthwash containing sodium salts like, sodium chloride and sodium bicarbonate. Sodium chloride acts as deodorant and makes the preparation isotonic. Sodium bicarbonate acts as deodorant, antacid (contols pH) and also dissolves the mucus. Both salts are readily soluble in peppermint water, hence mouthwash is prepared by simple solution method.

In this preparation, amaranth solution is used as coloring agent, to give an attractive colour to the mouthwash and peppermint water is used as a flavored vehicle.

Procedure:

1) Accurately weigh the sodium chloride and sodium bicarbonate and dissolve in ¾ th quantity of of peppermint water and transfer to a measure.
2) Add measured quantity of amaranth solution and mix well. Add more amount of peppermint water, to adjust the final volume.

Dispensing: Transfer this solution to a clear, fluted, narrow mouthed, glass or plastic bottle, close throughly with coloured plastic screw cap, polish and label.

Direction: Dilute with equal volume of warm water, before use and rinse the mouth every morning.

Storage: Store in a cool place.

Auxilliary label:
- FOR EXTERNAL USE ONLY.
- NOT TO BE SWALLOWED, IN LARGE QUANTITIES.

Uses: Compound sodium chloride mouthwash is used to clean and deodorize the buccal cavity. It is widely used in refreshing of buccal cavity, particularly to the bed ridden patients.

Note: Direction to patients before dispensing,

Patients should be directed to use about 15 ml (tablespoonful) diluted in equal volume of warm water before use, usually morning and night unless otherwise directed.

ZINC SULPHATE AND ZINC CHLORIDE MOUTHWASH B.P.C

Rx	
Zinci sulphatis	3 Vi
Zinci chloridi	3 iii
Acidi hydrochloridi diluti	M CL
Tartrazini liquor composite	M CL
Aquam chloroformi..q.s...	fl. dr CCL
Fiat : Collutorium	Mitte : fl.oz iii

Signa : Cum duplo viginti, aqua calidae pro utendum, et rinse oris mane et nocte.

Conversion :

3 Vi → 6 drachms	3 iii → 3 drachms
1 drachm = 4 g	1 drachm = 4 g
6 drachms = 24 g	3 drachms = 12 g
M CL → 150 minims	fl. dr CCL → 250 fl. dr
15 minims = 1 ml	1 fl. dr = 4 ml
150 minims = 10 ml	250 fl. dr = 1000 ml

Calculation : For fl.oz iii → 3 fl.oz = 90 ml

Zinc sulphate $= \frac{24}{1000} \times 90 = 2.16$ g

Zinc chloride $= \frac{12}{1000} \times 90 = 1.08$ g

Dilute hydrochloric acid $= \frac{10}{1000} \times 90 = 0.9$ ml

Compound tartrazine solution $= \frac{10}{1000} \times 90 = 0.9$ ml

Chloroform water...q.s..... = 90 ml

Type	Ingredients	Quantity in imperial	Quantity in metric	Quantity taken
Monophasic liquid, used only in mouth or buccal cavity.	Zinc sulphate	6 dr	24 g	2.16 g
	Zinc chloride	3 dr	12 g	1.08 g
	Dilute hydrochloric acid	150 minims	10 ml	0.9 ml
	Compound tartrazine solution	150 minims	10 ml	0.9 ml
	Chloroform water....q.s....	250 fl. dr	1000 ml	90 ml
	Make: Mouthwash	Send: 90 ml		
	Direction: Dilute with 20 times its volume of warm water, before use and rinse the mouth morning and night.			

Theory:

Both the salts, zinc sulphate and zinc chloride are freely soluble in water, hence the mouthwash is prepared by simple solution method. Zinc chloride is very deliquecent in nature and usually contains small amount of oxychloride, which makes the solution turbid. This turbidity will disappear, when dilute hydrochloric acid is added.

Since mouthwash is to be used in oral cavity, which will be in contact with mucous membrane, it should be free from irritant particles, which can be removed by filtration. Zinc chloride reacts with the filter paper, therefore sintered glass funnel should be used to filter or clarify the solution before making the final volume.

Compound tartarzine solution is used as coloring agent. Chloroform water provides palatability (good mouth feel) and also acts as a preservative.

Procedure:

1) Dissolve zinc sulphate and zinc chloride in ¾ th quantity of chloroform water.
2) To this solution add dilute hydrochloric acid and mix with continuous stirring until turbidity disappears. Filter the solution through sintered glass funnel.
3) Add compound tartrazine solution and adjust to the final volume with remaining amount of chloroform water.

Dispensing: Transfer this solution to a clear, fluted, narrow mouthed, glass or plastic bottle, close throughly with coloured plastic screw cap, polish and label.

Direction: Dilute with 20 times its volume of warm water before use and rinse the mouth morning and night. (i.e. Dilute15 ml with 300 ml of warm water or three 5 ml spoonfuls to be added to a tumbelreful of warm water before use).

Storage: Store in a cool place.

Auxiliary label:
- FOR EXTERNAL USE ONLY.
- NOT TO BE SWALLOWED IN LARGE QUANTITIES.

Uses: Both zinc sulphate and zinc chloride acts as astringents, therefore this mouthwash is used as astringent.

> **Note:** Zinc chloride is very deliquescent in nature, therefore it should be stored in desicator. A small quantity of zinc chloride should be crushed in a mortar before use, weighing and compounding should be done as quickly as possible.

PHENOL MOUTHWASH

Rx	
Liquoris phenolis	M VL
Liquor potassii hydroxidi	M VL
Liquore amaranthi	M XV
Aquam....q.s....	fl.oz iii
Fiat : Collutorium	Mitte : fl.oz iii

Signa : Cum duplo aqua calidae aequales, pro utendum et rinse oris quartis horis.

Conversion :

M VL → 45 Minims

15 minims = 1 ml

45 minims = 3 ml

M XV → 15 Minims = 1 ml

fl.oz iii → 3 fl. oz = 90 ml

Calculation : For fl.oz iii → 3 fl.oz = 90 ml

Liquified phenol = $\frac{3}{90} \times 90 = 3$ ml

Potassium hydroxide solution = $\frac{3}{90} \times 90 = 3$ ml

Amarauth solution = $\frac{1}{90} \times 90 = 1$ ml

Purified water ....q.s...... = 90 ml

Type	Ingredients	Quantity in imperial	Quantity in metric	Quantity taken
Monophasic liquid, used only in mouth or buccal cavity.	Liquified phenol	45 minims	3 ml	3 ml
	Potassium hydroxide solution	45 minims	3 ml	3 ml
	Amaranth solution	15 minims	1 ml	1 ml
	Purified water...q.s....	3 fl.oz	90 ml	90 ml
	Make: Mouthwash	Send: 90ml		
	Direction: Dilute with equal volume of warm water, before use and rinse the mouth every four hours.			

Theory:

Liquified phenol is just the melted phenol crystals at 41^{0}C. Phenol acts as a disinfectant against gram-positive and gram-negative bacteria, but aqueous solution of 0.2 to 1 % acts as bacteriostatic. Hence 0.2 to 0.5 % solution of alkali phenates is used in mouthwash. To get alkali phenates, alkalining agent like potassium hydroxide is used. Amaranth solution is used as a dye, to give a distinctive colour to the mouthwash.

Procedure:

1 Accurately measure the liquified phenol and potassium hydroxide solution separately and dissolve in ¾ th portion of purified water by stirring.

2. Add amaranth solution and mix well. Transfer this content to a measure and adjust the final volume, by adding sufficient purified water.

Dispensing: Transfer this solution to a clear, fluted, narrow mouthed, glass or plastic bottle, close throughly with coloured plastic screw cap, polish and label.

Direction: Dilute with equal volume of warm water, before use and rinse the mouth, every four hours.

Storage: Store in a cool place.

Auxilliary label:
- FOR EXTERNAL USE ONLY.
- SHOULD NOT TO BE SWALLOWED.(Since phenol is a disinfectant, this mouthwash should not be swallowed)

Uses: This mouthwash is used as bacteriostatic, in the treatment of mouth infections.

Note: Phenol at higher concentrations acts as disinfectant, which is effective against gram-positive and gram-negative bacteria. Aqueous solutions (diluted solution) of phenol at the concentration of 0.2 to 1 % acts as bacteriostatic and still stronger solutions are acts as bactericidal.

GLYCERIN TANNIC ACID MOUTHWASH

Rx	
Glycerini acidi tannici	fl. ʒ iii
Aquam chloroformi...q.s..	fl. ʒ xxv
Fiat : Collutorium	Mitte : fl.oz ii
Signa : Cum duplo aqua calidae aequales pro utendum, et rinse oris omni tertis - quartis horis.	

Conversion :

fl. ʒ iii → 3 fl. drachms

1 fl. drachm = 4 ml

3 fl. drachms = 12 ml

fl. ʒ xxv → 25 fl. drachms = 100 ml

Calculation : For fl.oz ii → 2 fl.oz = 60 ml

Glycerin of Tannic acid $= \frac{12}{100} \times 60 = 7.2$ ml

Chloroform water ...q.s... = 60 ml

Type	Ingredients	Quantity in imperial	Quantity in metric	Quantity taken
Monophasic liquid used only in mouth	Glycerin of Tannic acid	3 fl. dr	12 ml	7.2 ml
	Chloroform water....q.s...	25 fl. dr	100 ml	60 ml
	Make: Mouthwash	Send: 60ml		
	Direction: Dilute with equal volume of warm water before use and rinse the mouth, every three to four hours.			

Theory:

Tannic acid is slightly soluble in water, but aqueous solution of tannic acid decomposes during storage. Tannic acid is soluble in glycerin and solution does not decompose. Hence glycerin is used as excellent solvent (carrier) for tannic acid.

Tannic acid acts as an astringent and exerts a healing action (haemostatic action), therefore it is used in mouthwash, for the treatment of painful bleeding in the gums. Mouthwash of tannic acid can be prepared by mixing glycerin of tannic acid with chloroform water, which acts as vehicle and also as preservative.

Procedure:

1) Measure accurately glycerin of tannic acid and dissolve in ¾ th quantity of chloroform water by continuous stirring.
2) Transfer this content to a measure and add sufficient chloroform water to make up the final volume.

Dispensing: Transfer this solution to a clear, fluted, narrow mouthed, glass or plastic bottle, close throughly with coloured plastic screw cap, polish it and dispense with label.

Direction: Dilute with equal volume of warm water before use and rinse the mouth, at every 3 to 4 hours.

Storage: Store in a cool place.

Uses: Glycerin tannic acid mouthwash is used as astringent, in the treatment of bleeding gums.

Auxilliary label:
- FOR EXTERNAL USE ONLY.
- NOT TO BE SWALLOWED IN LARGE QUANTITIES.

Formula for Glycerin of tannic acid I.P.

Tannic acid	---	200 g
Sodium citrate	---	10 g
Dried sodium sulphite	---	2 g
Glycerin	---	788 g

Student's exercise:

1) What is collutorium?
2) Define mouthwashes, what is their importance?
3) What is the pH of Mouthwash and why?
4) Give examples for mouthwashes.
5) What types of medicaments are used in mouthwashes?
6) Comment : Mouthwashes should be diluted with warm water before use.
7) How will you dispense Mouthwashes?
8) Which auxilliary label is required for mouthwashes?
9) Differentiate between Mouthwashes and Gargles.
10) Define (a) Sailogogue (b) Antiseptic (c) Deodorant (d) Astringent with examples.
11) Which colouring agents are used in mouthwashes?

12) How can you avoid turbidity in zinc sulphate and zinc chloride mouthwash?

13) Comment : For filtration of Zinc chloride solution, filter paper is used.

14) What is liquified phenol? Why Phenol is used in this form?

15) Explain why tannic acid is used in the form of Glycerin of tannic acid. Give the formula for Glycerin of tannic acid IP.

16) What is the use of following mouthwashes :

   (a) Glycerin tannic acid mouthwash

   (b) Phenol mouthwash

   (c) Compound sodium chloride mouthwash.

17) Write label direction for phenol mouthwash.

11 GARGLES

Latin term: Gargarisma

Gargles are aqueous solutions of medicaments, used in the treatment of throat infections (specially pharynx and nasopharynx infections) by forcing the air from lungs through solution, which is held in the throat.

Gargles are intended, to bring the medicament into close contact with the mucous surface of the throat. Therefore gargles are used in the posterior region of the mouth cavity, by agitating (gargaling) the solution by forcing the air from lungs for certain while and then it is thrown out of the mouth. As the contact period of gargle and mucous membrane is short, the preparation must be fast acting.

Gargles are supplied in concentrated form, along with direction for dilution with warm water before use. Compared to the mouthwashes, gargles are highly medicated and pleasantly flavored with pH 5 to 9.5.

Gargles restore the tone of relaxed throat and stimulates the flow of saliva, which relives dryness of the mouth.

Gargles generally contains medicaments like,

1. Antiseptics : Borax.
2. Antibiotics : Flohexidine, Chloramphenicol.
3. Anti-inflammatory agents : Clove oil.
4. Bactericides : Phenol, Thymol.
5. Astringents : Potassium chlorate, Benzalkonium chlorate
6. Local anesthetics : Eugenol, Benzocaine.
7. Alkalining agents : Crestone, Sodium chloride

Examples for Gargles:

- Phenol gargle
- Phenol-glycerin gargle
- Potassium permanganate gargle
- Potassium chlorate and phenol gargle
- Thymol glycerin gargle

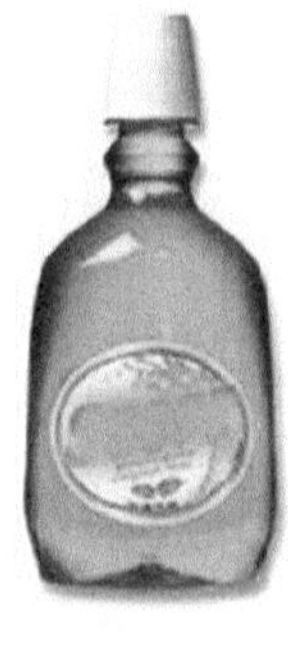

Example for gargles

Dispensing: Gargles should be dispensed in narrow mouthed, clear fluted glass or plastic bottles with coloured plastic screw cap, in order to distinguish them from the preparations meant for internal use. If ingredients are sensitive to the light, gargle should be stored in amber coloured bottles.

Direction: Gargles should contain direction to the patients like, Dilute with equal volume of warm water, before use.

Label: Label should bear all necessary requirements of liquid dosage forms, except dose. In addition, it should also contain auxilliary labels like:

- FOR EXTERNAL USE ONLY.
- DILUTION RATIO WITH WARM WATER.
- NOT TO BE SWALLOWED IN LARGE QUANTITIES.

Storage: Gargles should be stored in a cool place (at room temperature not exceding 25 ºC.)

PHENOL GARGLE B.P.C

Rx	
Glyerini phenolis	fl. 3 i s
Amaranthi liquor	M XV
Aquam...q.s...	fl. 3 xxv
Fiat : Gargarisma	Mitte : fl.oz i
Signa : Cum duplo aquae calidae aequales pro utendum, et utendus more dicto.	

Conversion :

fl. 3 i s → 1.25 fl. drachms — M XV → 15 Minims

1 fl. drachm = 4 ml — 15 minims = 1 ml

1.25 fl. drachms = 5 ml — fl. 3 xxv → 25 fl. drachms = 100 ml

Calculation : For fl.oz i → 1 fl.oz = 30 ml

$$\text{Phenol glycerin} = \frac{5}{100} \times 30 = 1.5 \text{ ml}$$

$$\text{Amaranth solution} = \frac{1}{100} \times 30 = 0.3 \text{ ml}$$

Water ....q.s....... = 30 ml

Type	Ingredients	Quantity in imperial	Quantity in metric	Quantity taken
Monophasic liquid, used only in mouth.	Phenol glycerin	1.25 fl. dr	5 ml	1.5 ml
	Amaranth solution	15 minims	1 ml	0.3 ml
	Purified water..q.s..	25 fl. dr	100 ml	30 ml
	Make: Gargle	Send: 30 ml		
	Direction: Dilute with equal volume of warm water, before use and use as directed.			

Theory :

Phenol glycerin contains 16 % w/w phenol and 84 % w/w glycerin, phenol which is present in phenol glycerin is sufficient to act as bactericide. Glycerin makes the preparation viscous, which helps the preparation to remain in contact with mucous membrane of the throat for longer time. It also has sweet taste and gives cooling sensation. Amaranth is used as a dye, to give distinctive colour to the gargle.

All the ingredients are water soluble. Hence gargle can be prepared easily by simple solution method.

Procedure :

1) Accurately measure phenol glycerin and amaranth solution separately.
2) Mix amaranth solution with small portion of purified water and add phenol glycerin by continuous stirring.
3) Transfer this content to a measure and add sufficient amount of purified water to produce final volume.

Dispensing: Phenol is sensitive to the light and glycerin is hygroscopic in nature, therefore transfer phenol gargle to a coloured, fluted, plastic or glass bottle, close it thoroughly with plastic screw cap, polish and label.

Direction: Dilute with equal volume of warm water, before use and use as directed.

Storage: Store in a cool and dark place.

Auxilliary label:
- FOR EXTERNAL USE ONLY.
- SHOULD NOT TO BE SWALLOWED.

Uses: 0.8 to 1.0 % of phenol present in this gargle act as bactericide, therefore Phenol gargle is used as a bactericide, in the treatment of pharynx and nasopharynx infections.

Note: Formula for phenol glycerin:

Phenol — 16 g

Glycerin — 84 g

Dissolve phenol in glycerin with the help of gentle heat, if necessary.

POTASSIUM CHLORATE AND PHENOL GARGLE BPC.

Rx	
Potassii chloratis	3 i
Liquoris phenolis	M xxx
Patent blue 'V' solution	q.s
Aquam...q.s...	fl. 3 xxv
Fiat : Gargarisma	Mitte : fl.oz ii
Signa : Cum duplo decem in aquae calidae, pro utendum et utendus more dicto.	

Conversion :

3 i → 1 drachm	M xxx → 30 minims
1 drachm = 4 g	15 minims= 1 ml
fl. 3 xxv → 25 fl. dr = 100 ml	30 minims = 2 ml

Calculation : For fl.oz ii → 2 fl.oz = 60 ml

Potassium chlorate = $\frac{4}{100} \times 60 = 2.4$ g

Liquefied phenol = $\frac{2}{100} \times 60 = 1.2$ g

Patent blue 'V' solution = ...q.s....

Water ...q.s...... = 60 ml

Type	Ingredients	Quantity in imperial	Quantity in metric	Quantity taken
Monophasic liquid, used only in mouth.	Potassium chlorate	3 dr	4 g	2.4 g
	Liquefied phenol	30 minims	2 ml	1.2 ml
	Patent blue 'V' solution	..q.s..	..q.s..	..q.s..
	Purified water ....q.s.....	25 fl. dr	100 ml	60 ml
	Make: Gargle Send: 60 ml Direction: Dilute with ten times its volume by warm water, before use and use as directed.			

Theory:

Potassium chlorate acts as sailogogue (Stimilates the flow of saliva), hence it is used in the form of gargle. Percentage of phenol (0.8 to 1.0%), which is present in liquified phenol is sufficient to act as bactericide.

Potassium chlorate and liquefied phenol are water soluble, hence gargle can be prepared by simple solution method. Since potassium chlorate is highly soluble in hot water, the solution can be heated, to enhance its dissolution. Patent blue 'V' solution is used as coloring agent, to give an attractive colour to the gargle.

Procedure:

1) Accurately weigh potassium chlorate and dissolve in ¾ th of purified water by heating, on a water bath.
2) To this solution, add liquefied phenol, mix well by stirring.
3) Transfer this content to a measure and add patent blue 'V', mix well and add sufficient amount of purified water to adjust the final volume.

Dispensing: Potassium chlorate is very sensitive to the light, hence transfer the solution to a coloured, fluted, plastic or glass bottle, close it thoroughly with plastic screw cap, polish and label.

Direction: Dilute with ten times of its volume with warm water, before use and use as directed.

Storage: Store in a cool and dark place.

Auxilliary label:
- FOR EXTERNAL USE ONLY.
- NOT TO BE SWALLOWED IN LARGE QUANTITIES.

Use: Potassium chlorate has week astringent effect, to tone up a relaxed throat and it also acts as sailogogue (it increase the flow of saliva), hence it stimulates the secretion of saliva, which relives the dryness of mouth.

Liquified phenol acts as bactericide. Therefore this gargle is used as sailogogue, astringent and bactericide.

> **Note:** Patent blue 'V' solution is prepared by dissolving 50 mg in 100 ml of water. From this solution required volume, which is equivalent to prescribed weight is taken.

Student's exercise:

1) What is the Latin term for Gargles?
2) Define Gargles : For what purpose it is used and how?
3) Comment : Gargles are highly medicated than mouthwashes.

4) What is the pH of gargles and why?
5) Enlist the medicaments used in gargles.
6) Give examples for gargles.
7) How will you dispense gargles? Explain with reaction.
8) Which label direction and auxilliary label is necessary for gargles?
9) What is phenol glycerin? What is its use and how it is prepared? (give its formula).
10) What is patent blue 'V' solution? Explain.
11) Differentiate bacterostatic and bactericide and give examples.
12) Comment: Gargles are dispensed in concentrated forms.

12 THROAT PAINTS

Latin term : Guttur pigmentum.

Throat paints are viscous solutions or dispersions of one or more medicaments, which are used in the treatment of mouth or throat infections. They made viscous because, they should remain in contact with mucous membrane, to exert its medicinal action for longer time. Therefore glycerin is commonly used as a base (vehicle), due to its viscous nature and its agreeable sweet taste and cooling effect.

If paints are applied externally to the skin, they are called simply as "paints" (skin paints). Paints should not be used as throat paints.

Throat paints are applied to the affected part with the help of camel hairbrush or by cotton plug, twisted at the tip of plastic stick. They should be applied as such, without dilution with water.

Medicaments used in Throat paints:

1) Astringents : Tannic acid, Boric acid
2) Antiseptics : Iodine, Crystal violet
3) Anti-infectives : Phenol
4) Analgesics : Clove oil, Potassium permanganate

Examples for Throat paints:

- Mandl's paint (Compound iodine paint)
- Tannic acid - glycerin throat paint
- Phenol - glycerin throat paint
- Boro- glycerin throat paint

Advantages:

1) Throat paints are useful in the treatment of pharyngitis, laryngitis, tonsilitis thrush, abscess of throat and ulcerative stomatitis.
2) Due to high viscous nature, they retain the drug for longer time on affected part of the throat.

Disadvantages:

1) Throat paints initiate salivation. Hence patient has to spit again and again till salivation subsides. This makes it uncomfortable to the patients.
2) As shown in the figure it is very difficult, to apply the throat paint to the inner parts of the mouth and throat by fingers. Hence always requires camel hairbrash or cotton plug, twisted at the tip of plastic stick, for application of throat paint. This makes it difficult and uncomfortable to the patients.

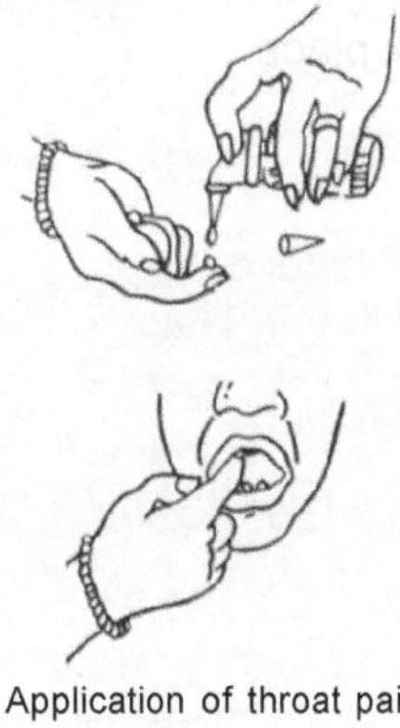

Application of throat paints

Formulation: Along with medicaments, it contains high proportion of glycerin and other additives like sweetening agents, flavouring agents, stabilizers and preservatives.

Method of preparation: They are prepared by simple solution method, with the aid of heat.

Dispensing: Throat paints should be dispensed in air tight, coloured (light resistant), narrow or wide mouthed bottle in order to distinguish them from the preparations meant for internal use and they should be supplied with camel hairbrush (Throat brush).

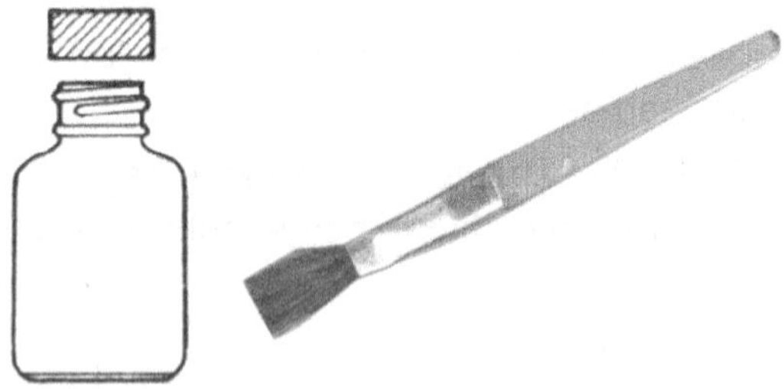

Container for Throat paint with camel hair brush

Direction: Throat paints should contain the direction to the patients as,

Apply with camel hairbrush, as directed.

Label: Label should bear all necessary requirements of liquid dosage forms, except dose. In addition, it should also contain auxilliary label like:

- FOR EXTERNAL USE ONLY.
- STORE IN A COOL PLACE.
- SHAKE WELL BEFORE USE.
- NOT TO BE SWALLOWED IN LARGE QUANTITIES.
- KEEP THE CONTAINER TIGHTLY CLOSED.

Storage: Throat paints usually contain volatile oils as flavouring agents. Therefore to prevent their volatalisation at higher temperature, they should be stored in a cool and dark place.

COMPOUND IODINE THROAT PAINT I.P.

Synonym: Mandl's paint

Rx	
Potassii Iodidi	3 vi
Iodi	3 iii
Alcoholis (96%)	fl. 3 x
Aquam	fl. 3 vi
Olei menthae piperitae	fl. 3 i
Glyerini...q.s....	fl. 3 CCL
Fiat : Guttur pigmentum	Mitte : fl.oz i
Signa : Cum penicillion applicandus, quartis horis.	

Conversion :

3 i → 1 drachm = 4 g — fl. 3 x → 10 fl. drachms = 40 ml

3 Vi → 6 drachms = 24 g — fl. 3 vi → 6 fl. drachms = 24 ml

3 iii → 3 drachms = 12 g — fl. 3 CCL → 250 fl. drachms = 1000 ml

Calculation : For fl.oz i →1 fl.oz = 30 ml

Potassium iodide $= \frac{24}{1000} \times 30 = 0.72$ g

Iodine $= \frac{12}{1000} \times 30 = 0.36$ g

Alcohol $= \frac{40}{1000} \times 30 = 1.2$ ml

Water $= \frac{24}{1000} \times 30 = 0.72$ ml

Peppermint oil $= \frac{4}{1000} \times 30 = 0.12$ ml

Glycerin ....q.s.... = 30 ml

Type	Ingredients	Quantity in imperial	Quantity in metric	Quantity taken
Monophasic liquid, used in throat.	Potassium iodide	6 dr	25 g	0.72 g
	Iodine	3 dr	12 g	0.36 g
	Alcohol (96%)	10 fl.dr	40 ml	1.2 ml
	Water	6 fl.dr	24 ml	0.72 ml
	Peppermint oil	1 fl.dr	4 ml	0.12 ml
	Glycerin........q.s...	250 fl.dr	1000 ml	30 ml
	Make:Throat paint	Send: 30 ml		
	Direction: Apply with camel hairbrush, every four hours.			

Theory:

Iodine is slightly soluble in water, but it is soluble in presence of potassium Iodide and forms polyiodides. These polyiodides are highly soluble in water and hence produce monophasic liquid.

I_2 +	KI	→ I_2.KI....................Pot. mono iodide	
Iodine	Pot.iodide		
$2I_2$ +	KI	→ $2I_2$.KI ....Pot. di iodide	
Iodine	Pot.iodide		
$3I_2$ +	KI	→ $3I_2$.KI ....Pot. tri iodide	
Iodine	Pot.iodide	Poly iodides	

Alcohol (90%) acts as cosolvent, to increase the solubility of iodine. It is also used to dissolve peppermint oil, which acts as flavouring agent. Glycerin is viscous in nature hence Mandl's paint will remain in contact with mucous membrane of throat for longer time, it also acts as humectant and soothing agent.

Procedure:

1) Triturate iodine in glass motor, to get fine powder and accuretly weigh the required amount of iodine.
2) Dissolve potassium iodine in water. To this solution, add iodine powder and dissolve by stirring.
3) Dissolve peppermint oil and half of the portion of glycerin in alcohol.
4) Add this solution to the above iodine and potassium iodide solution, with continuous stirring and adjust the final volume with remaining portion of glycerin.

Dispensing: Mandl's paint contains volatile ingredients like iodine, alcohol (90%) and peppermint oil. Iodine is sensitive to the light, hence transfer the paint to a light resistant, fluted wide mouthed, glass bottle, close it tightly with plastic screw cap (waxed - card lined), polish and label. Supply with camel hairbrush.

Direction: Apply with camel hairbrush, every four hours.

Auxilliary label:

- FOR EXTERNAL USE ONLY.
- KEEP THE CONTAINER TIGHTLY CLOSED.
- NOT TO BE SWALLOWED IN LARGE QUANTITIES.
- SHAKE WELL BEFORE USE -- (**Reason** - Since there are chances of separation of oil globules of peppermint oil, during storage)

Storage: Store in a cool and dark place.

Uses: Mandl's paint is used in the treatment of pharyngitis, laryngytis, tonsillitis and sore throat.

Note:

1) Iodine stains as brown colour to the skin, cloths, and containers made up of porcelain and metals. Therefore for the preparation of iodine solution, glass mortar should be used instead of porcelain.

2) Metal spatula should not be used for handling of iodine and metallic containers should not be used for storing of iodine preparations, because iodine being an oxidizing agent, it oxidizes iron and converts in to ferrous iodide.

$$Fe + I_2 \longrightarrow FeI_2$$

Hence plastic spoons are used for handling and containers made up of plastic or glass are used to store iodine preparations.

3) If necessary, iodine stain can be removed by using sodium thiosulphate solution.

TANNIC ACID - GLYCERIN THROAT PAINT I.P.

Rx	
Acidi tannici	3 v
Sodii citratis	gr xv
Siccci sodii sulphidi	gr iii
Glyerini ..q.s....	fl. 3 xxv
Fiat : Guttur pigmentum	Mitte : fl.oz i
Signa : Cum penicillion applicandum, s.o.s.	

Conversion :

3 v → 5 drachms — gr xv → 15 grains

1 drachm= 4 g — 15 grains = 1 g

5 drachms= 20 g — gr iii → 3 grains = 0.2 g

Calculation : For fl.oz i → 1 fl.oz = 30 ml

Tannic acid = $\frac{20}{100} \times 30 = 6\,g$

Sodium citrate = $\frac{1}{100} \times 30 = 0.3\,g$

Dried sodium sulphide = $\frac{0.2}{100} \times 30 = 0.06\,g$

Glycerin... q.s. ... = 30 ml.

Type	Ingredients	Quantity in imperial	Quantity in metric	Quantity taken
Monophasic liquid, used in throat.	Tannic acid	5 dr	20 g	6 g
	Sodium citrate	15 gr	1 g	0.3 g
	Dried sodium sulphide	3 gr	0.2 g	0.06 g
	Glycerin......q.s ...	25 fl. dr	100 ml	30 ml
	Make: Throat paint Send: 30 ml Direction: Apply with camel hairbrush, when ever necessary.			

Theory:

Tannic acid is slightly soluble in water (0.35 :1), but aqueous solution of tannic acid leads to decomposition during storage. Tannic acid is soluble in glycerin (1:1), hence glycerin is used as a vehicle to dissolve the tannic acid and because of its high viscous nature, it does not flow quickly and adhere to the mucous membrane of the throat for longer time. In addition, glycerin also acts as sweetening agent and gives cooling sensation.

Dried sodium sulphide and sodium citrate acts as stabilizers, which prevents the deterioration of tannic acid.

Procedure:

1) Separately weigh tannic acid, dried sodium sulphide and sodium citrate. Triturate them, to fine powder in a porcelain dish.
2) To this powder, add half of the portion of glycerin and triturate until a smooth mixture is produced, then add the remaining amount of glycerin and mix well.
3) Heat this mixture on a sand bath to a temperature between 115 to 120°C with occasional stirring, until a solution is formed and cool it to room temperature

Dispensing: Throat paint contains glycerin which is hygroscopic in nature, hence it should be protected from moisture. Therefore transfer the paint to a light resistant, wide mouthed, glass bottle, close it tightly with plastic screw cap, polish and label. Supply with camel hairbrush.

Direction: Apply with camel hairbrush, when ever necessary.

Storage: Store in a dry place.

Auxilliary label:
- FOR EXTERNAL USE ONLY.
- NOT TO BE SWALLOWED IN LARGE QUANTITY.
- KEEP THE CONTAINER TIGHTLY CLOSED.

Uses: It is used as an astringent in the treatment of soar throat and receding gums, because tannic acid precipitate the proteins. It also has haemostatic properties (i.e. its stop the bleeding in gums).

Student's exercise:

1) Comment : Throat paints consist of high percentage of glycerin.
2) Differentiate throat paints and paints.
3) For what purpose, throat paint is used?
4) How will to apply throat paints?
5) Comment : Throat paints are applied after suitable dilution.
6) Enlist the different types of medicaments used in throat paints.
7) What are the advantages and disadvantages of throat paints?
8) How will you dispense throat paints?
9) What direction and auxilliary label will you write on the label of throat paints.
10) What is the storage condition for throat paints and why ?
11) What is Mandl's paint ? What is the principle involved in its preparation.
12) How will you handle iodine and how will you store iodine preparations? Explain with reasons.
13) How will you remove the stains of iodine?
14) Define (1) Pharyngitis (2) Tonsillitis (3) Laryngitis (4) Sinusitis
15) What is the use of Dried sodium sulphide in paints?

13 THROAT SPRAYS

Latin term: Guttur nebula.

Throat sprays are the aqueous or alcoholic or glycerin solutions of medicaments, applied to the mucous membrane of the throat by means of nebulizer or automizer, which produce very fine droplets of drug solution, so as to reach the upper parts of the throat.

They are used for the treatment of the throat infections. They contain medicaments like antiseptics, deodorants and flavourants, which are employed to relieve conditions like sore throat, laryngitis or halitosis (foul - smelling breath).

In certain throat sprays glycerin is used, because it gives cooling and soothing effect and it also gives viscous nature to the droplets of the spray, to adhere for longer time on the mucous membrane of throat, to exert maximum therapeutic effect of the medicaments.

The purpose of using an atomizer or nebulizer is, to break up the solution into small droplets for effective action of the medicaments. Coarse droplets of throat spray are suitable for producing drug action in the upper part of the throat (upper respiratory tract).The type of automizer depends upon the viscosity of the spray solution. Hence a more viscous solution may need more powerful atomizer.

Dispensing: Throat sprays are dispensed in small coloured or clear, fluted glass bottle. Now-a-days, they are dispensed in plastic squeeze bottles, automizer or nebulizer or pressurized aerosol containers.

Direction: Use in a nebulizer as directed.

Storage: Since throat sprays consist volatile solvents, to prevent their volatalisation they should be stored in cool place and protected from light and flame (heat).

Label: Label should bear all necessary requirements of liquid dosage forms, except dose. In addition, it should also contain auxilliary label like,

- FOR EXTERNAL USE ONLY.
- STORE IN A COOL PLACE AWAY FROM LIGHT AND FLAME.
- KEEP AWAY FROM CHILDREN.

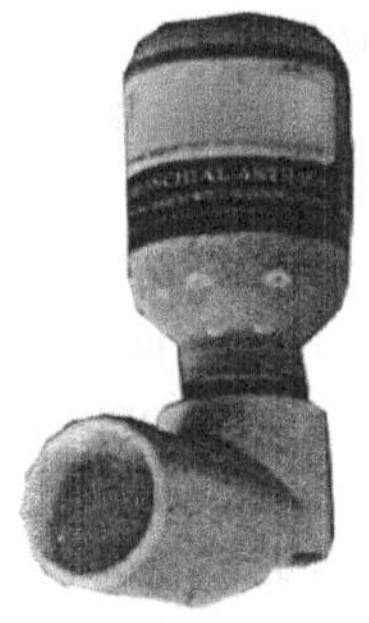

Container for throat sprays

BORAX – PHENOL THROAT SPRAY

Rx	
Boracis	gr xxxvii ss
Sodii benzoatis	gr xv
Phenolis glyerini	fl. 3 i s
Aquam....q.s...	fl. 3 xxv
Fiat : Guttur nebula	Mitte : fl.oz i
Signa : Utendus more dicto.	

Conversion :

gr XXXVii ss → 37.5 grains	3 i s → 1.25 fl. drachm
15 grains = 1 g	1 fl. drachm = 4 ml
37.5 grains = 2.5 g	1.25 fl. drachms = 5 ml
gr xv → 15 grains = 1 g	fl. 3 xxv → 25 fl. dr = 100 ml

Calculation : For fl.oz i → 1 fl.oz = 30 ml

Borax = $\frac{2.5}{100} \times 30 = 0.75$ g

Sodium benzoate = $\frac{1}{100} \times 30 = 0.3$ g

Phenol glycerin = $\frac{5}{100} \times 30 = 1.5$ ml

Water ...q.s..... = 30 ml

Type	Ingredients	Quantity in imperial	Quantity in metric	Quantity taken
Monophasic liquid, used in throat.	Borax	37.5 gr	2.5 g	0.75 g
	Sodium benzoate	15 gr	1 g	0.3 g
	Phenol glycerin	1.25 fl. dr	5 ml	1.5 ml
	Purified water.......q.s......	25 fl. dr	100 ml	30 ml
	Make: Throat spray Send: 30 ml Direction : To be used, as directed.			

Theory:

Borax acts as a bacteriostatic, phenol glycerin acts as bactericide. Sodium benzoate acts as a preservative. Glycerin present in phenol glycerin gives cooling and soothing effect and it also gives viscous nature to the droplets of the spray, to adhere on the mucous membrane of the throat for longer time, to exert maximum therapeutic effect of medicaments.

All the ingredients, borax, sodium benzoate and phenol glycerin are soluble in water. Hence spray solution is prepared by simple solution method, by mixing them in water.

Procedure:

1) Accurately weigh borax and sodium benzoate and dissolve in ¾th of total volume of water in a beaker.
2) Filter the solution through muslin cloth, to remove if any impurities present.
3) Pass 3 to 5 ml of water, through muslin cloth, to rinse it.
4) To the filtrate, add phenol glycerin and mix well.
5) Transfer this solution to a measure and make up the final volume with purified water.

Dispensing: Transfer this solution to a small, coloured, fluted, glass bottle or plastic squeeze bottle, close it tightly, polish and label.

Direction : To be used, as directed.

Storage: Store in a cool place away from flame or heat.

Auxilliary label:

- FOR EXTERNAL USE ONLY.
- STORE IN A COOL PLACE AWAY FROM LIGHT AND FLAME.
- KEEP AWAY FROM CHILDREN.

Uses: Borax – phenol throat spray is used as antiseptic and analgesic.

Student's exercise:

1) Define Throat sprays and for what purpose they are used?.
2) What are the advantages of glycerin in throat sprays?
3) What is the purpose of using drug in the form of throat spray and how ?
4) How will you dispense throat sprays?
5) Write auxilliary label for throat sprays.
6) What is borax? What is its use?
7) Differentiate between throat paints and throat sprays.

14 EYE DROPS

Latin term : Oculus guttae

Eye drops are sterile aqueous or oily solutions or suspensions of drugs, which are instilled into the eye with the help of dropper. They are usually instilled into the space between the eye ball and eye lids (cul-de-sac) or on to the corneal surface.

Eye drops should be sterile, isotonic with lacrymal secretions, suitably buffered and free from foreign particles, to prevent irritation to the eyes.

Eye drops are mainly used for anti-inflammatory, local anesthetic, antiseptic, mydriatic, miotic or diagnostic purpose.

Commonly used medicaments in eye drops are: -

1. Anti-microbial agents : Gentamycin, Framycetin, Sulphacetamide sodium
2. Anti-inflammatory agents : Corticosteroids
3. Miotic agents : Physostigmine sulphate
4. Mydriatic agents : Atropine sulphate
5. Astringents : Zinc sulphate, Silver nitrate
6. Local anesthetics : Cocaine hydrochloride, Amithocaine hydrochloride
7. Diagnostic agents : Flourocein sodium.

Formulation:

Sr.no	Ingredients type	Examples
1.	Vehicles	Sterile water, Sterile castor oil.
2.	Viscosity improving agents	Methylcellulose, Hydroxy propyl ethyl cellulose, Polyethylene glycol, Poly vinyl pyrrolidone, Poly vinyl alcohol.
3.	Buffers	Monophasic sodium phosphate solution, Dibasic sodium phosphate solution, Sodium chloride solution.
4.	Tonicity modifiers	Sodium chloride, Boric acid.
5.	Surfactants	Poly sorbate-20
6.	Anti-oxidants	Sodium-thiosulphate (0.1%), Sodium meta bisulphite (0.1%)
7.	Chelating agents	Disodium EDTA.
8.	Preservatives	Benzalkonium chloride (0.01% w/v), Chlorhexidine acetate (0.01% w/v), Phenyl mercuric nitrate (0.002% w/v), Phenyl mercuric acetate (0.002% w/v). Chlorbutol (0.5% w/v), Phenyl ethyl alcohol (0.5% w/v),

Method of preparation: Preparation of eye drops involves the following steps:

1. Dissolution of drug and additives in a suitable vehicle.
2. Preparation of a bactericidal vehicle.
3. Clarification (filtration).
4. Sterilization.
5. Packing and labeling.

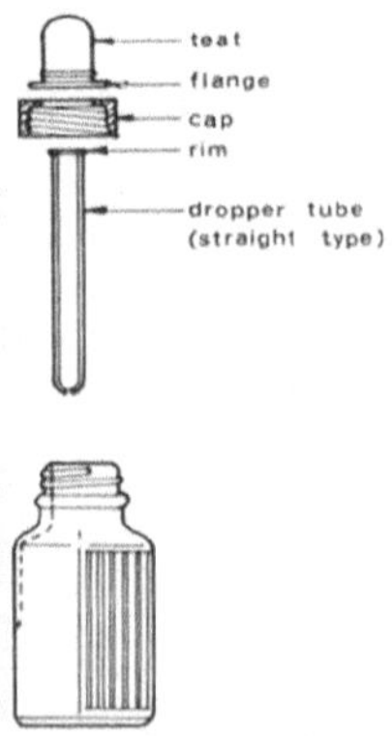

Eye drops dispensed in glass bottle with separate dropper

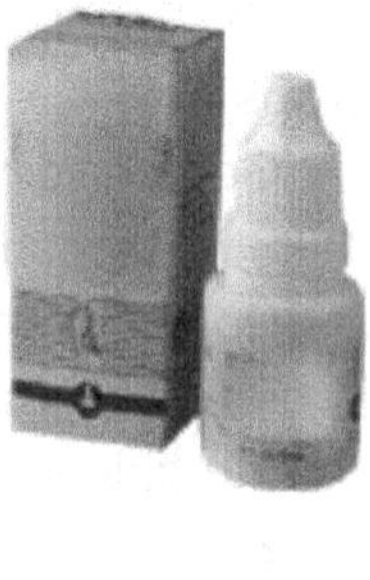

Flexible, plastic built in dropper for multi dose eyedrops

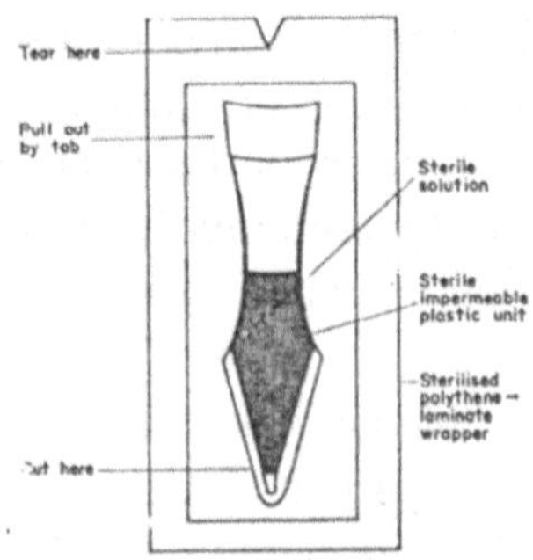

Single dose eyedrops

Dispensing: Eye drops are dispensed either in multidose or unit dose container

a) **Multi dose container:** Eye drops are supplied in small volume bottles of 10 –15 ml capacity with a separate (integral) dropper. Now-a-days, glass bottles are replaced with flexible plastic containers made of polyethylene or polypropylene with "built in dropper" (previously sealed dropping bottles), to prevent the contamination and for easy instillation.

   Eye drops are usually supplied in 10 ml quantities, to avoid use over a longer period of time (to avoid contamination).

b) **Single dose container:** In this type of container, only single dose of (one time applicable) eye drops is dispensed. These containers are disposable, pliable, tube like applicator made from polypropylene by ultrasonic sealing. It is dispensed with a nozzle, which is protected with cap. Unit dose packages are becoming more popular for dispensing eyedrops, because of its advantages.

Storage: Eye drops should be stored in a cool place and protected from light and contamination.

Since eye drops are sterile preparations, they should be protected from contamination during use and hence they must be used within four weeks (1 month) of opening the container (seal).

Label: Label of eye drops should bear necessary requirements of liquid dosage forms. In addition, it should contain auxilliary label like,

- FOR EXTERNAL USE ONLY **or** USE ONLY FOR EYES.
- NUMBER OF DROPS TO BE INSTILLED IN TO EYES.
- DO NOT TOUCH TIP OF THE DROPPER.
- NOT FOR INJECTION.
- NOT FOR EAR.
- NAME AND CONCENTRATION OF PRESERVATIVES USED IN EYEDROPS.

Direction: Label should bear suitable directions to the patients like,

1. If irritation persists, discontinue the use and consult the physician.
2. Discard the container, after 1 month of opening the seal.
3. If any visible particles are seen, discard the preparation.
4. If any change in colour, do not use.
5. After instillation of drops, do not close eyes tightly or blink more often (This may remove the medicine from the place, where it is nedded)

How to use Eyedrops: .

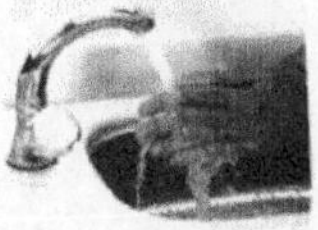

1. Clean hands prior to the use of eyedrops. Do not touch the tip of the bottle.

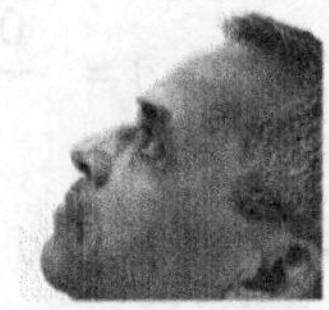

2. Lie down and look at the ceiling or sit down and tilt your head back.

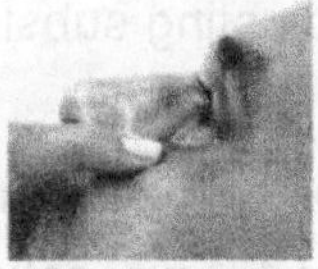

3. Pull down your lower eyelid with index finger making a pocket.

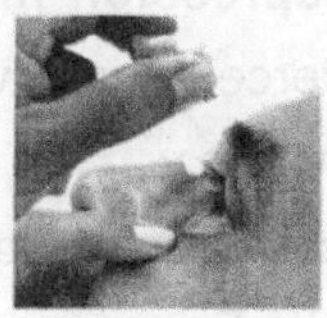

4. Look up and squeeze a drop into the pocket. Do not blink or wipe the eye.

Instruction For Use :

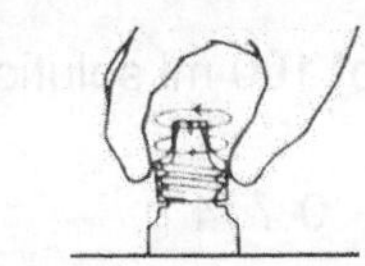

1. Tighten the cap on the nozzle by tuming it as shown. The spike in the cap will make a dispensing hole on the nozzle.

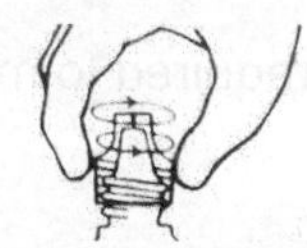

2. Remove the cap, by tuming it in the oppsite direction.

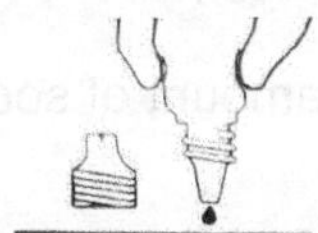

3. The bottle is now ready for use, turn it up side down. squeeze the walls of the bottle gently to deliver sterile drop into the eye.

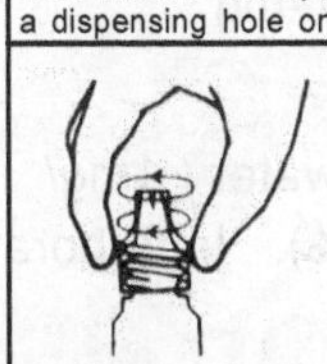

4. Replace the cap. Tighten it firmly and keep the bottle closed for subseqent use.

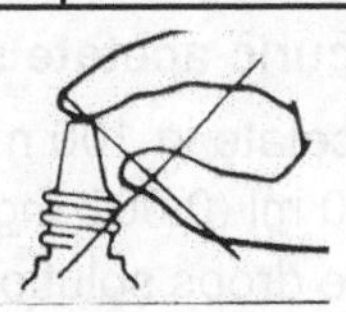

5. Do not touch the nozzle.

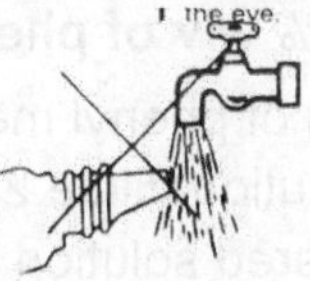

6. Do not rinse the nozzle.

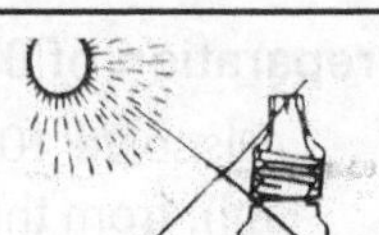

7. Do not expose to sunlight.

ATROPINE SULPHATE EYE DROPS

Rx	
Atropine sulphatis	gr XV
Aquam......q.s....	fl. 3 XXV
Fiat : Oculus guttae	Mitte : 3 ii ss
Signa : Duo guttae instillandus affectae oculus, mane et nocte.	

Conversion :

gr XV → 15 grains = 1 g

fl. 3 XXV → 25 fl. drachms = 100 ml

Calculation : For fl. 3 ii ss → 2.5 fl. drachms = 10 ml

Atropine sulphate $= \frac{1}{100} \times 10 = 0.1\text{g}$

Purified water ....q.s...... = 10 ml

Calculation of sodium chloride for adjustment of isotonicity, by freezing point depression method.

Percentage w/v of adjusting substance required = $\frac{0.52 - a}{b}$

Where,

'a' = Freezing point of 1% w/v solution of un-adjusted drug solution.

'b' = Freezing point of 1% w/v solution of the adjusting substance.

From literature,

Freezing point of lachrymal secretion = - 0.52 °C

Freezing point of 1% w/v solution of Atropine sulphate (a) = - 0.074 °C

Freezing point of 1% w/v solution of sodium chloride (b) = - 0.576 °C

∴ The amount of sodium chloride required to maintain isotonicity of 100 ml solution,

$$= \frac{0.52 - 0.074}{0.576} = 0.774 \text{ g}$$

But, for 10 ml solution $= \frac{0.774}{10} = 0.0774$ g = 77.4 mg or 78.0 mg

Preparation of 0.002% w/v of phenyl mercuric acetate solution :

Dissolve 100 mg of phenyl mercuric acetate in 100 ml of purified water (1mg/ ml), from this solution dilute 2 ml to 100 ml (0.002 mg/ml = 0.002%). Incorporate 2 ml of this prepared solution to the eye drops solution.

Revised formula for 10 ml:

Atropine sulphate	---	100 mg
Sodium chloride	---	78 mg

0.002% w/v Phenyl mercuric acetate solution --- 2 ml
Purified water .....q.s........ --- 10 ml

Type	Ingredients	Quantity in imperial	Quantity in metric	Quantity taken
Monophasic liquid, for ophthalmic use.	Atropine sulphate	15 gr	1 g	100 mg
	Purified water....q.s..	25 fl. dr	100 ml	10 ml
	Make: Eye drops	Send:10 ml		
	Direction: Two drops to be instilled in to affected eye, morning and night.			

Theory:

This eye drop consists of alkaloidal salt Atropine sulphate and it should be made isotonic with the tear secretions. The adjustment of isotonicity can be made by using several substances like sodium chloride, sodium sulphate, dextrose, boric acid etc.., but the most widely used substance is sodium chloride.

In this preparation, isotonicity adjustment is done by freezing point depression method. Phenyl mercuric acetate (0.002% w/v) is used as a preservative, it also helps in preserving sterility.

Procedure:

1) First calculate the amount of sodium chloride required for adjustment of isotonicity, by freezing point depression method.
2) Dissolve accurately weighed Atropine sulphate in ¾ th quantity of purified water.
3) To this solution add sodium chloride and measured amount of (2 ml) of 0.002 % of phenyl mercuric acetate solution and mix well.
4) Filter the solution through the sintered glass funnel to remove foreign particles, if present.

Dispensing: Atropine sulphate is sensitive to the light, hence transfer the eye drops solution to a 10 to 15 ml capacity, ambered coloured glass bottle, close it thoroughly with rubber closure and aluminium cap and sterilize in an autoclave at 121°C for 15 minutes at 15 lb p.s.i. pressure. After sterilization, cool it to room temperature, polish and label.

Direction: Two drops to be instilled in to affected eye, morning and night.

Storage: Store in a cool place and away from light.

Auxilliary label:
- FOR EXTERNAL USE ONLY **OR** FOR EYE USE ONLY.
- DO NOT TOUCH THE TIP OF DROPPER.
- IF IRRITATION PERSISTS DISCONTINUE THE USE AND CONSULT THE PHYSICIAN.
- DISCARD THE CONTAINER AFTER 1 MONTH OF OPENING THE SEAL.
- STORE IN A COOL AND DARK PLACE.

Uses: Atropine sulphate dilates the pupil and increases the intra ocular pressure, therefore Atropine sulphate eye drops is used as mydriatic and cycloplegic.

ZINC SULPHATE EYE DROPS

Rx	
Zinci sulphatis	0.25%
Aquam... q.s.....	fl. ʒ xxv
Fiat : Oculus guttae	Mitte : fl. ʒ ii ss
Signa:Duo guttae instillandus ana oculus, q.i.d.	

Calculation : For fl. ʒ ii ss → 2.5 fl. dr = 10 ml

Zinc sulphate ---- 0.25 % means, 250 mg in 100 ml

For 10 ml, ------- $\frac{250}{100} \times 10 = 25$ mg of zinc sulphate is required

But, 25 mg is not a weighable quantity. The minimum weighble quantity is 100 mg on dispensing balance.

∴ Dissolve 100 mg of zinc sulphate in 10 ml of purified water, which gives 100 mg / 10 ml.

1 ml of this solution contains 10 mg of zinc sulphate

For 25 mg of zinc sulphate = $\frac{1}{10} \times 25 = 2.5$ ml

Hence,

Take 2.5 ml of zinc sulphate solution, to prepare 10 ml of eye drops.

Calculation of sodium chloride for adjustment of isotonisity, by freezing point depression method.

Percentage w/v of adjusting substance required = $\frac{0.52 - a}{b}$

Where,

'a' = Freezing point depression of 1% w/v solution of un-adjusted drug solution.

'b' = Freezing point depression of 1% w/v solution of the adjusting substance.

From Literature,

Freezing point depression of Lacrymal secretion = - 0.52 °C

Freezing point depression of 1% w/v solution of zinc sulphate(a) = - 0.086 °C

Freezing point depression of 1% w/v solution of sodium chloride(b) = - 0.576 °C

The amount of sodium chloride required, to maintain isotonicity of 100 ml solution will be = = $\frac{0.52 - 0.086}{0.576} = 0.753$ g

But for 10 ml = = $\frac{0.753}{10} = 0.0753$ g $\cong$ 75 mg

Preparation of 0.002% w/v of phenyl mercuric acetate solution :

Dissolve 100 mg of phenyl mercuric acetate in 100 ml of purified water (1mg/ ml), from this solution dilute 2 ml to 100 ml (0.002 mg/ml = 0.002%). Incorporate 2 ml of this prepared solution to eye drops.

Revised formula for 10 ml :

Zinc sulphate solution	---	2.5 ml
Sodium chloride	---	75 mg
0.002% w/v phenyl mercuric acetate solution	---	2 ml
Purified water.........q.s........	---	10 ml

Type	Ingredients	Quantity in imperial	Quantity in metric	Quantity taken
Monophasic liquid, for ophthalmic use.	Zinc sulphate	0.25 %	0.25%	2.5 ml
	Purified water....q.s...	25 fl. dr	100 ml	10 ml
	Make: Eye drops. Send: 10 ml			
	Direction: Two drops to be instilled, to each eye, four times a day.			

Theory:

Zinc sulphate acts as an antiseptic, which is used to relieve chronic inflammation of cornea in conjunctivitis. It is freely soluble in water. Zinc sulphate solution is instilled in to the eyes, therefore it should be isotonic with lachrymal secretion. It should be made isotonic with the tear secretions. The adjustment of isotonicity can be made by using several substances like sodium chloride, sodium sulphate, dextrose, boric acid etc., but the most widely used substance is sodium chloride.

In this preparation, isotonicity adjustment is done by freezing point depression method. Prescribed formula says to prepare, 10 ml of 0.25% of zinc sulphate solution, means 25 mg in 10 ml, but it is not weighable quantity.

The minimum weighable quantity is 100 mg. Therefore accurate amount of zinc sulphate is calculated by dilution method. 0.002% w/v phenyl mercury acetate is used as a preservative, it also helps in preserving sterility.

Procedure:

1) First calculate the amount of sodium chloride required for adjustment of isotonicity, by freezing point depression method.
2) According to dilution method calculation, dissolve zinc sulphate in water and measure 2.5 ml of the solution.
3) To this solution, add sodium chloride and measured amount of (2 ml) of 0.002% of phenyl mercury acetate solution and mix well.
4) Adjust the final volume up to 10 ml by purified water and filter through sintered glass funnel, to remove foreign particles, if present.

Dispensing: Transfer the solution to a small glass bottle, close it thoroughly with rubber closure and aluminium cap and sterilize in an autoclave at 121°C, for 15 minute at 15 lb p.s.i. pressure. After sterilization, cool it to room temperature, polish and label.

Direction: Two drops to be instilled to each eye four times a day.

Storage: Store in a cool place.

Auxilliary label:

- FOR EXTERNAL USE ONLY **OR** FOR EYE USE ONLY.
- DO NOT TOUCH THE TIP OF DROPPER.
- IF IRRITATION PERSISTS DISCONTINUE THE USE AND CONSULT THE PHYSICIAN.
- DISCARD THE CONTAINER AFTER 1 MONTH OF OPENING THE SEAL (CONTAINER).

Uses: Zinc sulphate eye drops is used, to relieve the chronic inflammation of cornea in conjunctivitis.

Other examples of Eye drops

1) **Physostigmine sulphate eye drops**

Physostigmine sulphate	---	0.5 g
Sodium metabisulphite	---	0.2 g
Benzalkonium chloride solution	---	0.02 ml
Purified water....q.s...	----	100 ml

2) **Chloramphenicol eye drops**

Chloramphenicol	---	0.5 %
Phenyl mercuric nitrate	---	0.002 % w/w

3) **Framycetin sulphate eye drops**

Framycetin sulphate	---	5 mg
Phenyl mercuric nitrate	---	0.002 % w/w

Student's exercise:

1) Define eye drops. Why eye drops are used ?
2) List out the commonly used medicaments in eye drops.
3) Comment : Eye drops should be isotonic and sterile.
4) Explain in briefly, the formulation of eye drops.
5) Define isotonicity and give the examples for substances used for adjustment of isotonicity.

6) Which are the different methods used for adjustment of isotonicity of the solution? Explain.
7) How will you dispense eye drops?
8) Write the auxilliary label for eye drops.
9) Comment : Eye drops should be used within one month of opening the container (seal).
10) What is the freezing point of 2% solution of Atropine sulphate and Zinc sulphate.
11) Define mydriatic and miotic. Give examples.
12) Define cycloplegic and conjunctivitis.
13) What is cornea?

15 EYE LOTIONS

Latin term: Collyrium

Eye lotions are sterile aqueous solutions, used for washing (irrigating) the eyes or for impregnating the eye dressings. They are generally used to remove foreign materials from the eyes and to relieve eye irritation with the help of clean eye-bath or sterile fabric dressing or by directly flowing large volume of eye lotion, quickly over the eye.

Classification of eye lotions: They are of two types,

1) **Sterile aqueous solutions, without bactericide:** These are used for first aid purpose and used for once or within the period not more than 24 hours. They should be used as such, without diluting with water.
2) **Aqueous solutions, containing bactericide:** These are used for intermittent purpose, up to one week. These types of eye lotions are supplied in concentrated form and required to be dilute with equal volume of sterile or warm water immediately before use. After dilution they should be used immediately and should not be stored for longer time, to avoid the contamination from microorganisms.

   Eg: Sodium chloride eye lotion,
   Sodium bicarbonate eye lotion,
   Boric acid eye lotion.

Eye lotions should be,

1) Sterile
2) Isotonic with lachrymal secretion
3) Have neutral pH, to avoid any irritation and discomfort to the eyes.

The control of pH and tonicity in the eye lotions is more important. Therefore eye lotions should be formulated to have a neutral pH and to have tonicity equivalents to 0.9% solution of sodium chloride. Additives like buffers and isotonic salts are used for this purpose.

Formulation:

Vehicles	Sterile water, Purified water
Buffering agents	Monobasic sodium phosphate, Sodium chloride
Tonicity modifiers	Sodium chloride, Boric acid

Dispensing: Eye lotions should be dispensed in narrow mouthed, coloured fluted glass or plastic bottle with coloured plastic screw cap, to distinguish them from the preparations, which are meant for oral use.

Direction: Dilute with equal volume of warm water before use. Label should also give direction about, how to use (wash the eye) with figure.

Label: Label of eye lotions should bear necessary requirements of liquid dosage forms. In addition, it should contain auxilliary label like:

- FOR EYE USE ONLY.
- NOT TO BE TAKEN ORALLY.
- AVOID CONTAMINATION DURING USE.
- DISCARD ANY UNUSED PART, AFTER 24 HOURS OF OPENING OF THE CONTAINER **OR** DISCARD THE DILUTION AFTER 24 HOURS.

Storage: Eye lotions should be stored in a cool place.

BORIC ACID EYE LOTION

Rx	
Acidi borici	1 %
Aquam....q.s....	fl. 3 xxv
Fiat : Collyrium	Mitte : fl.oz iv
Signa : Cum duplo aquae calidae aequales pro utendum, et utendus more dicto.	

Calculation : For fl.oz iv → 4 fl.oz = 120 ml

Boric acid = $\frac{1}{100} \times 120 = 1.2$ g

Purified water ....q.s... = 120 ml

Calculation of sodium chloride for adjustment of isotonisity, by freezing point depression method.

Percentage w/v of adjusting substance required = $\frac{0.52 - a}{b}$

Where,

'a' = Freezing point depression of 1% w/v solution of un-adjusted drug solution.

'b' = Freezing point depression of 1% w/v solution of the adjusting substance.

From literature,

Freezing point depression of Lacrymal secretion = - 0.52 °C

Freezing point depression of 1% w/v solution of boric acid (a) = - 0.288 °C

Freezing point depression of 1% w/v solution of sodium chloride (b) = - 0.576 °C

The amount of sodium chloride requiredto maintain isotonicity of 100 ml solution will be

$= \frac{0.52 - 0.288}{0.576} = 0.4$ g = 400 mg

But, for 120 ml of solution requires = = 480 mg

Revised formula for 120 ml

Boric acid --- 1.2 g

Sodium chloride --- 480 mg

Purified water......q.s... --- 120 ml

Type	Ingredients	Quantity in imperial	Quantity in metric	Quantity taken
Monophasic liquid, for ophthalmic use- Eye lotion (wash).	Boric acid	1 %	1 g	1.2 g
	Purified water ...q.s..	25 fl. dr	100 ml	120 ml
	Make: Eye lotion Send: 120 ml			
	Direction: Dilute with equal volume of warm water, before use and to be used as directed.			

Theory:

Boric acid eye lotion is used for irrigation of eyes, hence it should be iso-osmotic (isotonic) with tears (Lachrymal secretion). Therefore isotonicity of eye lotion is adjusted by sodium chloride.

Boric acid acts as anti-infective (antibacterial and antifungal). Hence addition of extra preservative is not required.

Procedure:

1) Calculate the amount of sodium chloride required for adjustment of isotonicity by freezing point method.
2) Dissolve boric acid in water. To this solution, add sodium chloride and adjust the final volume with purified water.
3) Filter the solution through sintered glass funnel and transfer the filtrate to a suitable container.

Dispensing: Transfer the filtrate to a narrow mouthed, coloured, fluted glass or plastic bottel. Close it tightly with plastic screw cap and sterilize in autoclave at 121°C for 15 minutes at 15 lb p.s.i.. After the sterilization , cool it and dispense.

Direction: Dilute with equal volume of warm water, before use and to be used as directed.

Auxilliary label:

- DILUTE THE LOTION WITH EQUAL VOLUME OF WARM WATER BEFORE USE
- DISCARD ANY UNUSED SOLUTION AFTER 24 HOURS OF THE DILUTION
- FOR EXTERNAL USE ONLY

Storage: Store in a cool place.

Use : Boric acid acts as anti infective. Therefore Boric acid eye lotion is used, for irrigation of eyes during eye infection.

Other examples of Eye lotions

1) Boric acid-sodium chloride eye lotion

Boric acid	3.5 g
Sodium chloride	5 g
Glycerin	3 g
Camphor water	13 ml
Purified water ... q.s..	100 ml

2) Sodium chloride eye lotion

Sodium chloride	0.5 g
Purified water ...q.s....	100 ml

3) Sodium bicarbonate eye lotion

Sodium bicarbonate	3.5 g
Purified water... q.s...	100 ml

Student's exercise:

1) What is the Latin term for eye lotions?
2) Define eye lotions. What is the purpose of using eye lotions?
3) Classify the eye lotions, with examples.
4) How the isotonicity of eye lotion is adjusted ?
5) What should be the pH of eye lotion and why ?
6) Comment : Eye lotion should be isotonic with lachrymal secretion.
7) How will you dispense the eye lotions?
8) Which auxilliary label will you write on label of eye lotions?
9) Comment : Dilution of eye lotion should be discarded after 24 hours.
10) What is the use of boric acid eye lotion?

16 EAR DROPS

Latin term: Auristillae

Eardrops are medicated liquid preparations, which are instilled in to the ear with the help of a dropper. In these preparations, the drug is usually dissolved or suspended in a suitable solvent such as glycerin, propylene glycol, alcohol and water.

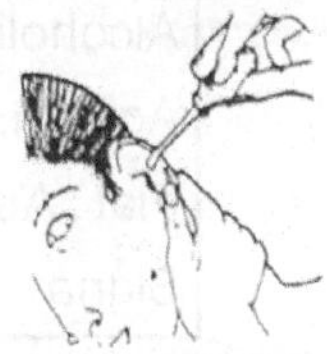

Instillation of ear drops to ears.

Eardrops are used,

1) For treating the mild infections in the ear.
2) For softening the earwax.
3) For cleansing the ear.
4) For drying the weeping surfaces of the ear.

The main classes of drugs used in the eardrops are,

Analgesics	Salicylic acid.
Antibiotics	Neomycin, Chloramphenicol, Framycetin sulphate.
Anti-inflammatory agents	Cortisone, Boric acid, Phenol, Sulphonamide, Neomycin
Astringents	Aluminium sulphate
Antiseptics	Phenol
For softening earwax	Hydrogen peroxide, Magnesium sulphate

Examples for ear drops:

- Boric acid ear drops.
- Chloramphenicol ear drops.
- Aluminium acetate ear drops.
- Phenol glycerin ear drops.
- Sodium bicarbonate ear drops.

Dispensing: Ear drops should be dispensed in small glass or plastic bottles of 10-15 ml capacity with a separate dropper or previously sealed dropping bottles.

Ear drops should be used with in one month (4 weeks) of the opening the seal of the container, to avoid the contamination with microorganisms, if we store for longer time.

Storage: Eardrops should be stored in a cool place.

Label: Label of eardrops should bear necessary requirements of liquid dosage forms. In addition, it should contain auxilliary labels like,

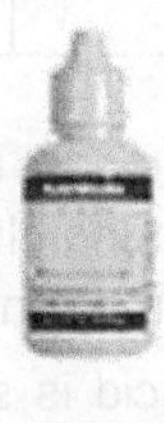

Flexible plastic built in dropper type container for eardrops

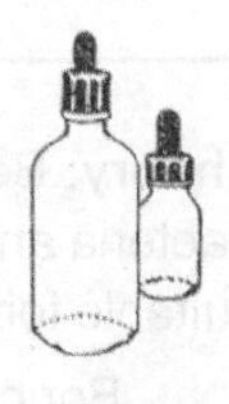

Glass container with seperate dropper

- FOR EXTERNAL USE ONLY **OR** FOR EAR USE ONLY **OR** DO NOT USE FOR EYE.
- NOT FOR INJECTION.
- NOT TO BE DILUTED WITH WATER.
- DISCARD AFTER ONE MONTH OF OPENING THE CONTAINER (SEAL).
- STORE IN COOL PLACE (AT TEMPERATURE NOT MORE THAN 25 ºC).

BORIC ACID EAR DROPS

Rx	
Acidi borici	gr iV ss
Alcoholis	M VL
Aquam......q.s.......	½ fl.oz
Fiat : Auristillae	Mitte : fl.oz ½
Signa : Instillandus duo-tries guttae auris, more dicto.	

Conversion :

gr iV → 4.5 grains — M VL → 45 minims

15 grains = 1 g — 15 minims = 1 ml

4.5 grains = 0.3 g — 45 minims = 3 ml

Calculation : For fl.oz ½ = 15 ml

Boric acid = $\frac{0.3}{15} \times 15 = 0.3$ g

Industrial alcohol = $\frac{3}{15} \times 15 = 3$ ml

Water....q.s... = 15 ml

Type	Ingredients	Quantity in imperial	Quantity in metric	Quantity taken
Monophasic liquid, instilled in to ear.	Boric acid	4.5 gr	300 mg	0.3 g
	Industrial alcohol	45 minims	3 ml	3 ml
	Purified water.....q.s....	fl.oz 1/2	15 ml	15 ml
	Make: Ear drops Send: 15 ml Direction: Two - three drops to be instilled in to ear, as directed.			

Theory: Boric acid is a weak germicide (antiseptic), which inhibits the growth of certain bacteria and fungi. It is also used as atorrhoea. It is non-irritating in nature. Therefore it is suitable for preparing eardrops.

Boric acid is slightly soluble in water. But it is freely soluble in Industrial alcohol (alcohol 95%). Therefore alcohol 95% is used, to enhance the solubility of boric acid in water. Alcohol also acts as a preservative.

Procedure:

1) Accurately weigh boric acid and dissolve in Industrial alcohol.
2) To the above solution, add ¾ th of total volume of purified water and mix thoroughly.

3) Filter the solution through muslin cloth to remove, if any foreign particles or any undissolved substances are present.
4) Transfer the content to a measure, add sufficient amount of water to adjust the final volume.

Dispensing: Transfer the solution to a small glass or plastic bottle of 10-15 ml capacity, close it thoroughly with rubber closure and aluminium cap, polish, label and supply with a dropper.

Direction: Two - three drops to be instilled in to ear, as directed.

Storage: Store in a cool place.

Auxilliary label:
- FOR EXTERNAL USE ONLY **OR** FOR EAR USE ONLY.
- NOT FOR INJECTION.
- NOT TO BE DILUTED WITH WATER BEFORE USE.
- KEEP AWAY FROM CHILDREN.

Uses: Boric acid eardrops is used as local anti-infective (germicide), in the treatment of infections in the ear.

CHLORAMPHENICOL EARDROPS

Rx	
Chloramphenicol	5 %
Propylene glycol....q.s....	fl. 3 XXV
Fiat : Auristillae	Mitte : fl. 3 ii ss
Signa : Instillandus tries guttae affectae auris, b.i.d in die.	

Conversion :

5% → 5 g in 100 ml

fl. 3 XXV → 25 fl. drachms = 100 ml

Calculation : For fl. 3 ii ss → 2.5 fl. dr = 10 ml.

Chloramphenicol $= \frac{5}{100} \times 10 = 0.5$ g

Propylene glycol .q.s.... = 10 ml

Type	Ingredients	Quantity in imperial	Quantity in metric	Quantity taken
Monophasic liquid, instilled in to ear.	Chloramphenicol	5 %	5 g	0.5 g
	Propylene glycol....q.s..	25 fl. dr	100 ml	10 ml
	Make: Ear drops Send: 10 ml Direction: Three drops to be instilled in to the affected ear, two times a day.			

Theory: Chloramphenicol acts as antibiotic and antiseptic, which is used in the treatment of chronic otorrhoea and chronic otitis. Chloramphenicol is sparingly soluble in water, but it is freely soluble in propylene glycol (1:7). Hence propylene glycol is used as a vehicle.

Ear drops is prepared by simple solution method, by dissolving chlormphenicol in propylene glycol.

Procedure:

1) Accurately weigh chloramphenicol and dissolve in ¾ th of propylene glycol.
2) Filter the solution through sintered glass funnel or muslin cloth to remove, if any foreign particles or any undissolved substances are present.
3) Transfer this content to a measure and adjust the final volume with propylene glycol.

Dispensing: Chloramphenicol is sensitive to the light, therefore transfer the solution to a amber coloured, small, glass or plastic bottle of 10-15 ml capacity, close it thoroughly with rubber closure and aluminium cap, polish, label and supply with a dropper.

Direction: Three drops to be instilled in to the affected ear, two times a day.

Storage: Store in a cool and dark place.

Auxilliary label:
- FOR EXTERNAL USE ONLY. **OR** FOR EAR USE ONLY.
- NOT TO BE TAKEN ORALLY.
- NOT TO BE DILUTED WITH WATER BEFORE USE.
- STORE IN A COOL AND DARK PLACE.
- KEEP AWAY FROM CHILDREN.

Uses: Chloramphenicol ear drops is used in the treatment of chronic otorrhoea and chronic otitis.

ALUMINIUM ACETATE EARDROPS B.P.

Synonym : Burow's solution

Rx	
Aluminii sulphatis	gr VL
Acetic acid	fl.3 Viii
Acidi tartraci	gr LXVii ss
Calcii carbonatis	3 iii s
Aquam.......q.s.....	fl. 3 XXV
Fiat : Auristillae	Mitte : fl.oz ½
Signa : Instillandus tries guttae auris, quartis horis.	

Conversion :

gr VL → 45 grains

15 grains = 1 g

45 grains = 3 g

gr LXVii ss → 67.5 grains = 4.5 g

fl. 3 Viii → 8 fl. drachms

1 fl. drachm = 4 ml

8 fl. drachms = 32 ml

3 iii s → 3.25 drachms = 13 g

Calculation : For fl.oz $\frac{1}{2}$ = 15 ml

Aluminium sulphate = $\frac{3}{100} \times 15 = 0.45$ g

Acetic acid = $\frac{32}{100} \times 15 = 4.8$ml

Tartaric acid = $\frac{4.5}{100}$ x $15 = 0.675$ g

Calcium carbonate = $\frac{13}{100} \times 15 = 1.95$ g

Purified water... q.s. ... = 15 ml

Type	Ingredients	Quantity in imperial	Quantity in Metric	Quantity Taken
Monophasic liquid, instilled in to ear.	Aluminium sulphate	45 gr	3 g	0.45 g
	Acetic acid (33%)	8 fl. dr	32 ml	4.8 ml
	Tartaric acid	67.5 gr	4.5 g	0.675 g
	Calcium carbonate	3.25 dr	13 g	1.95 g
	Purified water....q.s.....	25 fl. dr	100 ml	15 ml
	Make: Ear drops Send: 15 ml Direction: Three drops to be instilled in to ear, every four hours.			

Theory: This ear drops consists aluminium aceto tartarate. This is obtained by reaction between aluminium sulphate, acetic acid and tartaric acid, in a sequence. All the three ingredients are soluble in water, hence eardrops can be prepared by simple solution method.

Aluminium sulphate reacting with acetic acid forms aluminium acetate. To this suspension, calcium carbonate is added with stirring. The final suspension is left for 24hrs in cool place with occational agitation. During this period, the following reaction takes place.

$$\underset{\text{Aluminium sulphate}}{Al_2(SO_4)_3} + \underset{\text{Calcium carbonate}}{3\,CaCO_3} + \underset{\text{Acetic acid}}{4\,CH_3COOH} \longrightarrow \underset{\text{Basic aluminium acetate}}{2\,Al\,(CHCOO)_2\,OH} + 3\,CaSO_4 + 3CO_2\uparrow + H_2O$$

After 24 hrs, the solution obtained is filtered to remove the precipitate. To the filtrate, tartaric acid is added, to convert the basic aluminium acetate to aluminium aceto tartarate and then final volume is adjusted with water.

Aluminium sulphate is highly soluble in hot water, than cold water. Therefore hot water is used for the preparation of eardrops

Procedure:

1) Dissolve aluminium sulphate in ½ of portion of purified hot water, because it is highly soluble in hot water than cold water.
2) Prepare calcium carbonate suspension, in small portion of water.
3) To the aluminium sulphate solution, add calcium carbonate suspension and acetic acid with stirring. The obtained product (suspension) is allowed to stand for 24 hrs in a cool place, with occational stirring.
4) After 24 hrs, filter the preparation. To the filtrate add tartaric acid, mix well and adjust the final volume with water.

Dispensing: Transfer the solution to a small glass or plastic bottle of 15 ml capacity, close it thoroughly with rubber closure and aluminium cap, polish, label and supply with a dropper.

Direction: Three drops to be instilled in to ear, every four hours.

Storage: Store at room temperature, not exceeding 25°C.

Auxilliary label:
- FOR EXTERNAL USE ONLY **OR** FOR EAR USE ONLY.
- NOT TO BE TAKEN ORALLY **OR** NOT FOR INJECTION.
- NOT TO BE DILUTED WITH WATER BEFORE USE.
- KEEP AWAY FROM CHILDREN.

Uses: Aluminium acetate ear drops is used as antiseptic.

SODIUM BICARBONATE EAR DROPS B.P.

Rx	
Sodii bicarbonatis	3 i s
Glyerini	fl.oz i
Aquam......q.s.....	fl. 3 XXV
Fiat : Auristillae	Mitte : fl.oz ½
Signa : Instillandus duo-tries guttae auris, more dicto.	

Conversion :

3 i s → 1.25 drachms　　　fl.oz i → 1 fl.oz = 30 ml

1 drachm = 4 g

1.25 drachms = 5 g

fl. 3 XXV → 25 fl. dr = 100 ml

Calculation : For fl.oz ½ → 15 ml

Sodium bicarbonate $= \frac{5}{100} \times 15 = 0.75$ g

Glycerin $= \frac{30}{100} \times 15 = 4.5$ ml

Purified water ...... q.s..... = 15 ml

Type	Ingredients	Quantity in imperial	Quantity in metric	Quantity taken
Monophasic liquid, instilled in to ear.	Sodium bicarbonate	1.25 dr	5 g	0.75 g
	Glycerin	1 fl.oz	30 ml	4.5 ml
	Purified water (Freshly boiled and cooled)..q.s..	25 fl. dr	100 ml	15 ml
	Make: Ear drops　Send: 15ml Direction: Two - three drops to be instilled into ear, as directed.			

Theory: Sodium bicarbonate dissolves the earwax and removes it, from the auditory canal. It is readily soluble in water. Since glycerin and sodium bicarbonate are soluble in water, ear drops is prepared by simple solution method.

In this preparation, glycerin is used to improve softening capacity of the solution. Its hygroscopic and emollient nature diminishes the itching sensation and softens the wax.

Procedure:

1) Accurately weigh sodium bicarbonate and dissolve in ¾th quantity of freshly boiled and cooled water.
2) To the above solution, add glycerin, filter and adjust the final volume with water.

Dispensing: Transfer the solution to a small glass or plastic bottle of 15 ml capacity, close tightly with rubber closure and aluminium cap, polish, label and supply with a dropper.

Direction: Two – three drops to be instilled in to ear, as directed.

Storage: Store in a cool place.

Auxilliary label:
- FOR EXTERNAL USE ONLY **OR** FOR EAR USE ONLY.
- NOT TO BE TAKEN ORALLY **OR** NOT FOR INJECTION.
- NOT TO BE DILUTED WITH WATER BEFORE USE.
- KEEP AWAY FROM CHILDREN.

Uses: Sodium bicarbonate ear drops is used, for softening of the earwax.

PHENOL GLYCERIN EAR DROPS

Rx	
Phenolis glyerini	fl. 3 i
Glyerini......q.s...	fl. 3 ii ss
Fiat : Auristillae	Mitte : fl.oz ½
Signa : Instillandus duo guttae affectae auris, more dicto.	

Conversion :

3 i → 1 fl. drachm = 4 ml

3 ii ss → 2.5 fl. drachams =10 ml

Calculation : For fl.oz ½ = ½ fl.oz = 15 ml

Phenol glycerin = $\frac{4}{10} \times 15 = 6 \text{ ml}$

Glycerin.......q.s... = 15 ml

Type	Ingredients	Quantity in imperial	Quantity in metric	Quantity taken
Monophasic liquid, instilled in to ear.	Phenol glycerin	1 fl. dr	4 ml	6 ml
	Glycerin...q.s..	2.5 fl. dr	10 ml	15 ml
	Make: Ear drops	Send: 15 ml		
	Direction: Two drops to be instilled into affected ear, as directed.			

Theory: Phenol glycerin is too strong, hence it should be diluted with equal volume of glycerin, to use as antiseptic.

In this preparation water cannot be used as vehicle, due to the formation of phenoxy ions, the preparation becomes caustic. Therefore glycerin is used as vehicle and also as base, due to its hygroscopic and emollient nature diminishes itching sensation and softens the wax. Hence for the same reason eardrops should be prepared in dry apparatus.

Procedure:

1) Accurately measure phenol glycerin and glycerin.
2) In a dry container (beaker), mix them thoroughly by stirring.

Dispensing: Transfer the solution to a well-dried, small, glass or plastic bottle of 15 ml capacity, close throughly with rubber closure and aluminium cap, polish, label and supply with a dropper.

Direction: Two drops to be instilled into affected ear, as directed.

Storage: Store in a dry place.

Auxilliary label:

- FOR EXTERNAL USE ONLY **OR** FOR EAR USE ONLY.
- NOT TO BE TAKEN ORALLY **OR** NOT FOR INJECTION.
- NOT TO BE DILUTED WITH WATER
- STORE IN A DRY PLACE.
- KEEP AWAY FROM CHILDREN.

Uses: Phenol glycerin eardrops is used as local antiseptic, in the treatment of infection of the middle ear and boils in the ear.

> **Note:** Formula for phenol glycerin,
>
> Phenol – 16 g
>
> Glycerin – 84 g
>
> Dissolve the phenol in glycerin with the help of gentle heat, if necessary.

Another example for Eardrops:

Rx

Hydrogen peroxide solution (6%) 25 ml

Purified water (freshly boiled and cooled) 100 ml

Prepare: Eardrops Send:10 ml

Direction:- One to two drops to be instilled in to affected ear.

Uses: Hydrogen peroxide eardrops is used to remove wax from the ear. Because Hydrogen peroxide soften the wax. It also acts as antiseptic.

Student's exercise:

1) Define ear drops. For what purposes it is used ?
2) Give the examples for ear drops.
3) What is the Latin term, for ear drops ?
4) What type of containers should be used for ear drops?
5) Comments : Ear drops should be diluted with water before use.
6) Write the auxilliary label for ear drops.
7) What types of medicaments are used in eye drops? Give examples.

8) Write the uses of (a) Chloromphenical ear drops. (2) Boric acid ear drops. (3) Sodium bicarbonate ear drops.
9) What is Burow's solution ? Explain is the principle involved in its preparation.
10) Comment : Glycerin is used as one of the ingredients in ear drops.
11) Why hydrogen peroxide is used in ear drops?
12) Comment : Phenol ear drops should not be diluted before use.
13) Comment : Ear drops can also be used as eye drops.

17 NASAL DROPS

Latin term: Naristillae

Nasal drops are aqueous preparations of the drugs, intended for instillation into nostrils with the help of a dropper. They are generally used for their antiseptic, local analgesic or vasoconstriction properties.

Medicaments commonly used are,

1) Anti-inflammatory agents : Corticosteroids, Betamethasone.
2) Sympathomimetics : Ephedrine hydrochloride
3) Decongestants : Phenylephrine, Oxymetazole, Tetrahydrozoline hydrochloride, Xylomethazoline hydrochloride Oxymetazole hydrochloride

Nasal drops are generally formulated to resemble the nasal secretions. Hence nasal drops should be isotonic and slightly buffered, to maintain pH 5.5 to 7.5. The viscosity of nasal drops should be similar to the viscosity of the nasal secretions. Therefore viscosity of nasal drops is adjusted with the help of thickening agents like methylcellulose, hydroxy propyl methylcellulose.

For preparation of nasal drops, generally aqueous vehicle is used. Oils are not preferred as vehicles, because oily drops inhibit the ciliary movements of the nasal mucosa and even cause lipoidal pneumonia (drops of oil enter the lungs).

Since the nasal drops is instilled in to nasal cavity, that will be in contact with mucous membrane of nose, it should be clarified by passing through sintered glass funnel, before making the final volume with water.

Examples for Nasal drops:

- Ephedrine hydrochloride nasal drops,
- Phenylephrine nasal drops,
- Oxymetazoline nasal drops,
- Betamethasone nasal drops.

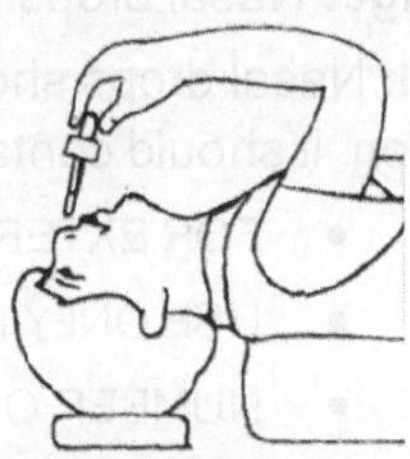

Instillation of Nasal drops to nostrils

Formulation:

Sr. No	Ingredients type	Examples
1	Vehicle	Purified water
2	For tonicity adjustment	Sodium chloride, Dextrose
3	Buffers	Phosphate buffer (pH – 6.5)
4	Preservatives	Chlorbutonol (0.5%) Benzalkonium chloride (0.01 to 0.05%) Aromatic alcohols (0.5 to 0.9%)

Method of preparation:

Simple solution method is employed for the preparation of nasal drops, because most of the drugs and additives used are water soluble.

Dispensing:

Nasal drops are generally dispensed in small (10-15 ml capacity) clear or amber coloured bottle with a dropper fitted with rubber teat. But now a days, nasal drops are dispensed in small, fluted plastic containers made up of polyethylene with "built in droppers" (Bottle previously sealed with dropper).

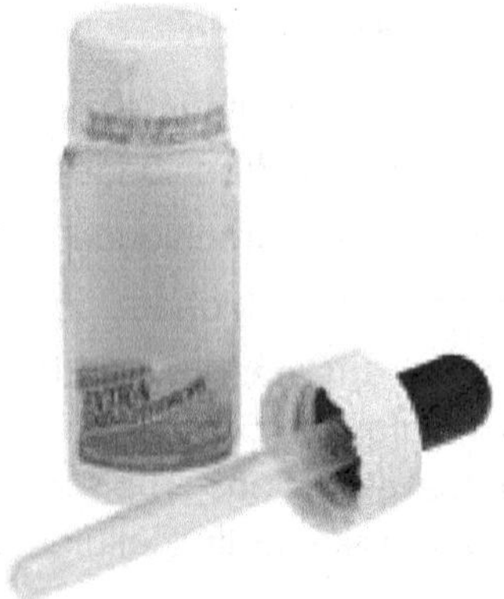

Nasal drops with separate dropper

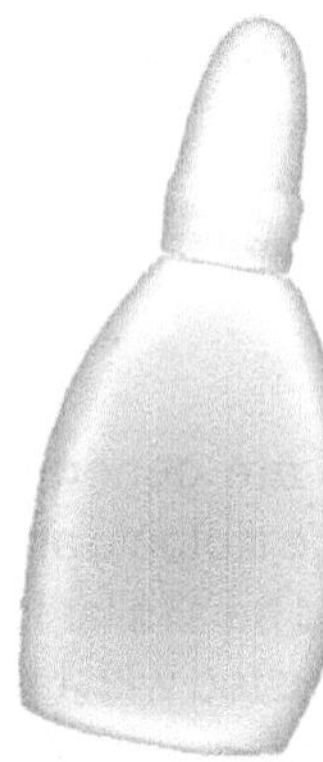

Flexible, plastic built -in-dropper for Nasal drops

Nasal drops should be used within one month (four weeks) after opening seal of the container. If any unused amount of nasal drops is present, that should be discarded after one month, to avoid contamination from microorganisms, if it is stored for longer time.

Storage: Nasal drops should be stored in a cool place.

Label: Nasal drops should bear necessary requirements of liquid dosage forms. In addition, it should contain auxilliary labels like,

- FOR EXTERNAL USE ONLY.
- USE ONLY IN THE NOSTRIL **OR** FOR NASAL USE ONLY.
- NUMBER OF DROPS TO BE INSTILLED PER SINGLE TIME.
- DISCARD THE CONTAINER AFTER ONE MONTH OF THE OPENING OF SEAL (CONTAINER).
- NOT FOR INJECTION.
- DO NOT TOUCH TIP OF THE DROPPER.
- DO NOT DILUTE WITH WATER BEFORE USE.
- KEEP AWAY FROM CHILDREN.

EPHEDRINE HYDROCHLORIDE NASAL DROPS B.P.C

Rx	
Ephedrine hydrochloridi	gr vii ss
Sodii chloridi	gr vii ss
Chlorbutol	gr vii ss
Aquam.....q.s......	fl. 3 xxv
Fiat : Naristillae	Mitte : fl. 3 ii ss
Signa : Instillandus duo guttae naso, more dicto.	

Conversion :

gr vii ss → 7.5 grains   fl. 3 xxv → 25 fl. drachms

15 grains = 1 g   1 fl. drachm = 4 ml

7.5 grains = 0.5 g   25 fl. drachms = 100 ml

Calculation : For fl. 3 ii ss → 2.5 fl. dr = 10 ml.

If, we calculate all the ingredients for 10 ml, the quantities comes below 100 mg. It is not a weighable quantity, on dispensing balance. Hence calculate for 20 ml, to obtain weighable quantities of the solid ingredients but dispense only 10 ml.

So, calculate the formula for 20 ml,

Ephedrine hydrochloride $= \frac{0.5}{100} \times 20 = 0.1$ g

Sodium chloride $= \frac{0.5}{100} \times 20 = 0.1$ g

Chlorbutol $= \frac{0.5}{100} \times 20 = 0.1$ g

Purified water ...q.s.... = 20 ml

Type	Ingredients	Quantity in imperial	Quantity in metric	Quantity taken
Monophasic liquid, instilled into nostrils.	Ephedrine hydrochloride	7.5 gr	0.5 g	0.1 g
	Sodium chloride	7.5 gr	0.5 g	0.1 g
	Chlorbutol	7.5 gr	0.5 g	0.1 g
	Water ...q.s.....	25 fl. dr	100 ml	20 ml
	Make: Nasal drops	Send: 10 ml		
	Direction: Two drops to be instilled into nostrils, as directed.			

Theory:

In this preparation, ephedrine hydrochloride acts as nasal decongestant. Sodium chloride is used to make nasal drops isotonic with nasal secretions. Chlorbutol is used as preservative.

Salts like ephedrine hydrochloride and sodium chloride are soluble in water, but chlorbutol is a volatile substance and it dissolves very slowly, in presence of salts at room temperature. Hence it requires vigorous shaking, with maximum amount of water.

In order to achieve rapid dissolution, first chlorbutol is dissolved in hot water. During dissolving, conical flask should be stoppered to prevent the volatalisation of chlorbutol. After cooling, other salts are dissolved and the solution should be passed through sintered glass funnel, before making the final volume with water.

Procedure:

1) Accurately weigh the chlorbutol and powder it.
2) Select a small conical flask with a suitable stopper.
3) In conical flask, take ¾ th quantity of water and heat to 60 °C without putting the stopper.
4) Add chlorbutol to the hot water and quickly insert the stopper, to prevent the volatalisation of chlorbutol and and shake until, solution completes.
5) Allow the solution to cool (room temperature) and add ephedrine hydrochloride and sodium chloride, dissolve them by stirring and filter the solution through sintered glass funnel or muslin cloth.
6) Transfer the filtrate to a measure and adjust the final volume with water.

Dispensing: Ephedrine hydrochloride is light sensitive, therefore transfer the solution to a amber coloured, small glass or plastic bottle of 10-15 ml capacity, close it thoroughly with rubber closure, polish, label and supply with a dropper.

Direction: Two drops to be instilled into nostril, as directed

Storage: Ephedrine hydrochloride is light sensitive and chlorbutol is volatile in nature, hence it should be stored in a cool and dark place.

Auxiliary label:

- FOR EXTERNAL USE ONLY **OR** FOR NASAL USE ONLY.
- NOT TO BE DILUTED WITH WATER BEFORE USE.
- DO NOT TOUCH THE DROPPER TIP.
- STORE IN A COOL AND DARK PLACE.
- KEEP AWAY FROM CHILDREN.

Uses: The local application of ephedrine hydrochloride to the mucous membrane of the nose stimulates the vasoconstrictor sympathetic nerve endings, hence produces a balancing of the area and a reduction in nasal secretions (Nasal congestions).

If the mucous surface is inflamed, ephedrine relieves symptoms of painful swelling. It also relieves allergic and vasomotor rhinitis and sinusitis, therefore Ephedrine hydrochloride nasal drops is used as nasal decongestant.

PHENYLEPHRINE HYDROCHLORIDE NASAL DROPS

Rx	
Phenylephrine hydrochloride	gr iii ss
Sodium metabisulphite	gr i ss
Sodium chloride	gr Viii
Chlorbutol	gr vi sss
Propylene glycol	M LXVii ss
Purified water......q.s.......	fl.oz iii
Fiat : Naristillae	Mitte : fl. 3 V
Signa : Instillandus guttae naso, more dicto.	

Conversion :

gr iii ss → 3.5 grains

15 grains = 1 g

3.5 grains = 0.23 g

gr i ss →1.5 grains = 0.1 g

gr Viii →8 grains = 0.53 g

gr vi sss → 6.75 grains = 0.45 g

M LXVii ss → 67.5 minims

15 minims = 1 ml

67.5 minims = 4.5 ml

fl.oz iii → 3 fl.oz = 90 ml

Calculation : For fl. 3 V → 5 fl.drachms = 20 ml

Phenylephrine hydrochloride = $\frac{0.23}{90} \times 20 = 0.051g$

Sodium metabisulphite = $\frac{0.1}{90} \times 20 = 0.02$ g

Sodium chloride = $\frac{0.53}{90} \times 20 = 0.12$ g

Chlorbutol = $\frac{0.45}{90} \times 20 = 0.1$ g

Propylene glycol = $\frac{4.5}{90} \times 20 = 1$ ml

Purified water... q.s. .... = 20 ml.

1) Phenylephrine hydrochloride required for 20 ml is 0.051 g ≅ 51 mg. But it is a potent medicament, hence its minimum weighble quantity on dispensing balance is 300 mg.

∴ Dissolve Phenyl ephedrine hydrochloride --- 300 mg
in water...q.s.. --- 10 ml
i.e. 300 mg of Phenylephrine hydrochloride is present in 10 ml of solution

For 51 mg of Phenylephrine hydrochloride = $\frac{51}{300} \times 10 = 1.7$ ml

2) For 20 ml, Sodium metabisulphite required is, 0.020 g (20 mg). Since it is a non-potent substance, its minimum weighble quantity on dispensing balance is 100 mg.

∴ Dissolve, Sodium metabisulphite --- 100 mg
in Water.......q.s... --- 10 ml
i.e. 100 mg of Sodium metabisulphite present in 10 ml of solution

For 20 mg of Sodium metabisulphate = $\frac{20}{100} \times 10 = 2$ ml solution is required.

Revised formula for 20 ml :

Phenylephrine hydrochloride solution --- 1.7 ml
Sodium metabisulphite solution --- 2 ml
Sodium chloride --- 0.12 g
Chlorbutol --- 0.1 g
Propylene glycol --- 1 ml
Purified water ....q.s... --- 20 ml

Type	Ingredients	Quantity in imperial	Quantity in metric	Quantity taken
Monophasic liquid, instilled into nostrils.	Phenylephrine hydrochloride	3.5 gr	0.23 g	1.7 ml
	Sodium metabisulphite	1.5 gr	0.1 g	2 ml
	Sodium chloride	8 gr	0.53 g	0.12 g
	Chlorbutol	6.75 gr	0.45 g	0.1 g
	Propylene glycol	67.5 minims	4.5 ml	1 ml
	Purified water...q.s..	fl.oz iii	90 ml	20 ml
	Prepare: Nasal drops Send: 20 ml. Direction : To be instilled into nostrils, as directed.			

Theory:

Phenylephrine hydrochloride is used as active drug, which acts as nasal decongestant. In this preparation salts like phenylephrine hydrochloride, sodium chloride and sodium metabisulphite are easily soluble in water. Phenylephrine is very sensitive to the light and atmospheric oxygen, hence it undergoes oxidation. Therefore, to prevent its oxidation, sodium metabisulphite is used as antioxidant.

Sodium chloride is used to adjust the isotonicity of the preparation and chlorbutol is used as preservative. Propylene glycol is used to give viscous nature to the drops and acts as cosolvent.

In presence of the salts like phenylephrine hydrochloride, sodium chloride and sodium metabisulphite, chlorbutol is very slowly soluble in water. Therefore solubility of chlorbutol is increased by dissolving it in the hot water (at 60 °C) and after cooling, the drug and other ingredients are dissolved, filter and final volume is adjusted with water.

Procedure:

1) Accurately weigh the chlorbutol and finely powder it by trituration.
2) Select a small conical flask with a suitable stopper.
3) In conical flask, take ¾ th quantity of water and heat to 60 °C without closing stopper.
4) Add chlorbutol to the hot water and quickly insert the stopper and shake until solution completes, to prevent the volatalisation of chlorbutol and allow the solution to cool (room temperature).
5) To the chlorbutol solution, incorporate phenylephrine hydrochloride, sodium chloride, sodium metabisulphite, propylene glycol in a sequence and make a solution.
6) Filter the solution through a muslin cloth or sintered glass funnel, to remove any foreign particles present or any undissolved ingredients if remaining.
7) Adjust the final volume by adding sufficient volume of water.

Dispensing: Phenylephrine is very sensitive to the atmospheric oxygen and light, hence it undergoes oxidation reaction. Therefore transfer the solution to a light resistant glass or plastic bottle of 10-15 ml capacity, close it tightly, label and supply with a dropper.

Direction: To be instilled into nostrils, as directed.

Storage: Store in a cool and dark place.

Auxilliary label:

- FOR EXTERNAL USE ONLY **OR** FOR NASAL USE ONLY.
- NOT TO BE DILUTED WITH WATER BEFORE USE.
- DO NOT TOUCH THE DROPPER TIP.
- STORE IN A COOL AND DARK PLACE.
- KEEP AWAY FROM CHILDREN.

Uses: Phenylephrine nasal drops is used as nasal decongestant.

Student's exercise:

1) Define nasal drops. What are its uses?
2) What should be the pH of nasal drops and why?
3) Comment : Nasal drops should be made isotonic.
4) Give the examples for drugs, which are used in nasal drops.
5) Comment : Oils are used as vehicles for preparation of nasal drops.
6) How will you adjust the viscosity of nasal drops?
7) Give the four examples for nasal drops with their uses.
8) What is the Latin term for nasal drops?
9) What is the meaning of (a) instillandus (b) Guttae
10) What is "lipoidal pneumonia"

18 NASAL SPRAYS AND NASAL WASH

Latin term: Nebula.

Nasal sprays are liquid preparations of medicaments in aqueous or alcoholic vehicle, which is sprayed into the nostrils in the form of fine mist, with the help of atomizer or nebulizer.

The main aim to prepare nasal spray is, to have the maximum drug action and to reach the drug solution up to nasal (respiratory) tract, in the form of fine droplets. They are used to relieve nasal congestion and to treat nasal infections.

Nasal sprays mainly contain medicaments like antibiotics, antihistaminics, sympathomimetic agents and bronchodilators. They should be isotonic with nasal secretion and buffered at pH 6.2.

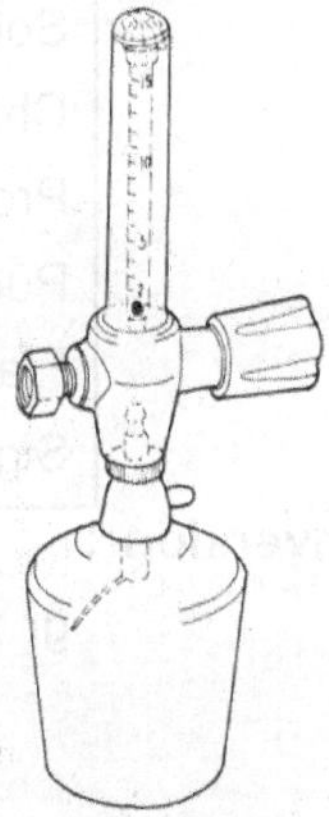

[Nebulizer]

Examples:

1) Compound adrenaline and atropine sulphate nasal spray.
2) Compound isoprenaline and papavarine nasal spray.

Dispensing:

Nasal sprays are dispensed in small, light resistant bottle, fitted with nebulizer or atomizer or squeeze like bottle. The purpose of using this type of container is to break up the nasal solution into small droplets, to reach into the respiratory tract for effective action. Because coarse droplets are suitable for producing drug action in upper respiratory tract, but fine droplets further penetrate into respiratory tract up to bronchi.

Storage: Nasal sprays should be stored in a cool place, away from light and flame.

Label: Label of nasal sprays should bear necessary requirements of liquid dosage forms. In addition, it should contain auxilliary label like,

- FOR NASAL USE ONLY.
- STORE IN A COOL AND DARK PLACE, AWAY FROM FLAME OR HEAT.
- KEEP AWAY FROM CHILDREN.

Advice for patients: Avoid excessive use. Avoid use in very young babies, unless under medical advice.

COMPOUND ADRENALINE AND ATROPINE NASALSPRAYB.P.C.

Rx	
Adrenaline acid tartrate	3 ii
Atropine methonitrate	gr xv
Papaverine hydrochloride	3 ii
Sodium metabisulphite	gr xv
Chlorbutol	3 i s
Propylene glycol	fl. 3 xii ss
Purified water......q.s.......	fl. 3 CCL
Fiat : Nebula	Mitte : fl.zo i
Signa : Nebulus naso, more dicto.	

Conversion :

gr xv → 15 grains = 1 g

3 ii → 2 drachms

1 drachm = 4 g

2 drachms = 8 g

fl. 3 xii ss →12.5 fl. drachms = 50 ml

3 i s → 1.25 dr = 5 g

fl.dr CCL → 250 fl.dr = 1000 ml

Calculation : For fl.oz i → 1 fl.oz = 30 ml

Adrenaline acid tartarate = $\frac{8}{1000} \times 30 = 0.24$ g

Atropine methonitrate = $\frac{1}{1000} \times 30 = 0.03$ g

Sodium metabisulphite = $\frac{1}{1000} \times 30 = 0.03$ g

Papaverine hydrochloride = $\frac{8}{1000} \times 30 = 0.24$ g

Chlorobutol = $\frac{5}{1000} \times 30 = 0.15$ g

Propylene glycol = $\frac{50}{1000} \times 30 = 1.5$ g

Purified water... q.s. ... = 30 ml

Adrenaline acid tartarate and Atropine salts are potent medicaments, since their maximum dose is less than 60 mg, therefore their minimum weighble quantity is 300 mg, on dispensing balance.

Hence, Adrenaline acid tartarate and Atropine salts are taken by "dilution method" as shown in the calculation.

1) Dissolve, Adrenaline acid tartarate - 300 mg

in Water.......q.s... - 10 ml

i.e. 300 mg Adrenaline acid tartarate present in 10 ml of solution

240 mg of Adrenaline acid tartarate is present in = $\frac{240}{300}$ x 10 = 8 ml

2) Dissolve, Atropine methonitrate - 300 mg

in Water.......q.s... - 10 ml

i.e. 300 mg Atropine methonitrate present in 10 ml of solution

30 mg of Atropine methonitrate is present in = $\frac{30}{300}$ x 10 = 1 ml

3) Since, Sodium metabisulphate is a non-potent substance. Its minimum weighble quantity, on dispensing balance is 100 mg.

Dissolve, Atropine methonitrate - 100 mg

in Water.......q.s... - 10 ml

i.e. 100 mg of Sodium metabisulphate present in 10 ml of solution

30 mg of Sodium metabisulphate is present in = $\frac{30}{100}$ x 10 = 3 ml

Revised formula :

Adrenaline acid tartrate solution --- 8 ml

Atropine methonitrate solution --- 1 ml

Sodium metabisulphite solution --- 3 ml

Papavarine hydrochloride --- 0.24 g

Chlorobutol --- 0.15 g

Propylene glycol --- 1.5 g

Purified water ....q.s... --- 30 ml

Type	Ingredients	Quantity in imperial	Quantity in metric	Quantity taken
Monophasic liquid, sprayed into nostrils.	Adrenaline acid tartrate	2 dr	8 g	0.24 g
	Atropine methonitrate	15 gr	1 g	0.03 g
	Sodium metabisulphite	15 gr	1 g	0.03 g
	Papavarine hydrochloride	2 dr	8 g	0.24 g
	Chlorobutol	1.25 dr	5 g	0.15 g
	Propylene glycol	12.5 dr	50 ml	1.5 g
	Purified water ..q.s..	250 fl.dr	1000 ml	30 ml
	Make: Nasal Spray Send: 30 ml Direction: Spray to the nostrils, as directed.			

Theory:

Adrenaline acid tartrate and atropine methonitrate acts as bronchodilators. Papavarine hydrochloride, acts as smooth muscle relaxant. Combination of all these drugs is used, in the treatment of asthma.

All the active ingredients are in salt form, therefore they are freely soluble in water, hence nasal solution is prepared by simple solution method. Sodium metabisulphite is used as an antioxidant to prevent the oxidation of adrenaline acid tartrate and chlorbutol is used as preservative. Polyethylene glycol is used as co-solvent for dissolving chlorbutol.

Procedure:

Use the sterile water for preparation of nasal spray, otherwise boil the purified water for 10 minutes, to remove dissolved oxygen and to destroy vegetative bacteria and mould spores. Cool and use for the preparation of nasal spray.

1) Accurately weigh adrenaline acid tartrate, atropine methonitrate and sodium metabisulphite.
2) Do the proper dilution, according to calculation. Take the required amount of all these solutions and dissolve them in a small portion of boiled and cold water. Add papavarine hydrochloride to this mixture.
3) Dissolve chlorbutol in propylene glycol and mix with the above solution thoroughly.
4) Filter the solution, to remove foreign particles.
5) Transfer the solution to a measure and adjust the final volume with water.

Dispensing: Adrenaline is sensitive to the oxygen and light, hence preparation undergoes oxidation. Therefore transfer nasal spray solution to a small, amber coloured, fluted glass bottle, close it tightly with plastic screw cap, polish and label.

Direction: Spray to the nostrils, as directed.

Storage: Store in a cool place and protect from light.

Auxilliary label:
- FOR NASAL USE ONLY.
- STORE IN COOL AND DARK PLACE, AWAY FROM FLAME.
- KEEP AWAY FROM CHILDREN.

Uses: This nasal spray is used in the treatment of asthma.

ISOPRENALINE SULPHATE NASAL SPRAY B.P.C.

Rx	
Isoprenaline sulphate	3 ii ss
Propylene glycol	fl. 3 xii ss
Sodium metabisulphite	gr xv
Purified water......q.s.......	fl. 3 CCL
Fiat : Nebula	Mitte : fl.oz i
Signa : Nebulus naso, more dicto.	

Conversion :

3 ii ss → 2.5 drachms	fl. 3 xii ss → 12.5 fl. drachms
1 drachm = 4 g	1 fl. drachm = 4 ml
2.5 drachms = 10 g	12.5 fl. drachms = 50 ml
gr xv → 15 grains = 1 g	fl. 3 CCL → 250 fl.dr = 1000 ml

Calculation : For fl.oz i → 1 fl.oz = 30 ml

Isoprenaline sulphate $= \frac{10}{1000} \times 30 = 0.3$ g

Propylene glycol $= \frac{50}{1000} \times 30 = 1.5$ ml

Sodium metabisulphite $= \frac{1}{1000} \times 30 = 0.03$ g

Purified water... q.s. ... = 30 ml

(**Note** - Since, Sodium metabisulphate is a non-potent substance. Its minimum weighble quantity on dispensing balance is 100 mg.

Dissolve, Sodium metabisulphite - 100 mg

in Water.......q.s... - 10 ml

i.e. 100 mg of Sodium metabisulphite present in 10 ml of solution

30 mg of Sodium metabisulphite is present in $= \frac{30}{100} \times 10 = 3$ ml)

Type	Ingredients	Quantity in imperial	Quantity in metric	Quantity taken
Monophasic liquid, sprayed into nostrils.	Isoprenaline sulphate	2.5 dr	10 g	0.3 g
	Propylene glycol	12.5 fl. dr	50 ml	1.5 ml
	Sodium metabisulphite	15 gr	1 g	3 ml
	Purified water......q.s......	250 fl. dr	1000 ml	30 ml
	Make: Nasal spray Send: 30 ml Direction: Spray to the nostris as directed.			

Theory:

Isoprenaline sulphate is a sympathomimetic, beta-receptor agonist, which acts as potent bronchodilator. Propylene glycol is used as co-solvent, to dissolve isoprenaline sulphate. Sodium metabisulphite is used as antioxidant. All the ingredients are soluble in water, hence the nasal solution is prepared by simple solution method.

Procedure:

1) Accurately weigh isoprenaline sulphate and dissolve in purified water. To this solution, add propylene glycol and mix uniformly.
2) Add sodium metabisulphite to the above mixture and dissolve by stirring.
3) Make up the final volume with purified water.

Dispensing: Isoprenaline sulphate is sensitive to the light, hence preparation undergoes degradation. Therefore transfer nasal spray solution to a small, amber coloured, fluted glass bottle, close it tightly with plastic screw cap, polish and label.

Direction: Spray to the nostrils, as directed.

Storage: Store in a cool place and protect from light.

Auxilliary label:
- FOR NASAL USE ONLY.
- STORE IN A COOL PLACE, AWAY FROM FLAME OR HEAT.
- KEEP AWAY FROM CHILDREN.

Uses: It is used as bronchodilator, in the treatment of asthma.

Another example for Nasal spray

Rx

Sodium bicarbonate	---	2 g
Borax	---	2 g
Glycerin	---	30 ml
Phenol	---	0.72 ml
Water.....q.s....	---	90 ml

(Note: This spray solution involves evaluation of CO_2. Therefore for further details, see the chemical incompability page no.- 531)

BORAX – GLYCERIN NASAL WASH

Rx	
Boracis -glyerini	fl.oz i
Sodii bicarbonatis	3 i
Aquam... q.s. ...	fl.oz vi
Fiat : Collunarium	Mitte : fl.oz i
Signa : Cum duplo aquae calidae aequales pro utendum, et utendus more dicto.	

Conversion :

fl.oz i → 1 fl.oz = 30 ml   3 i → 1 drachm = 4 g

fl.oz vi → 6 fl.oz = 180 ml

Calculation : For fl.oz i → 1 fl.oz = 30 ml

Borax -glycerin = $\frac{30}{180} \times 30 = 5$ ml

Sodium bicarbonate = $\frac{4}{180} \times 30 = 0.66$ g

Purified water... q.s. ... = 30 ml.

Type	Ingredients	Quantity in imperial	Quantity in metric	Quantity taken
Monophasic liquid, for external use (For nostril).	Borax - glycerin	fl.oz i	30 ml	5 ml
	Sodium bicarbonate	3 i	4 g	0.66 g
	Water.....q.s......	fl.oz vi	180 ml	30 ml
	Make: Nasal wash	Send: 30 ml		
	Direction: Dilute with equal volume of warm water, before use and to be used as directed.			

Theory:

Borax is a white crystalline powder and effloresces in dry air. It is sparingly soluble in water (1 in 16 parts), but it is freely soluble in glycerin. Hence glycerin is used as carrier (vehicle) for borax.

$$Na_2B_4O_7 + 3H_2O \longrightarrow Na_2B_2O_4 + 2H_3BO_3$$

Borax → Sodium meta borate + Boric acid

$$3H_3BO_3 + 2C_3H_5(OH)_3 \longrightarrow (C_3H_6)_2 \cdot (HBO_3)_3 + 6H_2O$$

Boric acid Glycerin → Glyceryl boric acid

Glycerin is soluble in water and acts as bacteriostatic. This preparation shows evolution of carbon dioxide gas due to acid-base reaction i.e. when borax glycerin and sodium bicarbonate are mixed together in the presence of water, borax hydrolyses into boric acid and sodium meta per borate. The liberated boric acid reacts with glycerin and coverts into monobasic glycerol boric acid which is strong acidic in nature. When glyceryl-boric acid reacts with alkali like, sodium bicarbonate, it causes effervescence due to the liberation of carbon dioxide gas.

If this reaction mixture is dispensed as such, without complete evolution of carbon dioxide and mixture is transferred immediately to the bottle and closed, there are chances of explosion with bursting of the bottle, due to excessively increased pressure of gas, inside the bottle.

Procedure:

A) Preparation of Borax - glycerin:

Accurately weigh borax and powder it by triturating in a mortar. Dissolve it in glycerin by gentle heating on waterbath, with constant stirring until solution is affected and filter, if necessary.

Formula for Borax-glycerin:

Borax	1.2 g
Glycerin	8.8 g
	10 g

B) Preparation of Borax - glycerin nasal wash:

1) Measure the borax-glycerin and mix with sodium bicarbonate in an open vessel (beaker) until effervescence ceases completely.
2) To this solution, add sufficient water to produce final volume.

Dispensing: Transfer the solution to a narrow mouthed, clear, fluted plastic bottle, close it thoroughly, with plastic screw cap, polish and label.

Direction: Dilute with equal volume of warm water, before use and to be used as directed.

Storage: Store in a cool place.

Auxilliary label : FOR EXTERNAL USE ONLY **OR** FOR NASAL USE ONLY.

Uses: Borax-glycerin nasal wash is used as antiseptic (bacteriostatic) in the treatment of nasal infections.

Similar example for Nasal wash:

Rx

Borax	---	2 g
Sodium bicarbonate	---	2 g
Phenol	---	0.5 ml
Sucrose	---	4 g
Water.....q.s....	---	90 ml

COMPOUND SODIUM CHLORIDE NASAL WASH (DOUCHE)

Rx	
Sodii chloridi	gr XV
Sodii bicarbonatis	gr XV
Sodii perboratis	gr XV
Aquam...... q.s. ...	fl.oz ii
Fiat : Collunarium	Mitte : fl.oz ii
Signa : Cum duplo aquae calidae aequales pro utendum, more dicto.	

Conversion :

gr XV → 15 grains   fl.oz ii → 2 fl.oz

15 grains = 1 g   1 fl.oz = 30 ml

2 fl.oz = 60 ml

Calculation : For fl.oz ii → 2 fl.oz = 60 ml

Sodium chloride = $\frac{1}{60} \times 60 = 1$ g

Sodium bicarbonate = $\frac{1}{60} \times 60 = 1$ g

Sodium perborate = $\frac{1}{60} \times 60 = 1$ g

Purified water... q.s. ... = 60 ml

Type	Ingredients	Quantity in imperial	Quantity in metric	Quantity taken
Monophasic liquid, for nose.	Sodium chloride	15 gr	1 g	1 g
	Sodium bicarbonate	15 gr	1 g	1 g
	Sodium perborate	15 gr	1 g	1 g
	Water....q.s......	fl.oz ii	60 ml	60 ml
	Make: Nasal wash Send: 60 ml Direction: Dilute with equal volume of warm water, before use and to be used as directed.			

Theory:

Sodium bicarbonate dissolves the mucous of nasal tract. Sodium perborate acts as mild antiseptic and deodorant, it also acts as preservative. Sodium chloride is used to adjust the isotonicity of the solution. All the ingredients are soluble in water, hence the nasal solution is prepared by simple solution method.

Procedure:

1) Accurately weigh sodium bicarbonate, sodium chloride and sodium perborate and dissolve in ¾th of total volume of water, in the ascending order of their weights by continuous stirring.
2) Filter the solution, to remove if any impurities present.
3) Transfer the solution to a measure, adjust the final volume with purified water.

Dispensing: Transfer the solution to a narrow mouthed, clear, fluted plastic bottle, close it thoroughly with plastic screw cap, polish and label.

Direction: Dilute with equal volume of warm water, before use and to be used as directed.

Storage: Store in a cool place.

Auxilliary label: FOR EXTERNAL USE ONLY **OR** FOR NASAL USE ONLY.

Uses: It is used as antiseptic and deodorant.

Student's exercise:

1) Explain why nasal drops are formulated as nasal sprays.
2) What is nebula, and why it is used ?
3) Why drugs are formulated in the form of nasal sprays?
4) What should be the pH of Nasal spray?
5) How will you dispense nasal sprays?
6) What should be the auxilliary label for nasal sprays?
7) Which type of medicaments used in nasal sprays?
8) What is the use of (a) Isoprenaline sulphate nasal spray (b) Compound Adrenaline and Atropine nasal sprays?
9) What are the differences between nasal drops and nasal sprays?
10) Explain why nasal wash is used? Give examples for nasal wash
11) What is collunarium and collutorium?
12) What is the use of borax-glycerin in nasal wash?
13) How will you supply collunarium?

19 INHALATIONS

Latin term : Inhalatio

Inhalations are solutions or suspensions of volatile substances, administered by nasal or oral respiratory route in the form of vapour. They are used to relieve, nasal congestion and inflammation of the respiratory tract. They are administered for local action on the bronchial tree or for their systemic effect through absorption from lungs.

Administration:

1) Some inhalations contain ingredients, which are highly volatile at room temperature, they are administered by placing them on handkerchief or absorbent pad and inhaled.
2) Some inhalations are added to the hot water (about 65 °C) but not boil water and vapour (steam) is inhaled for few minutes (5-10 minutes). Now-a-days apparatus like "vaporizer" is used for inhalation.

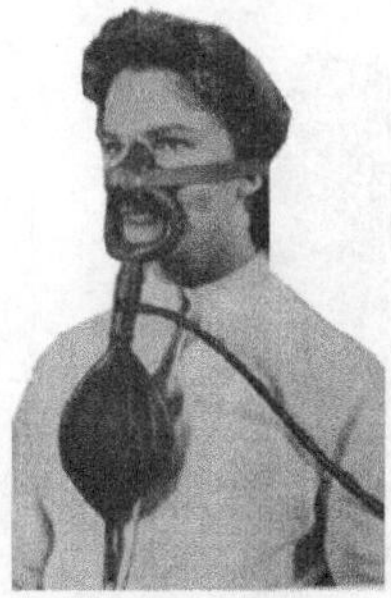

The nasal inhalation

Examples for Inhalations:

1) Benzoin inhalation
2) Menthol – benzoin inhalation
3) Menthol and eucalyptus oil inhalation
4) Epinephrine inhalation USP
5) Isoproterenol hydrochloride inhalation USP.

Preparation:

Some inhalations consist of one or more volatile oils like eucalyptus oil or pine oil. These oils are immiscible in aqueous vehicle. Hence they are uniformly distributed in aqueous vehicle by using an adsorbent, which is diffusible in nature.

eg. Magnesium carbonate.

Magnesium carbonate acts as distributing agent. i.e. subdivides the oil, sufficiently, to ensure its uniform dispersion upon shaking.

Method:

The volatile oils are triturated with adsorbent, because trituration helps to breakdown oils into fine globules, which will get easily adsorb on the adsorbent. When such inhalation (dispersion) is added to the hot water, a free vaporization of volatile oil takes place.

Compare to the emulsification method, this method is found to be better for dispersion of the oil, because adsorbent never interferes with free vaporization of oil and emulsification process may retard (slows down) the vaporisation.

If the quantity of adsorbent is not mentioned in the formula, following quantities can be used.

1) For volatile oils: for each 2 ml of oil, 1 gm of light magnesium carbonate can be used.
2) For volatile substances: for each 2 gm of volatile substance, 1 gm of light magnesium carbonate can be used.

Dispensing:

Because of high volatile nature of Inhalations, they should be dispensed in tightly closed, amber coloured, fluted glass bottle closed with plastic screw cap, to distinguish them from the preparations meant for internal use.

Now-a-days inhalations are dispensed in aerosol containers. (Inhalers)

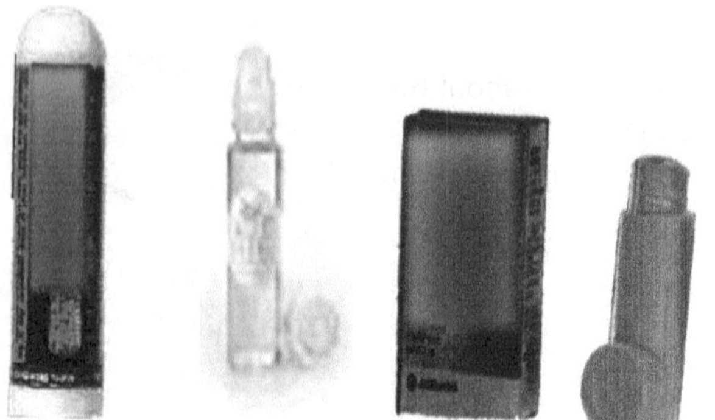

Different types of Inhaler

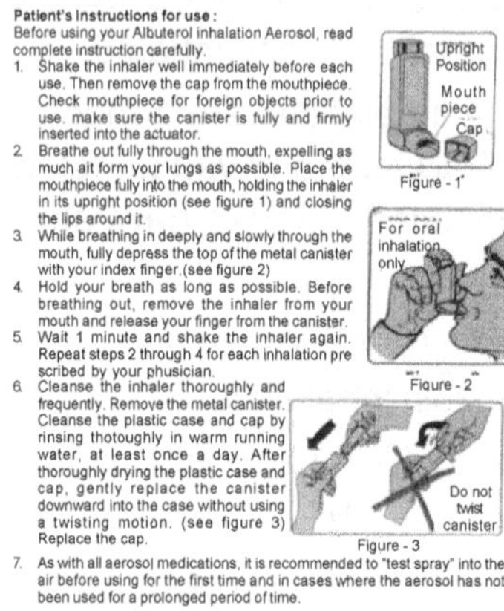

Patient's Instructions for use :
Before using your Albuterol inhalation Aerosol, read complete instruction carefully.

1. Shake the inhaler well immediately before each use. Then remove the cap from the mouthpiece. Check mouthpiece for foreign objects prior to use. make sure the canister is fully and firmly inserted into the actuator.
2. Breathe out fully through the mouth, expelling as much ait form your lungs as possible. Place the mouthpiece fully into the mouth, holding the inhaler in its upright position (see figure 1) and closing the lips around it.
3. While breathing in deeply and slowly through the mouth, fully depress the top of the metal canister with your index finger.(see figure 2)
4. Hold your breath as long as possible. Before breathing out, remove the inhaler from your mouth and release your finger from the canister.
5. Wait 1 minute and shake the inhaler again. Repeat steps 2 through 4 for each inhalation pre scribed by your phusician.
6. Cleanse the inhaler thoroughly and frequently. Remove the metal canister. Cleanse the plastic case and cap by rinsing thotoughly in warm running water, at least once a day. After thoroughly drying the plastic case and cap, gently replace the canister downward into the case without using a twisting motion. (see figure 3) Replace the cap.
7. As with all aerosol medications, it is recommended to "test spray" into the air before using for the first time and in cases where the aerosol has not been used for a prolonged period of time.

Storage:

Higher temperature leads to the volatilization (vaporization) of volatile substances, hence inhalations should be stored in a cool place.

Label: Label of Inhalation, should bear necessary requirements of liquid dosage forms. In addition it should contain auxilliary label like,

- FOR EXTERNAL USE ONLY **OR** FOR NASAL USE ONLY.
- SHAKE WELL BEFORE USE.
- QUANTITY REQUIRED TO BE ADDED IN THE HOT WATER.
- STORE IN A COOL PLACE.

Advice for patients: The patient should be advised, to "Add one teaspoonful of inhalation to one pint of hot water (not boiling water). A towel should be placed over the head and the vapour is inhaled for 5-10 minutes".

MENTHOL – EUCALYPTUS OIL INHALATION B.P.C.

(Aqueous inhalation)

Rx

Mentholis	gr VL
Olei eucalypti	fl. ʒ ii
Aquam.....q.s.......	fl. ʒ XXV
Fiat : Inhalatio	Mitte : fl.oz i

Signa : Cochleare minimum inhalatio addendus ad demid litrum aquae calide, inhalatus vapori, more dicto.

Conversion :

gr VL → 45 grains	fl. ʒ ii → 2 fl. drachms
15 grains = 1 g	1 fl. drachm = 4 ml
45 grains = 3 g	2 fl. drachms = 8 ml

Calculation : For fl.oz i → fl.oz = 30 ml

Menthol $= \frac{3}{100} \times 30 = 0.9$ g

Eucalyptus oil $= \frac{8}{100} \times 30 = 2.4$ ml

Water ...q.s.... = 30 ml

Calculation for Light magnesium carbonate:

Since, Menthol is a volatile substance,

2 g of menthol requires 1 g of Magnesium carbonate

0.9 g of menthol $= \frac{1 \times 0.9}{2} = 0.45$ g Magnesium carbonate

Where as,

Eucalyptus oil is volatile oil,

2 ml of Eucalyptus oil reequires 1 g of Magnesium carbonate

2.4 ml of Eucalyptus oil $= \frac{2.4 \times 1}{2} = 1.2$ g Magnesium carbonate

So, total quantity of light magnesium carbonate is required for 30 ml.

For Menthol	0. 45 g
For Eucalyptus oil	1.20 g

	1.65 g

Revised formula:

Menthol	--- 0.9 g
Eucalyptus oil	--- 2.4 ml
Magnesium carbonate	--- 1.65 g
Water.....q.s.......	--- 30 ml

Type	Ingredients	Quantity in imperial	Quantity in metric	Quantity taken
Monophasic liquid, used as vapour	Menthol	45 gr	3 g	0.9 g
	Eucalyptus oil	2 fl. dr	8 ml	2.4 ml
	Water.......q.s.......	25 fl.dr	100 ml	30 ml
	Light magnesium carbonate	--	--	1.65 g
	Make: Inhalation	Send: 30 ml		
	Direction: Add one teaspoonful linhalation, to half liter of hot water and inhale the vapor, as directed.			

Theory:

This inhalation is a suspension containing volatile ingredients like menthol and eucalyptus oil. Menthol is freely soluble in eucalyptus oil, but eucalyptus oil is not miscible with water. Hence it is uniformly distributed in water using adsorbent like, light magnesium carbonate.

Light magnesium carbonate is diffusible in nature and adsorbs the volatile oil, which helps to ensure a uniform dispersion. This adsorbent never interferes with free vaporization of oil, when inhalation is added to hot water.

Procedure:

1) Accurately weigh the menthol and finely powder it in a glass mortar and dissolve in eucalyptus oil.
2) To the above solution, add magnesium carbonate in small portions and mix well.
3) Gradually add water to produce a pourable suspension, transfer to a measure and adjust the final volume with water.

Dispensing: Transfer the solution to a amber coloured, fluted glass bottle and close it tightly with plastic screw cap, polish and label.

Direction: Add one teaspoonful, to half liter of hot water and inhale the vapor, as directed.

Storage: Store in a cool place.

Auxiliary label:

- FOR EXTERNAL USE ONLY **OR** FOR NASAL USE ONLY.
- SHAKE WELL BEFORE USE. (SINCE THERE ARE CHANCES OF SEPARATION OF OIL GLOBULES OF EUCALYPTUS OIL DURING STORAGE)
- QUANTITY REQUIRED TO BE ADDED IN TO HOT WATER.
- STORE IN A COOL PLACE.

Uses: Menthol acts as local anodyne and eucalyptus oil is used in the treatment of bronchitis and also acts as antiseptic, counter-irritant, therefore this inhalation is used for the relief of nasal congestion.

BENZOIN INHALATION

Rx	
Benzoin (crushed)	3 ii ss
Prepared Storax	3 i sss
Alcohol (95%) or Specially denatured spirit.....q.s....	fl. 3 xxv
Fiat: Inhalatio	Mitte : fl.oz. i
Signa: Addendus inhalatio super linteum, et inhelature lente, more dicto.	

Conversion :

3 ii ss → 2.5 drachms   fl. 3 xxv → 25 fl. dr =100 ml

1 drachm = 4 g

2.5 drachms =10 g

3 i sss → 1.75 drachms = 7 g

Calculation: For fl.oz i → fl.oz = 30 ml

Benzoin = $\frac{10}{100} \times 30 = 3$ g

Prepared Storax = $\frac{7}{100} \times 30 = 2.1$ g

Alcohol 95% or Specially denatured spirit…q.s… = 30 ml

Type	Ingredients	Quantity in imperial	Quantity in metric	Quantity taken
Monophasic liquid, used as inhalation.	Benzoin (crushed)	2.5 dr	10 g	3 g
	Prepared Storax	1.75 dr	7 g	2.1 g
	Alcohol 95% or Specially denatured spirit ...q.s....	25 fl. dr	100 ml	30 ml
	Prepare: Inhalation Send : 30 ml Direction: Place inhalation upon lint and to be inhaled slowly, as directed.			

Theory:

Benzoin is a resin, obtained from the incisions of stem Storax benzoin (Sumatra benzoin). Benzoin consists free balsamic acids like, cinnamic and benzoic acid and oily aromatic principles. These acids acts as antiseptic, expectorant and carminative.

Prepared Storax is a balsam, obtained from the trunk of Liquidambar orientalis. It acts as antiseptic, expectorant and stimulant.

Inhalation is prepared by maceration of crushed benzoin and prepared storax with alcohol (95%) for 24 hours.

Procedure:

1) Crush the benzoin into small pieces.
2) Accurately weigh benzoin and prepared Storax and macerate them with ¾ th quantity of alcohol (95%) in a closed vessel for 24 hours.
3) After 24 hours filter and pass the sufficient amount of alcohol (95%) through filter to produce the final volume and mix well.

Dispensing: Transfer the inhalation to an amber coloured, narrow mouthed, glass bottle, Close it tightly with plastic screw cap, polish and label.

Direction: Place inhalation upon lint and to be inhaled slowly, as directed.

Storage: Store in a cool place.

Auxillary label: FOR EXTERNAL USE ONLY **OR** FOR NASAL USE ONLY.

Uses: Benzoin inhalation is used as expectorant and anti-inflammatory agent, for the treatment of throat and bronchial inflammation.

Other examples for Inhalations

1. **Eucalyptus oil inhalation**

Rx

Oil of pine	1 fl. dr
Eucalyptus oil	1 fl. dr
Compound benzoin tincture...q.s..	6 fl. drachms

Uses: This inhalation is used as expectorant and also in the treatment of upper respiratory tract infection.

2. **Menthol inhalation**

Rx

Menthol	1 g
Specially denatured spirit...q.s..	50 ml

Uses: This inhalation can be used as anti pruritic agent, for nasal decongestion, headache and neuralgia.

Student's exercise:

1) Define inhalation. How it is administered?
2) Give the examples for inhalations.
3) Comment : Inhalations should be stored in a cool place.
4) Why an adsorbent is required for preparation of inhalations and in what proportions should be used?
5) Comment : Inhalation should not be added to boiling water.
6) What is the purpose to use inhalation ?
7) What is Benzoin Storax? What is its use?
8) Why Menthol and Eucalyptus oil are used in the preparation of inhalations ?
9) How will you administer (use) the Benzoin inhalation ?
10) Write the direction for the Menthol - Eucalyptus oil Inhalation.

20 DOUCHES

Douches are medicated aqueous solutions, used for rinsing of body surfaces or body cavities like eye, ear, nose, pharynx, bladder, rectum and vagina. But the term 'Douche' is most commonly used for vaginal douche.

Douches are generally used for their cleansing, antiseptic or astringent actions.

Medicaments commonly used in douches are,

1) Antiseptics : Potassium permanganate, Mercurous chloride, Chlorhexidine, Lactic acid, Chloroxylenol.
2) Astringents : Tannic acid, Zinc sulphate, Alum.
3) Cleansing agents : Sodium chloride, Sodium bicarbonate, Boric acid, Saponated cresol.
4) Soothing agent : Glycerin

According to the uses of douches in different body cavities, they will be called as,

1) Eye : Eye douches
2) Nose : Nasal douches
3) Pharnyx : Pharyngeal douches
4) Bladder : Bladder douches (Irrigations)
5) Vagina : Vaginal douches (Douches)
6) Rectum : Rectal douches (Enemas)

Vaginal douches are used for rinsing (cleansing) of vaginal cavity, after child birth or any surgery of vaginal region, therefore they should be sterile and have pH - 5.5.

Douches used for bladder (Irrigations) should be always sterile and they are administered into the bladder using a thin, soft, sterile rubber or plastic tube which is called as catheter.

Dispensing: Douches are generally dispensed as concentrated solutions, with direction "to dilute it with specific quantity of warm water before use". They are introduced to the body cavities, by gravitational flow by using "Douche can".

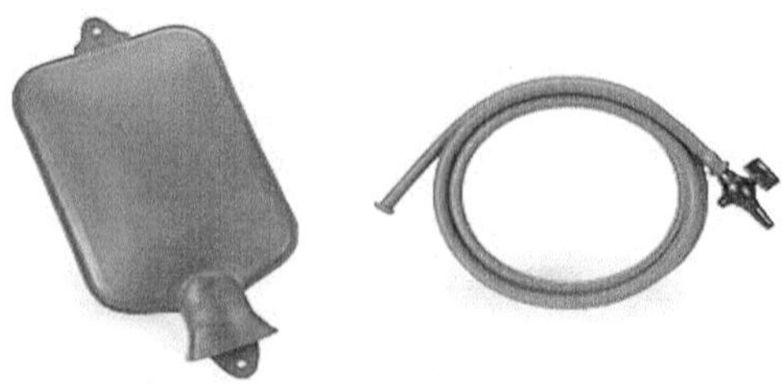

Douch can with long rubber tube

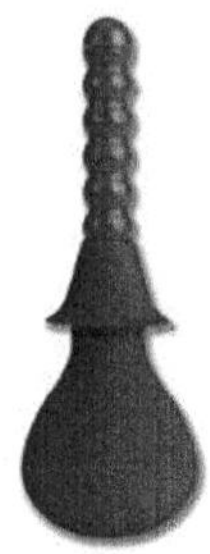

Rectal nozzle

"Douche can" is a rigid polyvinyl chloride container, and a rubber tube of about 2 meter long along with a nozzle attached with it. Generally 1-2 liter of solution is used as douche.

But now-a-way days douches are supplied with disposable polyvinyl chloride bags, with suitable rubber syringe with a specially designed nozzle. The syringe should be lubricated before introducing in to vagina, to facilitate easy movement.

Douches are also supplied in the form of powder or tablets with specific directions for dissolving in a specific quantity of warm water. They are supplied in suitable plastic boxes or in the aluminium strips.

Eg - Liquid phenol-Boric acid douche (powder).

Label : Along with general requirements of label, douches should contain auxilliary label like,

- FOR EXTERNAL USE ONLY **or** FOR VAGINAL USE ONLY.
- LUBRICATE THE NOZZEL BEFORE USE.
- STORE IN A COOL PLACE.

Direction: Direction should be given to the patients about,

a) Dilution with warm water before use and how to use. OR

b) Quantity of powder or tablet to be dissolved in a specified quantity of warm water and how to use.

Storage: Douches should be stored in a cool place.

Examples for Douches:

1) Potassium permanganate douche.
2) Boric acid douche.
3) Chlorhexidine douche.

POTASSIUM PERMANGANATE DOUCHE

Rx	
Potassium permanganate	gr xv
Aquam....q.s....	fl. 3 CCL
Fiat : Douche	Mitte : fl. 3 CXXV
Signa : Utendus more dicto.	

Conversion :

gr xv → 15 grains — fl. 3 CCL → 250 fl.dr

15 grain = 1 g — 1 fl.dr = 4 ml

250 fl.dr = 1000 ml

Calculation : For fl. 3 CXXV → 125 fl.dr = 500 ml, but calculate for (500+10) = 510 ml

$$\text{Potassium permanganate} = \frac{1}{1000} \times 510 = 0.51 \text{ g}$$

Purified water.....q.s.... = 510 ml

Type	Ingredients	Quantity in imperial	Quantity in metric	Quantity taken
Monophasic	Potassium permanganate	15 gr	1 g	0.51 g
liquid,	Purified water...q.s..	250 fl. dr	1000 ml	510 ml
used in vagina.	Make: Douche Send:500 ml of 0.1% of potassium permanganate			
	Direction: To be used, as directed.			

Theory: Potassium permanganate is soluble (1:15) in water, hence it forms a solution easily. It acts as disinfectant, due to its oxidizing action.

Potassium permanganate stains the surfaces of plastic and reacts with oxidisable residues of the containers, hence turns to brown colour with loss of strength. Therefore appropriate container (glass bottle) should be used for dispensing.

Procedure: Calculate the ingredients for 10 ml extra, than prescribed volume, to compensate the loss of preparation during administration.

1) Triturate potassium permanganate to fine powder in a glass mortar and then triturate with small portion of purified water.
2) Allow the undissolved solid to settle down and transfer the supernatant solution to another container.
3) Add small portion of water again to the mortar, to triturate the remaining undissolved solid. Transfer the supernatant solution to the container.
4) Repeat this procedure, until the entire potassium permanganate completely dissolves.

5) Filter the final solution through cleaned sintered glass, into a measuring cylinder. Add purified water to adjust the final volume.

Dispensing: Potassium permanganate undergoes oxidation reaction with atmospheric oxygen and turns to brown colour with loss of strength. Therefore transfer the solution to a amber coloured glass bottle and close it tightly, polish and label.

Direction: Direction should be given to the patients about, dilution with warm water, before use.

Auxillary label:

- FOR EXTERNAL USE ONLY.
- FOR VAGINAL USE ONLY.
- STORE IN A COOL PLACE.

Storage: Store in a cool place.

Uses: Potassium permanganate douche is used as irrigating solution, in the treatment of vaginal infections.

BORIC ACID DOUCHE

Rx	
Acidi borici	3 v
Aquam....q.s....	fl. 3 CCL
Fiat : Douche	Mitte : fl. 3 CXXV
Signa : Cum duplo aquae calidae pro utendus, more dicto utendus.	

Conversion :

3 v → 5 drachms — fl. 3 CCL → 250 fl.dr

1 drachm = 4 g — 1 fl.dr = 4 ml

5 drachms = 20 g — 250 fl.dr = 1000 ml

Calculation : For fl. 3 CXXV → 125 fl.dr = 500 ml, but calculate for (500+10) = 510 ml

Potassium permanganate = $\frac{5}{1000} \times 510 = 2.55$ g

Purified water.....q.s.... = 510 ml

Type	Ingredients	Quantity in imperial	Quantity in metric	Quantity taken
Monophasic liquid, used in vagina.	Boric acid	5 dr	20 g	2.55 g
	Purified water...q.s...	250 fl. dr	1000 ml	510 ml
	Make: Douche	Send: 500 ml		
	Direction: Dilute with warm water before use and tobe used as directed.			

Theory:

Boric acid acts as antiseptic. It is soluble in water (1 in 18 parts),but it is highly soluble in hot water and hence it dissolves and forms mono phasic solution. This solution is non-irritating, therefore it can be safely used as a douche.

Procedure: Calculate the ingredients for 10 ml extra, than prescribed volume, to compensate the loss of preparation during administration.

1) Dissolve boric acid, in sufficient amount of purified water.
2) To enhance the solubility of boric acid, heat the solution on a waterbath at 80 to 90°C.
3) Filter the solution, if any foreign particles or undissolved substances are there.

Dispensing: Transfer the solution to a amber coloured glass bottle and close it tightly, polish and label.

Direction: Dilute with warm water before use and to be used as directed.

Auxillary label:
- FOR VAGINAL USE ONLY.
- DILUTION WITH WARM WATER BEFORE USE.
- LUBRICATE THE NOZZEL BEFORE USE.

Storage: Store in a cool place.

Uses: It is used as antiseptic, in the treatment of vaginal infections.

LIQUID PHENOL-BORIC ACID DOUCHE (POWDER)

Rx	
Liquoris phenolis	M xxx
Mentholis	3 i s
Alum	3 vii ss
Acidi borici	3 viii s
Fiat : Douche	Mitte : 3 V

Signa : Solve cochleare minimum pulvis unus litare aqua calidae at, more dicto utendus.

Conversion :

3 i s → 1.25 drachms	M xxx → 30 minims
1 drachm = 4 g	15 minims = 1 ml
1.25 drachms = 5 g	30 minims = 2 ml
3 vii ss → 7.5 drachms = 30 g	3 viii s → 8.25 drachms = 33 g

Calculation : For 3 V → 5 dr = 20 g, but calculate for (20 + 2) = 22 g

Liquified phenol $= \frac{2}{70} \times 22 = 0.62$ ml

Menthol $= \frac{5}{70} \times 22 = 1.57$ g

Alum $= \frac{30}{70} \times 22 = 9.42$ g

Boric acid $= \frac{33}{70} \times 22 = 10.37$ g

Type	Ingredients	Quantity in imperial	Quantity in metric	Quantity taken
Powder intended for irrigation. (Powder douche)	Liquified phenol	30 minims	2 ml	0.62 ml
	Menthol	1.25 dr	5 g	1.57 g
	Alum	7.5 dr	30 g	9.42 g
	Boric acid	8.25 dr	33 g	10.37 g
	Make: Douche (powder) Send: 20 g Direction: Dissolve one teaspoonful of powder, in one liter of warm water and to be used as directed.			

Theory:

Liquified phenol is nothing but liquid carbolic acid. This is a solution of phenol in water. Phenol acts as disinfectant but aqueous solution of phenol at lower concentration of 0.2 to 1% acts as bactericide (antiseptic).

Menthol acts as counter irritant and local anodyne. Boric acid acts as antiseptic. Alum (potassium aluminium sulphate) acts as astringent.

Procedure:

1) Accurately weigh menthol, alum and boric acid.
2) Powder the each ingredient separately into a fine state, in a mortar by trituration.
3) Mix the alum and boric acid with trituration.
4) To the above triturate, add menthol, with further trituration till no lumps remain.
5) Accurately measure liquid phenol and add drop by drop, to the above powdered mixture, with continuous trituration.

Dispensing: This powder douche contains volatile substance-menthol, therefore transfer the prescribed amount of powder to air tight, wide mouthed, a plastic box, close it tightly with coloured plastic screw cap, label and supply with a small measure or teaspoon to measure.

Direction: Dissolve one teaspoonful of powder, in one liter of warm water and to be used as directed.

Auxilliary label :

- FOR VAGINAL USE ONLY.
- STORE IN A COOL PLACE.

Storage: Store in a cool place.

Uses: This powder douche is used as astringent, bactericide and antiseptic.

Other examples of Douche:

1) **Rx**

Menthol	1 g
Camphor	1 g
Zinc sulphate	8 g
Boric acid	48 g

2) **Rx**

Alum	4 g
Zinc sulphate	5 g
Liquified phenol	6 ml
Glycerin	125 ml
Purified water...q.s..	1000 ml

Student's exercise:

1) Define Douches.
2) Write the different types of douches.
3) Give the examples for medicaments, used in douches.
4) How will you dispense the douches ?
5) Comment : Nozzle should be lubricated before administration of douches.
6) Which Auxilliary label is required for douches?
7) Give the examples for douches.

21 ENEMAS

Enemas are aqueous or oily solutions or suspensions or o/w type emulsions, which are intended to introduce into rectum for cleansing, therapeutic or diagnostic purposes. They are also used to cause evacuation and for local or systemic and therapeutic action of the medicaments.

Types of enemas: There are three types of enemas,

1) **Cleansing enemas (Evacuating enemas):** are used to evacuate faeces in constipation and before any surgery of the gut. Cleansing enemas acts by three ways.

a) By stimulating peristalsis movement: (Large volume enemas):

The large volume enemas (500 ml to 1000 ml) are used, to stimulate the peristaltic movement of colon. The stimulation action may be obtained, due to the large volume of enema. Volume of enema is depending upon the age and condition of the patient. The large volume enemas should be warmed to body temperature (37^{0}C), before administration to prevent cold shock.

Eg:
- Plain water
- Turpentine enema
- Soft soap enema

b) By osmotic retention (Retention enemas):

This type of enemas contains small volume of about 100-200 ml, which acts by causing osmotic retention of water in the bowel.

Eg:
- Paraldehyde enema
- Magnesium sulphate enema
- Sodium chloride enema
- Sorbitol enema
- Sodium phosphate enema

The small volume enemas are used as such, without warming to body temperature (37^{0}C).

c) By lubricating impacted faeces (Lubricating enemas):

This type of enemas act by lubricating the impacted (hard) faeces during constipation, hence provides smooth passage in bowel.

They are smaller in volume 100-200 ml.

Eg:
- Castor oil enema
- Olive oil enema
- Arachis oil enema
- Glycerin enema

2) **Therapeutic (medicated) enemas:** These enemas are used to produce medicated effects in the bowel or in lower part of the colon in children and comatose patients. This action may be obtained by its local action (as in the case of piles, ulcerative colitis and inflammatory bowel disease) or systemic (therapeutic) action.

They contain therapeutic agents like,

Sedatives	: Chloral hydrate, paraldehyde
Anthalmintics	: Quassia (for thread warms)
Anti-inflammatory agents	: Corticosteroids (for ulcerative colitis)
Nutrients	: Vitamins, Minerals

3) **Diagnostic enemas:** They contain radio opaque substances, which are used for X-ray examination of lower bowel or colon part.

   Eg: • Barium sulphate suspension

Dispensing: Enemas are dispensed in coloured, fluted glass bottle along with rectal nozzle. Now-a-days enemas are supplied in single use, squeeze plastic bottles or disposable polyethylene or polyvinyl chloride bags sealed with rectal nozzle, which should be lubricated before administration. On the container, expiry date of only 2 days after issue, should be mentioned.

Lubrication of rectal nozzel, is usally done by lubricating jellies like,

Eg:
- Sodium alginate lubricating jelly,
- Sodium carboxy methyl cellulose lubricating jelly,

Direction: Warm up to the body temperature (37° C), before use (only for large volume enemas) and administer as directed.

Storage: Enemas should be stored in a cool and dark place.

Label: Label should bear all necessary requirements of liquid dosage forms, except dose. In addition, it should contain auxilliary label like,

- FOR RECTAL USE ONLY.
- LUBRICATE THE NOZZLE BEFORE USE.
- WARM TO THE BODY TEMPERATURE BEFORE USE.— (ONLY FOR LARGE VOLUME ENEMAS).
- STORE IN A COOL AND DARK PLACE.
- USE WITH IN TWO DAYS AFTER ISSUE **OR** DISCARD THE REMAINING PORTION AFTER TWO DAYS OF ISSUING.

CASTOR OIL ENEMA

Rx	
Olei ricini	fl. 3 XV
Aquam....q.s........	fl. 3 L
Fiat : Enema	Mitte : fl. 3 XXV
Signa : Utendus, more dicto.	

Conversion :

fl. 3 XV → 15 fl. drachms = 60 ml

fl. 3 L → 50 fl. drachms = 200 ml

Calculation : For fl. 3 XXV → 25 fl. dr = 100 ml but, calculate for 100 + 10 ml =110 ml

Castor oil = $\frac{60}{200} \times 110 = 33$ ml

Water ...q.s.... = 110 ml

<table>
<tr><th>Type</th><th>Ingredients</th><th>Quantity in imperial</th><th>Quantity in metric</th><th>Quantity taken</th></tr>
<tr><td rowspan="3">O/W type of emulsion, for rectal use. (Small volume enema)</td><td>Castor oil</td><td>15 fl. dr</td><td>60 ml</td><td>33 ml</td></tr>
<tr><td>Purified water......q.s......</td><td>50 fl. dr</td><td>200 ml</td><td>110 ml</td></tr>
<tr><td colspan="4">Make Enema. Send: 100 ml
Direction: To be used, as directed.</td></tr>
</table>

Theory:

Castor oil is a fixed oil, it acts as laxative (mild purgative). It is insoluble in water, hence a biphasic system of caster oil in water (emulsion) is prepared by using starch mucilage as an emulsifying agent.

Generally, starch or starch mucilage is not widely used as emulsifying agent, because it does not form a true emulsion, but it forms suspension of large globules. These globules may aggregate with each other and there is a chance of separation of oil and water phase. This problem can be prevented by maintaining high viscosity of dispersion medium (water) by using starch mucilage.

Procedure:

1) Calculate the ingredients for 10 ml extra, than prescribed volume, to compensate the loss of preparation during administration.
2) Accurately weigh starch and triturate in mortar, with a littel quantity of water to form a smooth cream.

3) To this cream add 15 to 20 ml of water and triturate to mix uniformly.
4) Transfer this suspension(mixture) to a measure.
5) Rinse the mortar and pestle, with little quantity of water and transfer to the measure. Adjust the volume to 70 ml with water.
6) Transfer this suspension to a 250 ml beakar. Mark the volume on the beaker and heat to boiling with frequent agitation, until the starch has get gelatinised and forms a mucilage.
7) Once the mucilage of starch is formed, remove the beaker from heat and immediately cool the beaker by holding to a stream of cold water.
8) Adjust the original (previous) volume by adding water (because during heating, loss of water takes place, due to evaporation).
9) Add the measured amount of castor oil, to the beaker and mix well by vigarous stirring.

Dispensing: Transfer the content to a coloured, fluted, narrow mouthed glass bottle or single use plastic squeeze bottle, close it thoroughly, polish and label.

Direction: To be used, as directed.

Storage: Store in a cool and dark place.

Auxilliary label:
- FOR RECTAL USE ONLY.
- LUBRICATE THE NOZZLE BEFORE USE.
- STORE IN A DARK PLACE.
- USE WITH IN TWO DAYS AFTER ISSUE AND DISCARD UNUSED PORTION.

Uses: Castor oil gets hydrolyzed by pancreatic lipase and liberates recinolic acid (racino-oleate), which is irritant in nature and produces laxative (mild purgative) effect. Therefore it is used as a lubricating enema, for easy evacuation of hard feces during constipation.

It also gives lubricating effect, therefore used for emptying the bowel , before delivery or any surgery, at lower concentration.

It is also useful for emptying the bowel in diarrhoea, due to food poisoning.

PARALDEHYDE ENAEMA

Rx	
Paraldehyde	fl. 3 ii ss
Benzyl alcohol	M XV
Sodium chloride solution..q.s..	fl. 3 XXV
Fiat : Enema	Mitte : 3 XXV
Signa : Utendus, more dicto.	

Conversion :

fl. 3 ii ss → 2.5 fl. drachms   M XV → 15 minims

1 fl. drachm = 4 ml   15 minims = 1 ml

2.5 fl. drachms = 10 ml

fl. 3 XXV → 25 fl. drachms = 100 ml

Calculation : For fl. 3 XXV → 25 fl. dr = 100 ml but, calculate for 100 + 10 ml = 110 ml

Paraldehyde = $\frac{10}{100} \times 110 = 11$ ml

Benzyl alcohol = $\frac{1}{100} \times 110 = 1.1$ ml

Sodium chloride solution...q.s.... = 110 ml

Type	Ingredients	Quantity in imperial	Quantity in metric	Quantity taken
Monophasic liquid, for rectal use.	Paraldehyde	2.5 fl. dr	10 ml	11 ml
	Benzyl alcohol	15 minims	1 ml	1.1 ml
	Sodium chloride solution (0.9% w/w)......q.s....	25 fl. dr	100 ml	110 ml
(Small volume enema)	Make: Enema Send: 110 ml For 5 years old child, weighing 20 kg Direction: To be used, as directed.			

Theory:

Paraldehyde is a trimer of acetaldehyde, it is colourless, transparent liquid with strong characteristic odour. It is used as sedative, hypnotic and anticonvulsant. For rectal administration, 10% enema in physiological saline (sodium chloride 0.9 % w/w) is used, because it is iso-osmotic with body fluids. Paraldehyde is freely soluble in cold water than hot water. Therefore for preparation of enema, sodium chloride solution should be freshly prepared and chilled overnight.

For preparation of enema, paraldehyde should be directly measured into a final container, which is previously marked to an appropriate final volume. To this container chilled sodium chloride solution is added, almost to the final volume and shaken vigorously to dissolve paraldehyde.

Enema is used in rectal cavity, which will be in contact with mucous membrane. Hence it should be free from irritant particles, which can be removed by filtration through sintered glass funnel by applying vacuum. Benzyl alcohol is incorporated, to reduce the local irritation, caused by the paraldehyde to the rectal mucosa.

Procedure:

1) Calculate the ingredients for 10 ml extra than prescribed volume, to compensate the loss of preparation during administration.
2) Accurately weigh sodium chloride and dissolve in overnight chilled purified water to get 0.9% w/w of sodium chloride solution (saline). Filter the solution through sintered glass funnel.
3) Calibrate a amber colored, narrow mouthed, glass bottle at required volume (110 ml.). Transfer a measured amount of paraldehyde and adjust the final volume with chilled 0.9% w/v sodium chloride solution, close it thoroughly with a plastic screw cap and shake vigorously until solution completes, polish and label.
   (**Note:** The completed enema should not be filtered, to avoid excessive exposure of paraldehyde to air)

Dispensing: Paraldehyde is very sensitive to the light and atmospheric air, because it reacts with air (O_2) and decomposes into acetic acid, which is having brownish yellow colour and sharp penetrating odour of acetic acid. Administration of partially decomposed paraldehyde is dangerous to the health.

Therefore this enema should be dispensed in air tight, well filled, small amber coloured glass bottle or disposable polyethylene bag, which is sealed with rectal nozzle.

Note: Paraldehyde reacts with cork and certain types of plastics, which are used for screw cap therefore wads of polyethylene are used as closures.

Direction: To be used, as directed.

Storage: Paraldehyde has instability (i.e. separates out as crystals) at higher temperature, therefore this enema should be stored in a cool place, in complete darkness.

Auxilliary label:
- FOR RECTAL USE ONLY.
- LUBRICATE THE NOZZLE BEFORE USE.
- STORE IN A COOL AND DARK PLACE.
- USE WITHIN 2 DAYS, AFTER ISSUE AND DISCARD UNUSED PORTION.

Uses: Paraldehyde enema is used as medicated enema as sedative, hypnotic and anticonvulsant.

Note: Paraldehyde enema **should not be** warmed to body temperature before administration because,

1) Paraldehyde separates out as crystalline mass due, to its lower solubility at higher temperature.
2) It is small volume enema, hence it does not require warming.

GLYCERIN ENEMA

Rx	
Glyerini	fl. 3 xii ss
Aquam..........q.s....	fl. 3 XXV
Fiat : Enema	Mitte : fl. 3 XXV
Signa : Utendus, more dicto.	

Conversion :

fl. 3 xii ss → 12.5 fl. drachms

1 fl. drachm = 4 ml

12.5 fl. drachms =50 ml

25 fl. drachms =100 ml

Calculation : For fl. 3 XXV → 25 fl. dr = 100 ml but, calculate for 100 + 10 ml = 110 ml

Glycerin $= \frac{50}{100} \times 110 = 55$ ml

Water...q.s.... = 110 ml

<table>
<tr><th>Type</th><th>Ingredients</th><th>Quantity in imperial</th><th>Quantity in metric</th><th>Quantity taken</th></tr>
<tr><td rowspan="3">Monophasic liquid, for rectal use. (Small volume enema)</td><td>Glycerin</td><td>12.5 fl. dr</td><td>50 ml</td><td>55 ml</td></tr>
<tr><td>Purified water......q.s.........</td><td>25 fl. dr</td><td>100 ml</td><td>110 ml</td></tr>
<tr><td colspan="4">Make: Enema Send: 100 ml
Direction: To be used, as directed.</td></tr>
</table>

Theory:

Glycerin acts as a stimulant laxative, because glycerin is hygroscopic in nature, when it comes in contact with rectal mucous membrane, it absorbs (withdraws) moisture and causes temporary irritation to the bowel. Hence promotes peristaltic movement and evacuation of feacal discharge.

Glycerin also lubricates and softens the hard feacal material. Due to both stimulating and lubricating nature of glycerin, it helps in the easy evacuation of bowels from colon.

Glycerin is miscible with water, hence enema is prepared by simple solution method. Glycerin is comparatively highly soluble in warm water than cold water, hence warm water is used for the preparation of enema.

Procedure:

1) Calculate the ingredients for 10 ml extra than prescribed volume, to compensate the loss of the preparation during administration.
2) Calibrate an amber colored, narrow mouthed glass bottle at required volume (110 ml). Transfer a measured amount of glycerin and adjust the final volume with warm water, close it thoroughly with plastic screw cap and shake vigorously, until glycerin completely miscible with water, polish and label.

Direction: To be used, as directed.

Storage: Store in a cool and dark place.

Auxilliary label:
- FOR RECTAL USE ONLY.
- LUBRICATE THE NOZZLE BEFORE USE.
- STORE IN A COOL AND DARK PLACE.
- USE WITHIN 2 DAYS AFTER ISSUE AND DISCARD UNUSED PORTION.

Uses: Glycerin enema is used as evacuating enema, during constipation.

SOFT SOAP ENEMA

Rx	
Soft soap	3 xii ss
Purified water......q.s.....	fl. 3 xxv
Fiat : Enema	Mitte : fl. 3 CXXV
Signa: Utendus more dicto.	

Conversion :

3 xii ss → 12.5 drachms — fl. 3 xxv → 25 fl. drachms

1 drachm = 4 g — 1 fl. drachm = 4 ml

12.5 drachms = 50 g — 25 fl. drachms = 100 ml

fl. 3 CXXV →125 fl. dr = 500 ml

Calculation : For fl. 3 CXXV →125 fl. dr = 500 ml but, calculate for 500 + 10 ml = 510 ml

Soft soap = $\frac{50}{100} \times 510 = 255\,g$

Purified water ....q.s..... = 510 ml

Type	Ingredients	Quantity in imperial	Quantity in metric	Quantity taken
Monophasic liquid, for rectal use (Large volume enema)	Soft soap	12.5 dr	50 g	255 g
	Purified water....q.s......	25 fl. dr	100 ml	510 ml
	Make: Enema.	Send: 500 ml		
	Direction: To be used, as directed.			

Theory:

Soft soap is soluble in water, hence it forms a homogenous solution. Soft soap solution has lubricant and irritant effect on mucous surface, hence it stimulates the peristaltic movement of the colon for easy evacuation of hard (inspissated) feacal material.

Large volume of the enema may also exerts stimulation effect on the colon. Since it is a large volume enema, it should be warmed to body temperature (37 °C), before administration to avoid cold shock.

Procedure:

1) Calculate the ingredients for 10 ml extra than prescribed volume, to compensate the loss of preparation during administration.
2) Calibrate the bottle to the required volume (510 ml).
3) Accurately weigh soft soap and transfer into a suitable beaker.
4) Add ¾ th of warm water and dissolve the soap by stirring until, it completely dissolves.

5) Transfer this soap solution to a measure, make up the final volume with purified water.

Dispensing: Transfer the soft soap enema in to an amber colored, narrow mouthed, fluted glass bottle, close it thoroughly with plastic screw cap, polish and label.

Direction: To be used as, directed.

Storage: Store in a cool and dark place.

Auxilliary label:
- FOR RECTAL USE ONLY.
- LUBRICATE THE NOZZLE BEFORE USE.
- WARM TO THE BODY TEMPERATURE BEFORE USE.
- STORE IN A COOL AND DARK PLACE.
- USE WITHIN 2 DAYS AFTER ISSUE AND DISCARD UNUSED PORTION.

Uses: Soft soap enema is used for evacuation of hard feacal material, during constipation.

Student's exercise:

1) Define enema and classify them.
2) What are large volume enemas? Give examples.
3) What is the mechanism of Soap enemas?
4) How lubricating enemas acts? Give examples.
5) Comment : Large volume enemas should be administered, after warming to body temperature.
6) How castor oil acts as purgative ?
7) Give the example for diagnostic enema.
8) Give the examples for medicaments (substances) used in therapeutic enemas.
9) How will you supply the enemas?
10) Write the auxilliary label for enemas.
11) Which label direction is necessary for enemas?
12) What is the difference between laxative and purgative? Give examples.
13) Comments : Lubricate the nozzle before administration of enemas.
14) What is paraldehyde? What is its use?
15) Comment : Paraldehyde enema should not be warmed to body temperature, before use.
16) Why glycerin is used for the preparation of enemas?
17) Differentiate between Enemas and Douches.

22 LOTIONS

Latin term: Lotio

Lotions are liquid or semi liquid preparations, meant for external application to the skin, without rubbing (friction). They may be aqueous or alcoholic solutions or suspensions in aqueous medium. If lotion is in suspension form, then it is called as "shake lotion".

Lotions are used to provide cooling, soothing or protective action to the skin. Lotions generally consist of medicaments like antiseptics, astringents, anesthetics, germicides, protective or screening agents for prevention or treatment of various skin diseases.

Lotions usually consist alcohol and glycerin as common ingredients. Because alcohol hastens (increases) the drying and produces cooling sensation. Glycerin acts as a humectant, hence it keeps the skin moist, for sufficiently longer time and does not allow the preparation, to dry out quickly.

Lotions are directly applied to the skin (affected part), without rubbing or dabbing on the skin or applied with the help of suitable absorbent material like cotton wool or gauze (dressing), which is soaked with the lotion.

Examples for Lotions:

- Calamine lotion
- Zinc sulphate lotion
- Cetrimide lotion
- Acriflavine lotion
- Dichloroxylenol lotion
- White lotion
- Salicylic acid lotion
- Boric acid lotion
- Gentian violet lotion

Formulation :

Sr.No	Ingredients type	Examples
1	Vehicles	Purified water, Alcohol and Iso-propyl alcohol In case of oily lotions, Liquid paraffin, Isopropyl myristate and other synthetic esters are used, as vehicles.
2	Co-solvents	Glycerin, Propylene glycol, Poly ethylene glycol (low molecular weight PEG like PEG 400, PEG 600)
3	Flavouring agents	Rose water
4	Preservatives	Methyl paraben, Propyl paraben.

In some lotions microorganisms (bacteria and moulds) may grow, if they do not contain preservatives. If lotions are alcoholic or hydroalcoholic (contain more than 20% of alcohol), they do not need any preservatives. If lotions are absolutely aqueous, then suitable preservatives should be incorporated. Even though a preservative is added, care must be taken, to avoid contamination during the preparation and its use.

Dispensing: Lotions should be dispensed in well closed, narrow mouthed, coloured, fluted plastic bottle, closed with coloured plastic screw cap, to distinguish them from the preparations, which are meant for internal administration. These containers should have adequate air space above the lotion, to permit adequate shaking before its use.

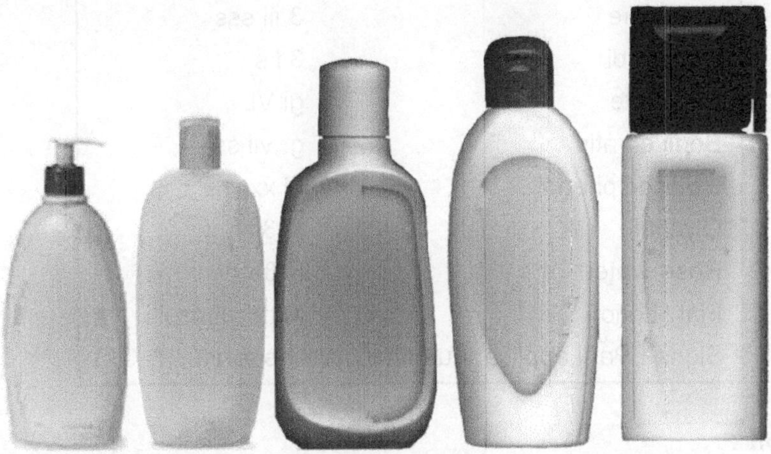

Different fluted, narrow mouthed plastic containers for lotions

Storage: Since lotions consist of highly volatile and inflammable solvents like alcohol (95%) or industrial methylated spirit, they should be stored in a cool place, away from flame or heat.

Label: Label of lotions should bear necessary requirements of liquid dosage forms. In addition, it should contain auxilliary labels like,

- FOR EXTERNAL USE ONLY.
- SHAKE WELL BEFORE USE.
- STORE IN A COOL PLACE.

Direction: Apply without rubbing or friction.

CALAMINE LOTION I.P.

Rx	
Calamine	3 iii sss
Zinci oxidi	3 i s
Bentonite	gr VL
Sodii citratis	gr vii ss
Liquified phenol	M xxii ss
Glyerini	fl. 3 i s
Rose water....q.s...	fl. 3 xxv
Fiat : Lotio	Mitte : fl.oz ii
Signa : Parti applicandus affectae sine teratur, S.O.S.	

Conversion :

3 iii sss → 3.75 drachms	gr VL → 45 grains
1 drachm = 4 g	15 grains = 1 g
3.75 drachms = 15 g	45 grains = 3 g
3 i s → 1.25 drachms = 5 g	gr vii ss → 7.5 grains = 0.5 g
fl. 3 i s → 1.25 fl. dr	M xxii ss → 22.5 minims
1 fl. dr = 4 ml	15 minims = 1 ml
1.25 fl. dr = 5 ml	22.5 minims = 1.5 ml

Calculation : For fl.oz ii → 2 fl.oz = 60 ml

Calamine = $\frac{15}{100} \times 60 = 9$ g

Zink oxide = $\frac{5}{100} \times 60 = 3$ g

Benzonite = $\frac{3}{100} \times 60 = 1.8$ g

Sodium citrate = $\frac{0.5}{100} \times 60 = 0.3$ g

Liquified phenol = $\frac{1.5}{100} \times 60 = 0.9$ ml

Glycerin = $\frac{5}{100} \times 60 = 3$ ml

Rose water ...q.s... = 60 ml

Type	Ingredients	Quantity in imperial	Quantity in metric	Quantity taken
Biphasic liquid,	Calamine	3.75 dr	15 g	9 g
for external use.	Zinc oxide	1.25 dr	5 g	3 g
	Bentonite	45 gr	3 g	1.8 g
Suspension.	Sodium citrate	7.5 gr	0.5 g	0.3 g
	Liquid phenol	15.5 minims	1.5 ml	0.9 ml
Lotion	Glycerin	1.25 fl. dr	5 ml	3 ml
containing,	Rose water......q.s.....	25 fl. dr	100 ml	60 ml
indiffusible	Prepared: Lotion	Send: 60 ml		
substances.	Direction: Apply to the affecet part, without rubbing, when ever necessary.			

Theory:

It is a suspension containing indiffusible solids like calamine and zinc oxide. Calamine is a mixture of 98% zinc oxide with small portion of ferric oxide. Ferric oxide imparts a distinctive pink colour to the zinc oxide, to give flesh (Buff) like colour to the lotion. Calamine acts as an astringent, soothing and protective agent. Zinc oxide acts as astringent and antiseptic. Both calamine and zinc oxide are indiffusible in nature, hence to make them diffusible uniformly in the vehicle, bentonite is used as a suspending agent.

Bentonite is a natural colloidal hydrated aluminium silicate, it is insoluble in water, but swells up and forms magma with little higher viscosity. When bentonite swells up, it makes the preparation viscous, so that it is difficult to pour from the container. Hence sodium citrate is incorporated, which causes partial deflocculation of the calamine and also transforms the bentonite, from gel to a solution form and hence reduces the viscosity of the preparation.

Sodium citrate is also used as a chelating agent, to chelate free iron of ferric oxide, because free iron can change the colour of the preparation. It also acts as buffer and maintains the pH appropriate for the skin and it also prevents the excessive frothing, formed upon shaking of the lotion.

Liquid phenol is used as antiseptic and preservative. Glycerin is used as humectant to keep the skin moist and to give cooling sensation and soothing effect to the skin. It does not allow the preparation to dry out fast. Rose water is used as perfume to give pleasant aroma to the lotion.

Procedure:

1) Dissolve sodium citrate in ¼ th of total volume of purified water.
2) Triturate the calamine, zinc oxide and bentonite (bentonite magma) with sodium citrate solution, until to get a smooth cream.

3) A smooth cream of indiffusible solid is prepared, to prevent the floating of powder, due to the presence of air in the interstices of powder. Dilute the cream with water, to make it pourable.
4) Transfer this mixture to a measure, add liquid phenol and glycerin, mix well. Adjust the final volume with the purified water.

Dispensing: Transfer calamine lotion to a narrow mouthed, coloured, fluted plastic bottle, close it thoroughly with plastic screw cap, polish and label.

Direction: Apply to the affeceted part, without rubbing, when ever necessary.

Storage: Store in a cool place.

Auxilliary label:
- FOR EXTERNAL USE ONLY.
- SHAKE WELL BEFORE USE.

Uses: Calamine lotion is used as skin protective and also used as soothing lotion for the relief of itching due to sunburns, prickly heat, insect bites, minor skin irritations.

> **Note:** Calamine lotion I.P is similar to Calamine lotion B.P except that, Calamine lotion I.P contains rose water as vehicle, where as Calamine lotion B.P contains purified water as vehicle.

SALICYLIC ACID LOTION B.P

Rx	
Acidi salicylici	gr xxx
Olei ricini	M xv
Alcoholis (96%)...q.s..	fl. ʒ xxv
Fiat : Lotio	Mitte : fl.oz i
Signa : Applicandus parti affecte S.O.S, sine teratur.	

Conversion :

gr xxx → 30 grains   fl. ʒ xxv → 25 fl.drachms

15 grains = 1 g   1 fl.drachm = 4 ml

30 grains = 2 g   25 fl.drachms = 100 ml

M xv → 15 minims = 1 ml

Calculation : For fl.oz i → 1 fl.oz = 30 ml

Salicylic acid = $\frac{2}{100}$ x 30 = 0.6 g

Castor oil = $\frac{1}{100}$ x 30 = 0.3 ml

Ethanol (96%) ...q.s.... = 30 ml

Type	Ingredients	Quantity in imperial	Quantity in metric	Quantity taken
Monophasic	Salicylic acid	30 gr	2 g	0.6 g
liquid, for	Castor oil	15 minims	1 ml	0.3 ml
external	Ethanol (96%)...q.s...	25 fl. dr	100 ml	30 ml
use.	Prepare: Lotion	Send: 30 ml		
Lotion.	Direction: Apply to the affected part when necessary, without rubbing.			

Theory:

Salicylic acid and castor oil are insoluble in water, but both are soluble in alcohol (96%), in the proportions of (1 in 4 parts) and (1 in 2.5 parts) respectively. Therefore they form a monophasic liquid, which is used as lotion for external use as keratolytic, bacteriostatic and germicide.

Castor oil acts as an emollient and gives viscous nature to the preparation, for easy application.

Since the preparation is for external use only, ethanol 96% may be replaced with industrial methylated spirit.

Procedure:

1) Dissolve salicylic acid in ¾ th of total volume of the ethanol (96%).
2) Add castor oil and dissolve it well by continuous stirring and transfer to a measure.
3) Add ethanol (96%) sufficiently, to adjust the final volume and mix well.

Dispensing: Due to the presence of highly volatile and inflammable alcohol (96%), transfer salicylic acid lotion to a narrow mouthed, coloured, fluted plastic bottle, close it thoroughly with plastic screw cap, polish and label.

Direction: Apply to the affected part when necessary, without rubbing.

Storage: Store in a cool place and away from flame or heat.

Auxilliary label:

- FOR EXTERNAL USE ONLY.
- SHAKE WELL BEFORE USE.
- STORE IN A COOL PLACE AWAY FROM NAKED FLAME.

Uses: Salicylic acid has bacteriostatic and germicidal properties. Hence it is externally used for the treatment of dandruff, psoriasis, eczema and parasitic skin diseases.

Salicylic acid also has keratolytic properties, it works by breaking down of the keratin, (an important protein of skin structure) which result in the destruction of epithelium and shedding of skin cells, from the effected area. Hence it is used in the treatment of warts and corns.

ZINC SULPHATE – SULPHURATED POTASH LOTION B.P.C.

Synonym : White Lotion N.F., Sulphite lotion B.P.C.

Rx	
Zinci sulphatis	ʒ i
Potassae sulphuratae	ʒ i
Aquam.....q.s.....	fl.ʒ xxv
Fiat : Lotio	Mitte : fl.oz ii
Signa : Parti affectae applicandus bis ad ter in die sine teratur.	

Conversion :

ʒ i → 1 drachm　　fl.ʒ xxv → 25 fl.drachms = 100 ml

1 drachm = 4 g

Calculation : For fl.oz ii → 2 fl.oz = 60 ml

Zinc sulphate $= \frac{4}{100} \times 60 = 2.4$ g

Sulphuated potash $= \frac{4}{100} \times 60 = 2.4$ g

Purified water ....q.s......... = 60 ml

Type	Ingredients	Quantity in imperial	Quantity in metric	Quantity taken
Biphasic liquid, for external use. Suspension.	Zinc sulphate	1 dr	4 g	2.4 g
	Sulphurated potash	1 dr	4 g	2.4 g
	Purified water....q.s..	25 fl. dr	100 ml	60 ml
	Make: Lotion	Send: 60 ml		
	Direction: Apply two to three times a day, to the affected part, without rubbing.			

Theory:

White lotion is a suspension prepared by chemical reaction between zinc sulphate and sulphurated potash. Sulphurated potash is a mixture of potassium polysulphites and potassium thiosulphate.

Lotion is prepared by adding dilute solution of sulphurated potash to the dilute solution of zinc sulphate, slowly with continuous stirring. When they are reacting with each other, forms a finely divided precipitate of zinc sulphide, which is diffusible in nature as shown in the following reaction.

$ZnSO_4$	+	K_2S	$\longrightarrow$	K_2SO_4	+	ZnS
Zinc sulphate		Sulphurated potash		Potassium sulphate		Zinc sulphide (Precipitate)

Zinc sulphate solution should not be added to the solution of sulphurated potash, because it causes formation of basic zinc salts and zinc hydrocxide rather than zinc sulfide.

The fine precipitate of zinc sulphide settles at the bottom upon standing (during storage) and forms a cake, it can not be dispersed uniformly in the vehicle, even after shaking. Therefore this lotion should be freshly prepared, to ensure uniformity. In some formulations bentonite is used as suspending agent, to prevent the cake formation of the precipitate.

Procedure:

1) Accurately weigh zinc sulphate and sulphurated potash and dissolve them separately, in each 20 ml of purified water.
2) Add dilute solution of sulphurated potash, to the dilute solution of zinc sulphate slowly, with constant stirring.
3) Transfer the content to a measure and make up the final volume with water.

Dispensing: Transfer the lotion to a narrow mouthed, coloured, fluted plastic or glass bottle, close it thoroughly with plastic screw cap. Shake vigorously to make fine precipitate of zinc sulphide, polish and label.

Direction: Apply two to three times a day, to the effected part, without rubbing.

Storage: Store in a cool place

Auxilliary label:
- FOR EXTERNAL USE ONLY.
- SHAKE WELL BEFORE USE.

Uses: Both zinc sulphate and sulphurated potash acts as astringents. Therefore White lotion is used as local astringent and protective. It is also used as an antiseptic, in the treatment of acne (pimples) and seborrhea.

PRECIPITATED SULPHUR LOTION

Rx	
Sulphuris precipitati	3 i s
Glyerini	fl. 3 i s
Sodium lauryl sulphate	gr iii sss
Alcoholis	fl. 3 iii sss
Aquam rosae...q.s......	fl. 3 xxv
Fiat : Lotio	Mitte : fl.oz i
Signa : Applicandus dolentiparti, sine teratur.	

Conversion :

3 i s → 1.25 drachms — gr iii sss → 3.75 grains

1 drachm = 4 g — 15 grains = 1 g

1.25 drachms = 5 g — 3.75 grains = 0.25 g

fl. 3 iii sss → 3.75 fl. dr = 15 ml

fl. 3 i s → 1.25 fl. dr = 5 ml — fl. 3 xxv → 25 fl. dr = 100 ml

Calculation : For fl.oz i → 1 fl.oz = 30 ml

Precipitated sulphur $= \frac{5}{100} \times 30 = 1.5$ g

Glycerin $= \frac{5}{100} \times 30 = 1.5$ ml

Sodium lauryl sulphate $= \frac{0.25}{100} \times 30 = 0.075$ g

Alcohol $= \frac{15}{100} \times 30 = 4.5$ ml

Rose water... q.s. ... = 30 ml

Type	Ingredients	Quantity in imperial	Quantity in metric	Quantity taken
Biphasic liquid,	Precipitated sulphur	1.25 dr	5 g	1.5 g
for external	Glycerin	1.25 fl. dr	5 ml	1.5 ml
use.	Sodium lauryl sulphate	3.75 gr	0.25 g	0.075 g
	Alcohol (95%)	3.75 fl. dr	15 ml	4.5 ml
Suspension.	Rose water.....q.s.....	25 fl. dr	100 ml	30 ml
	Make: lotion Send: 30 ml			
Shake lotion.	Direction: Apply to the effected part, without rubbing.			

Theory :

Precipitated sulphur lotion is an example for "shake lotion" i.e. aqueous suspension is prepared without a suspending agent, but it is prepared by using a surfactant, sodium lauryl sulphate and wetting agent like glycerin.

Precipitated sulphur is hydrophobic in nature, hence it is poorly miscible and wetted by water. Therefore surfactant like sodium lauryl sulphate is used, which reduces the surface tension.

Glycerin improves the wettability of precipitated sulphur and makes uniform dispersion in the rose water. Glycerin also acts as humectant and soothing agent. Alcohol gives cooling sensation, due to evaporation after its application. Rose water is used as vehicle and also as flavouring agent, to give a pleasant odour to the lotion.

Since the preparation is for external use only, Industrial methylated spirit may be used instead of alcohol (95%).

Procedure:

1) Mix glycerin, sodium lauryl sulphate and alcohol together by stirring.
2) Triturate the precipitated sulphur with the above mixture, in a mortar by adding drop by drop, to achieve maximum wetting, before aqueous solution is added.
3) Add rose water to make it pourable. Transfer to a measure, rinse the mortar and pestle with rose water, add to the measure and make up the final volume by adding sufficient amount of rose water.

Dispensing: Sulphur is sensitive to the light and contains highly volatile solvent like alcohol (95%). Hence transfer the lotion to a amber coloured, narrow mouthed, fluted glass bottle, close thoroughly with plastic screw cap, polish and label.

Direction: Apply to the effected part, without rubbing.

Storage: It should be stored in a cool and dark place away from naked flame, because it contains highly inflammable alcohol (95%).

Auxilliary label:

- FOR EXTERNAL USE ONLY.
- SHAKE WELL BEFORE USE.
- STORE IN A COOL AND DARK PLACE, AWAY FROM FLAME.

Uses: Precipitated sulphur acts as antiseptic and astringent. Therefore this lotion is used in the treatment of seborrhoea, psoriasis, acne (pimples) scabies and as a mild astringent and keratolytic agent.

Advice for patient when dispensed:

Clean the skin before use and apply to the affected area. The treatment should be discontinued, if excessive dryness or irritation occurs.

Other examples for Lotions

1) Cetrimide lotion:

Cetrimide	1 mg
Purified water... q.s...	100 ml

Uses: This lotion is used as antibacterial.

2) Gentian violet lotion:

Gentian violet	1 g
Ethanol (95%)	10 ml
Purified water..q.s..	100 ml

Uses: This lotion is used as antiseptic.

3) Zinc sulphate lotion:

Zinc sulphate	1 g
Amaranth solution	1 ml
Purified water q.s	100 ml

Uses: This lotion is used as astringent and protective.

4) Copper and zinc sulphate lotion:

Copper sulphate	9.14 g
Zinc sulphate	13.7 g
Camphor water..q.s.	1000 ml

Uses: This lotion useful for the treatment of impetigo, due to the astringent action of both Copper and Zinc sulphate.

5) Salicylic acid and mercuric chloride lotion:

Salicylic acid	2 g
Mercuric chloride	0.1 g
Castor oil	1 ml
Acetone	12.5 ml
Alcohol (95%)..q.s.	100 ml

Uses: This lotion is used as astringent, keratolytic and antiseptic.

Student's exercise:

1) Define lotions and how will you apply lotion?
2) Why Glycerin is used as a common ingredient in lotions?
3) What is humectant? Give example.
4) What types of medicaments are used in lotions ? give examples.
5) What is the meaning of "Shake lotions"?
6) What type of containers should be used for lotions and why ?
7) What is "White Lotion"? Write its ingredients and use.
8) What is calamine? Why calamine lotion is in pink colour ?
9) What is bentonite? Why it is used in calamine lotion ?
10) What are functions of sodium citrate in calamine lotion?
11) What is the meaning of S.O.S.?
12) What is the use of Salicylic acid?
13) Explain in brief, the principle involved in "White lotion".
14) Differentiate between lotions and liniments.
15) Why glycerin is used in precipitated sulphur lotion ?
16) Comments : Lotions require auxilliary label " Shake well before use" on their label.

23 LINIMENTS

Latin term: Linimentum

Liniments are alcoholic or oily liquid preparations or emulsions meant for external application to the unbroken skin. They are generally used for their rubifacient, counter irritant, mild astringent, analgesic, stimulating and penetrating effects of drugs, on the external parts of the body. Mostly they are rubbed into the skin but some are applied on a warm dressing or with a brush.

Liniments may be alcoholic or oily preparations. The type of liniment depends on the vehicle used for its preparation. Two types of vehicles are used for liniment preparations.

1) Alcohol: (Alcoholic liniments)

In this type of liniment, alcohol is used as a vehicle, which also acts as permeation enhancer to increase the penetration of medicaments into the skin and also has counter irritant, rubificient action. Therefore alcoholic liniments are used when rubifacient, counter irritant, penetrating or stimulating effect is required (essentiial).

Eg :
- Aconite liniment,
- Soap liniment.

Alcoholic liniments are irritant in nature, due to the presence of high percentage of alcohol. Hence these should not be applied to the broken skin. In certain cases, spreading of alcoholic liniment is improved by using soap.

2) Oils: (Oily liniments)

In this type of liniments, oil is used as vehicle. These liniments are used when the milder action or just massage is required, on the affected part.

Fixed oils like arachis oil, almond oil, seasame oil and cottonseed oil are used in oily liniments. Oily liniments are less irritant than alcoholic liniments and spread more easily.

Eg :
- Camphor liniment,
- Methyl salicylate liniment.

Perfumes: Since liniments are externally used preparations, their aesthetic characteristics can be improved by adding some pleasantly flavored oils like – Jasmine oil, Lemon oil.

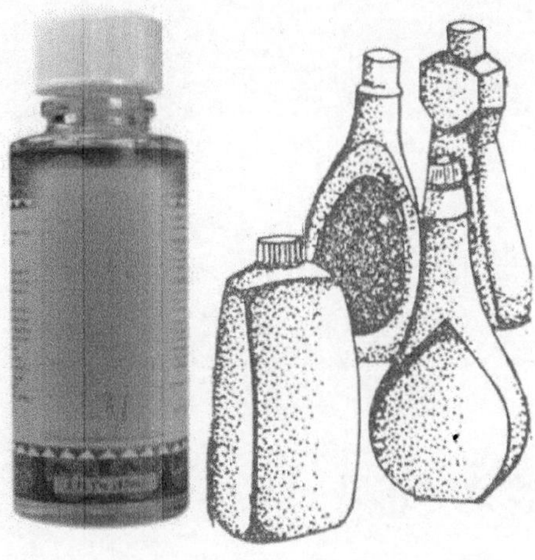

Containers for Liniments

Dispensing: Liniments should be dispensed in amber coloured, narrow mouthed bottle, tightly closed with coloured plastic screw cap, to distinguish them from preparations, which are meant for internal (oral) use. If liniment has semisolid consistency, that should be dispensed in wide mouthed bottle and supply with an applicator.

Label: Label of liniments should bear necessary requirements of liquid dosage forms. In addition, it should contain auxilliary label like,

- FOR EXTERNAL USE ONLY,
- NOT TO BE APPLIED ON BROKEN SKIN,
- SHAKE WELL BEFORE USE,
- STORE IN A COOL AND DARK PLACE, AWAY FROM FLAME,

OR

- HIGHLY INFLAMMABLE.

Storage: Liniments contain volatile ingredients and alcohol, hence it should be stored in a cool and dark place and keep away from flame.

TURPENTINE LINIMENT

Rx

Soft soap	3 ii s
Camphorae	3 i s
Olei terebinthinae	fl.oz ii
Aquam.....q.s....	fl. 3 xxv
Fiat : Linimentum	Mitte: fl.oz i

Signa : Infricandus parti affectae, dolore urgente.

Conversion :

3 ii s → 2.25 drachms	fl.oz ii → 2 fl.oz
1 drachm = 4 g	1 fl.oz = 30 ml
2.25 drachms = 9 g	2 fl.oz = 60 ml
3 i s → 1.25 drachms = 5 g	fl. 3 xxv → 25 fl. dr = 100 ml

Calculation : For fl.oz i → 1 fl.oz = 30 ml

Soft soap $= \frac{9}{100} \times 30 = 2.7$ g

Camphor $= \frac{5}{100} \times 30 = 1.5$ g

Turpentine oil $= \frac{60}{100} \times 30 = 18$ ml

Water ....q.s......... = 30 ml

Type	Ingredients	Quantity in imperial	Quantity in metric	Quantity taken
O/W type of emulsion.	Soft soap	2.25 dr	9 g	2.7 g
	Camphor	1.25 dr	5 g	1.5 g
	Turpentine oil	2 fl.oz	60 ml	18 ml
	Purified water....q.s...	25 fl. dr	100 ml	30 ml
	Make: Liniment Send: 30 ml			
	Direction: To be rubbed on affected part, if pain is sever.			

Theory :

Turpentine oil is a volatile oil, obtained from distillation of turpentine, which is an oleo-resin obtained from various species of pinus. Turpentine oil is not miscible with water and it doesn't contain any free fatty acids, hence it cannot form soap with alkaline substances. Therefore soft soap has been used, which is a monovalent soap, alkaline in nature and acts as an emulsifying agent.

Camphor is a volatile substance, it is insoluble in water but soluble in turpentine oil. Hence biphasic system like emulsion can be prepared using soft soap, which produces (o/w) type of emulsion. In this preparation, turpentine oil remains as dispersed phase and water as continuous phase. Due to the formation of viscous emulsion (oily liniment), it will be easy for rubbing on the skin.

Procedure:

1) In a dry container (dry measure) dissolve camphor in turpentine oil.
2) Take the required quantity of soft soap in a mortar, add water and triturate. Make a soapy solution. To this solution gradually add, the camphor solution with trituration until a thick creamy emulsion is formed. Allow it to stand for few minutes, for the separation of air bubbles.
3) Add sufficient purified water to produce final volume.

Dispensing: Both turpentine oil and camphor are volatile in nature. Turpentine oil undergoes rapid change, when come in contact with air and moisture. Therefore transfer the preparation to a narrow mouthed, light resistant glass bottle, close it tightly with a plastic screw cap, polish, label and supply with an applicator.

Direction: To be rubbed on affected part, if pain is sever.

Storage: Store in a dry place and protect from light.

Auxilliary label:
- FOR EXTERNAL USE ONLY.
- NOT TO BE APPLIED ON BROKEN SKIN.
- SHAKE WELL BEFORE USE.
- STORE IN A DRY PLACE, AWAY FROM LIGHT.

Uses:

1) Turpentine oil: acts as counter irritant and rubeficient.
2) Camphor: Externally it acts as a mild analgesic and rubeficient (It acts as a local *anodyne* by producing coolness). Hence used as counter irritant in the treatment of fibrositis and neuralgia.

   Internally it acts as a carminative.
3) Soft soap: It is an alkaline soap, acts as (o/w) type of emulsifying agent.

   Turpentine liniment is used as counter irritant and rubeficient. It is mainly used by the patients suffering from Arthralgia (pain in the joints),

   Myalgia (muscular pain),

   Fibrositis (ligamental pain) and Sprain.

Note:

1) Turpentine liniment (emulsion) tends to become aerated, after keeping aside for some time, then the volume occupied by it may be considerably more. Therefore strain through muslin cloth, which helps to remove air bubbles. But it is still good to keep the product aside, for some time before final adjustment of the volume.
2) Turpentine oil on exposure to air, under goes rapid changes, specially in presence of moisture and becomes viscous yellow and takes place acidic reaction, therefore freshly rectified oil should be used, for the preparation of liniment.

CAMPHOR LINIMENT I.P.

Rx

Camphorae	3 v
Arachis oil....q.s...	fl. 3 xx
Fiat : Linimentum	Mitte : fl.oz i
Signa : Infricandus dolenti parti S.O.S.	

Conversion :

3 v → 5 drachms	fl. 3 xx → 20 fl. dr
1 drachm = 4 g	1 fl. drachm = 4 ml
5 drachms = 20 g	20 fl. drachms = 80 ml

Calculation : For fl.oz i → 1 fl.oz = 30 ml

Camphor $= \frac{20}{100} \times 30 = 6$ g

Arachis oil... q.s. .... = 30 ml

Type	Ingredients	Quantity in imperial	Quantity in metric	Quantity taken
O/W type of emulsion	Camphor	5 dr	20 g	6 g
	Arachis oil....q.s....	20 fl. dr	80 ml	30 ml
	Make: Liniment Send: 30 ml Direction: To be rubbed on affected part, when ever necessary.			

Theory:

Camphor liniment contains 20 % w/w of camphor. Camphor is a volatile substance, obtained from wood of Cinnamonum camphora. It is available as colorless or white crystals, granules or crystalline mass. It is insoluble in water, but soluble in alcohol, chloroform, volatile oils and fixed oils.

In this preparation, arachis oil is used as a vehicle to dissolve camphor and to get a viscous preparation, which is suitable to spread (apply) on the skin.

Solubility of camphor in arachis oil is further increased, by heating (warming) on a warm water bath.

Procedure:

1) Accurately weigh camphor and dissolve in arachis oil, in a closed container by agitation.
2) Immerse the container in a warm water bath and constantly agitate, to increase the solubility of camphor in araches oil.

Dispensing: Camphor is volatile in nature, therefore transfer the preparation to a narrow mouthed, light resistant glass bottle, close it tightly with a plastic screw cap, polish, label and supply with an applicator.

Direction: To be rubbed on affected part, when ever necessary.

Storage: Since camphor is volatile in nature, high temperature may cause the volatilization of camphor. Hence it should be stored in a cool place,

Auxilliary label:

- FOR EXTERNAL USE ONLY.
- NOT TO BE APPLIED ON WOUNDS AND BROKEN SKIN.
- SHAKE WELL BEFORE USE.
- STORE IN A COOL PLACE.

Uses: Camphor liniment is used as an antipruritic and rubificient. It is also used as a counter irritant for inflammed joints, sprains, rheumatic and other inflammatory conditions such as cold in the throat and chest.

WHITE LINIMENT B.P. / B.P.C.

Synonym : Ammonium soap emulsion

Rx	
Acidi oleici	fl. 3 ii
Ammonii chloridi	M xx
Diluti liquoris ammoniae	fl. 3 i
Olei terebinthinae	fl. 3 vi
Aquam......q.s......	fl. 3 xxv
Fiat : Linimentum	Mitte : fl. oz i
Signa : Infricandus dolentiparti, dolere urgente.	

Conversion :

M xx → 20 minims — fl. 3 ii → 2 fl. drachms

15 minims = 1 ml — 1 fl. drachm = 4 g

20 minims = 1.2 ml — 2 fl. drachms = 8 g

fl. 3 vi → 6 fl. drachms = 24 ml

fl. 3 xxv → 25 fl. drachms = 100 ml

Calculation : For fl. oz i → 1 fl.oz = 30 ml

Oleic acid $= \frac{2}{100} \times 30 = 2.4$ ml

Ammonium chloride $= \frac{1.2}{100} \times 30 = 0.36$ ml

Dilute solution of ammonia $= \frac{4}{100} \times 30 = 1.2$ ml

Turpentine oil $= \frac{24}{100} \times 30 = 7.2$ ml

Purified water.....q.s.... = 30 ml

Type	Ingredients	Quantity in imperial	Quantity in metric	Quantity taken
O/W type of emulsion.	Oleic acid	2 fl. dr	8 ml	2.4 ml
	Ammonium chloride	20 minims	1.25 ml	0.36 ml
	Dilute ammonia solution	1 fl. dr	4 ml	1.2 ml
	Turpentine oil	6 fl. dr	24 ml	7.2 ml
	Water......q.s......	25 fl. dr	100 ml	30 ml
	Make: Liniment Send: 30 ml Direction: To be rubbed to the affected part, if pain is sever.			

Theory:

Turpentine oil does not contain any free fatty acids, hence it cannot form soap with alkaline substance. Therefore in this preparation, oleic acid is used, which consists sufficient free fatty acids, hence forms soap with alkali like dilute solution of ammonia and produces the soap --- ammonium oleate.

Ammonium oleate acts as an emulsifying agent and produces (o/w) type of emulsion. But due to the presence of ammonium chloride, which produce common ion effect and depresses the ionization of the soap and also decreases its solubility in water. This along with the high percentage of turpentine oil in the liniment, causes phase inversion and produces water in oil type of emulsion.

Procedure:

1) Measure turpentine oil, oleic acid and dilute solution of ammonia separately.
2) Mix turpentine oil and oleic acid in a large glass bottle. (i.e. 50 % larger than the prescribed volume).
3) Warm the water to 50°C. Add an equal volume of warm water, to the dilute ammonia solution.
4) Add this dilute ammonia solution, in small portion to the above oily mixture and shake vigorously after each addition, in the bottle.
5) Dissolve ammonium chloride in the remaining amount of purified water, add this solution to the above emulsion and shake the bottle vigorously, untill a homogenous emulsion is produced.

Dispensing: Turpentine oil is volatile in nature, therefore transfer the preparation to a narrow mouthed, light resistant (blue or amber coloured) bottle, close it tightly with a plastic screw cap, polish, label and supply with an applicator.

Direction: To be rubbed to the affected part, if pain is sever.

Storage: Since turpentine oil is volatile in nature, high temperature may cause the volatilization. Therefore it should be stored in a cool place, away from light and flame.

Auxilliary label:

- FOR EXTERNAL USE ONLY,
- NOT TO BE APPLIED ON BROKEN SKIN,
- SHAKE WELL BEFORE USE,
- STORE IN A COOL PLACE AWAY FROM LIGHT AND FLAME.

Uses: It is used as a rubificient and counter irritant, for relief of rheumatic pains and stiffness.

AMMONIATED CAMPHOR LINIMENT

Rx	
Olei eucalypti	M vii ss
Camphorae	3 iii
Liquoris ammoniae fortis	fl. 3 vi
Alcoholis...q.s...	fl. 3 xxv
Fiat : Linimentum	Mitte : fl.oz ii
Signa : Infricandus dolentiparti S.O.S.	

Conversion :

M vii ss → 7.5 minims	fl. 3 vi → 6 fl. drachms
15 minims = 1 ml	1 fl. drachms = 4 ml
7.5 minims = 0.5 ml	6 fl. drachms = 24 ml
fl. 3 xxv →25 fl. dr = 100 ml	3 iii → 3 drachms
	1 drachm = 4 g
	4 drachms = 12 g

Calculation : For fl.oz → 2 fl.oz = 60 ml

Eucalyptus oil $= \frac{0.5}{100} \times 60 = 0.3\,ml$

Camphor $= \frac{12}{100} \times 60 = 7.2\,g$

Ammonia solution strong $= \frac{24}{100} \times 60 = 14.4\,ml$

Alcohol......q.s.... = 60 ml

Type	Ingredients	Quantity in imperial	Quantity in metric	Quantity taken
O/W type of emulsion.	Eucalyptus oil	7.5 minims	0.5 ml	0.3 ml
	Camphor	3 dr	12.0 g	7.2 g
	Ammonia solution strong	6 fl. dr	24 ml	14.4 ml
	Alcohol (90%)....q.s....	25 fl. dr	100 ml	60 ml
	Make: Liniment Send: 60ml			
	Direction: To be rubbed on the affected part, whenever necessary.			

Theory:

Eucalyptus oil is a volatile oil obtained by distillation from, fresh leaves of Eucalyptus globulus. Both eucalyptus oil and camphor are not soluble in water. But they are soluble in alcohol (90%). Hence alcohol is used as a vehicle and also as permeation enhancer, to increase the penetration power of the preparation, through the skin.

Strong ammonia solution acts as a counter irritant and rubificient. Eucalyptus oil is used as a flavouring agent and rubificient.

In this preparation, camphor and eucalyptus oil are dissolved in major part of alcohol and then to this solution, aqueous solution of strong ammonia is added gradually with shaking after each addition. After addition of ammonia solution, a part of camphor will be precipitate out, but it is diffusible in nature, hence it will be redissolved after shaking.

Procedure:

1) Dissolve eucalyptus oil and camphor in 3/4th of total volume of alcohol 90%, in a closed vessel by shaking.
2) Add the strong ammonia solution and shake vigorously, to get uniform mixture.
3) Add the remaining portion of alcohol (90%), to adjust the final volume and mix it well

Dispensing: Eucalyptus oil, camphor and ammonia solution all are volatile in nature. Therefore to prevent their volatilazation, transfer the preparation to a narrow mouthed, light resistant glass bottle, close it tightly with a plastic screw cap, polish and label.

Direction: To be rubbed on the affected part, whenever necessary.

Storage: Store in a cool place.

Auxilliary label:
- FOR EXTERNAL USE ONLY.
- NOT TO BE APPLIED ON WOUNDS AND BROKEN SKIN.
- SHAKE WELL BEFORE USE.
- STORE IN A COOL AND DARK PLACE.

Uses: Eucalyptus oil acts as rubificient and flavouring agent, it also gives a sensation of cold. Camphor acts as a counter irritant and rubificient. Alcohol acts as vehicle and also as permeation enhancer, therefore Ammoniated camphor liniment is used as counter irritant and rubificient.

Student's exercise:

1) Define liniments.
2) Classify the liniments with examples.
3) Comment : Liniments are applied with rubbing (friction).
4) What types of drugs are used in liniments?
5) Define: Counter irritants, Irritants, Rubifacients and Stimulants with examples.
6) Comment : Liniments can be applied to the open wounds and cut parts.
7) Why oily liniments are preferred, than alcoholic liniments?
8) How will supply the liniments?
9) Comment: Liniments are flavoured using flavouring oil.
10) What auxilliary label you will mention on the label of liniment ?

11) Write the uses of camphor and terpentine oil in terpentine liniment.
12) Define myalgia and arthritis.
13) Comment: For preparation of Terpentine liniment, freshly rectified terpentine oil should be used.
14) Comment : Liniments should be stored in air tight containers.
15) What is White liniment? Write its ingredients and use.
16) Why oleic acid is used in white liniment ?
17) What is the use of Eucalyptus oil in liniment ?
18) Differentiate lotions and liniments.

24 COLLODIONS

Latin term: Collodium

Collodions are clear or slightly opalescent liquid preparations, meant for external application to the skin. Collodion consists a film forming substance, nitrocellulose (pyroxylin) in volatile solvents like alcohol, ether and acetone. After application of collodion, volatile solvent evaporates and leaves a thin, flexible transparent protective covering film on the affected part (site of application).

Collodions are applied to the skin, to close the small wounds, abrasions and cuts. It is also used to hold surgical dressings (wound dressings) in place and to keep medicaments in contact with the skin, for longer time (for sustained release or prolonged release of medicament). Collodions are applied either by brush or applicator.

Classification: Collodions are of two types,

1) **Non medicated collodions:** Contain only the collodion base, which is called as "Flexible collodion" or "Collodion base". It is a solution of pyroxylin, colophony and castor oil in a mixture of ether and alcohol. These collodions are used only, for protecting small cuts and abrasions.

2) **Medicated collodions:** These collodions contain medicament along with collodion base (flexible collodion). They provide prolonged contact between the skin and the medicament. These collodions are used to provide sustained source of keratolytic agents like, Salicylic acid in the treatment of corns and wrats.

   eg. Salicylic acid collodion.

Dispensing: Collodions are dispensed in small, light resistant, well closed containers, because they contain highly volatile solvents like ether and alcohol. The container should be small (capacity 5 to 10 ml) and closure must be air-tight, because in a larger bottle, the loss of solvent occurs when each time the cap is removed, which leads to a significant change in the concentration and solidification, before the preparation has been completely used. The cap should be fitted with a brush or a glass/plastic applicator.

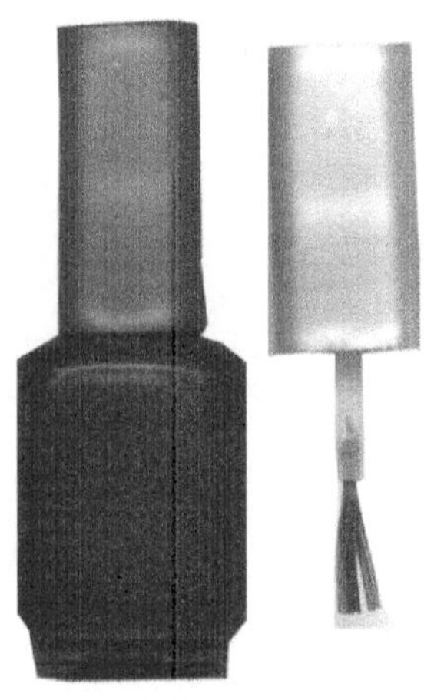

Container for collodion

Collodions contain pyroxylin, which is highly inflammable and they also contain highly volatile and inflammable solvents like alcohol and ether. Hence it is kept moist with industrial methylated spirit and stored in well closed container.

Storage: Store in a cool and completely darkness and away from flame.

Examples: There are only two collodions are official,

1. Flexible collodion B.P.
2. Salicylic acid collodion BPC.

FLEXIBLE COLLODION B.P.

Formula for collodion :

Rx	
Pyroxillin	3 ii ss
Alcoholis (90%)	fl. 3 v ss
Solvent ether...q.s...	fl. 3 xxv
Fiat : Collodium	Mitte : 3 ii ss
Signa : Use as base for preparation of flexible collodion.	

Conversion :

3 ii ss $\rightarrow$ 2.5 drachms   fl. 3 v ss $\rightarrow$ 5.5 fl.dr = 22 ml

1 drachm = 4 g   fl. 3 xxv $\rightarrow$ 25 fl.dr =100 ml

2.5 drachms = 10 g

Calculation for collodion : For fl. 3 ii ss $\rightarrow$ 2.5 fl. drachms = 10 ml

Pyroxillin $= \frac{10}{100} \times 10 = 1$ g

Alcohol $= \frac{22}{100} \times 10 = 2.2$ ml

Solvent ether......q.s.... = 10 ml

Formula for Flexible collodion :

Rx	
Colophony	gr xxxvii ss
Olei recini	M xxxvii ss
Collodium...q.s...	3 xxv
Fiat : Flexible collodium	Mitte : 3 ii ss
Signa: Cum penicillo parti affectae applicandus.	

Conversion :

M xxxvii ss $\rightarrow$ 37.5 minims   gr xxxvii ss $\rightarrow$ 37.5 gr

15 minims = 1 ml   15 grains = 1 g

37.5 minims = 2.5 ml   37.5 grains = 2.5 g

Calculation for Flexible collodion : For fl. 3 ii ss $\rightarrow$ 2.5 fl.drachms = 10 ml

Colophony $= \frac{2.5}{100} \times 10 = 0.25$g

Castor oil $= \frac{2.5}{100} \times 10 = 0.25$ ml

Collodion........q.s...... = 10 ml

Type	Ingredients	Quantity in imperial	Quantity in metric	Quantity taken
Monophasic liquid for external use	Colophony	37.5 dr	2.5 g	0.25 g
	Castor oil	37.5 minims	2.5 ml	0.25 ml
	Collodion ...q.s....	25 fl. dr	100 ml	10 ml
	Make: Collodion	Send: 10 ml		
	Direction: Apply with brush to the affected part, as directed.			

Theory:

Flexible collodion is a solution of colophony in a mixture of castor oil and collodion.

This is a non-medicated collodion, used for giving protective covering to small cuts and abrasions or to hold any dressing or applied medicament, for longer time.

Pyroxylin is a nitrocellulose obtained by treating defatted cotton (raw cotton) with a mixture of nitric acid and sulphuric acid at 15 °C.

$$\underset{\text{Cellulose (Cotten wool)}}{C_{12}H_{14}O_4(OH)_6} + \underset{\text{Nitric acid}}{4HNO_3} \xrightarrow{H_2SO_4} \underset{\text{Nitro cellulose}}{C_{12}H_{14}O_4(NO_3)_4(OH)_2} + 4H_2O$$

Pyroxylin resembles cotton wool but it is harsher to touch. It is also called as 'collodion cotton', 'soluble gun cotton', 'nitrocellulose' or 'cellulose tetra nitrate'. It is highly inflammable in nature.

Collodion is prepared by dissolving pyroxylin in a mixture of alcohol (90%) and solvent ether. This collodion is used as a base (vehicle) for preparation of flexible collodion.

When only collodion is applied to the skin, it forms an inflexible film and it may not stick on the applied part for longer time. Hence to stick on the applied part for longer time, flexible collodion is prepared by incorporating castor oil and colophony with collodion base.

Castor oil gives flexibility to the film. Colophony helps in sticking of the film to the skin and it also makes the preparation water proof. Hence this preparation is called as "Flexible collodion".

Procedure:

A) Preparation of collodion:

Formula for collodion	Quantity given	Quantity taken for 10 ml
Pyroxylin	10 g	1 g
Alcohol (90%)	22 ml	2.2 ml
Solvent ether..q.s...	100 ml	10 ml

1) In a container, take accurately weighed amount of pyroxylin.
2) To this, add measured amount of alcohol (90%) and solvent ether. Close the container thoroughly and shake vigorously until pyroxylin dissolves.

3) Keep the solution aside for few days, to allow settling of impurities of pyroxylin. Since preparation is highly volatile in nature, impurities cannot be removed by filtration. Therefore decant the supernatant liquid and cool the collodion.

B) Preparation of Flexible collodion :

1) In a container, take accurately weighed amount of colophony.
2) To this, add measured amount of castor oil and dissolve by stirring.
3) Measure the required amount of collodion and add to the above content, close the container thoroughly and shake well, until colophony dissolves completely.
4) Keep the preparation aside for certain time, to allow the impurities to settle down.

Dispensing: Decant the supernatant liquid and immediately transfer to a light resistant (amber coloured), small volume (capacity 5-10 ml) bottle. Close throughly with cap, which is fitted with a brush or an applicator made up of glass or plastic, should be supplied separately.

Direction: Apply with brush to the affected part, as directed.

Storage: Flexible collodion contains highly inflammable pyroxylin and volatile solvents like ether and alcohol (90%). Hence it should be kept moist with 25% w/w of Industrial methylated spirit and stored at low temperature not exceeding 25 ºC, in completely dark place, away from flames.

Auxilliary label:
- FOR EXTERNAL USE ONLY
- STORE IN A COOL AND DARK PLACE.
- HIGHLY INFLAMMABLE
- KEEP AWAY FROM NAKED FLAMES

Uses: Flexible collodion is used as topical protectant, to cover the small cuts and abrasions. It is also used to hold surgical dressings in place, for prolonged action of the medicaments.

Note: Formula for preparation of pyroxillin

Cotton	--- 10 g
Sulphuric acid	--- 100 ml
Nitric acid	--- 100 ml

SALICYLIC ACID COLLODION B.P.

Rx	
Acidi salicylici	3 ii ss
Flexible collodium...q.s..	fl. 3 xxv
Fiat : Collodium	Mitte : fl. 3 ii ss
Signa : Cum penicillo, parti affectae applicandus, more dicto.	

Conversion :

3 ii ss → 2.5 drachms — fl. 3 xxv → 25 fl. dr

1 drachm = 4 g — 1 fl. dr = 4 ml

2.5 drachms = 10 g — 25 fl. dr = 100 ml

Calculation : For fl. 3 ii ss → 2.5 fl. dr = 10 ml

Salicylic acid = $\frac{10}{100} \times 10 = 1$ g

Flexible collodion ....q.s.... = 10 ml

Type	Ingredients	Quantity in imperial	Quantity in metric	Quantity taken
Monophasic liquid, for external use	Salicylic acid	2.5 dr	10 g	1 g
	Flexible collodion...q.s...	25 fl.dr	100 ml	10 ml
	Make: Collodion	Send: 10 ml		
	Direction: Apply to the affected part, with brush as directed.			

Theory:

Salicylic acid collodion contains 10% solution of salicylic acid, in flexible collodion. It is used as keratolytic in the treatment of warts and carns. Salicylic acid works by breaking down keratin(keratin is a protein, which forms a part of the skin structure). This results in shedding of skin cells from the affected area. In the treatment of wrats, the effect of salicylic acid is to remove the affected skin over a period of time, and then new healthy skin cells will grow underneath.

Salicylic acid is miscible with flexible collodion, due to the presence of high proportions of volatile solvents like ether and alcohol in it. Hence this collodion is prepared by simple solution method in a closed, light resistant container.

Procedure:

1) Accurately weigh salicylic acid and transfer to a previously calibrated amber coloured (light resistant) glass bottle.
2) To the above, add accurately measured quantity of flexible collodion and cap the bottle thoroughly.
3) Shake the bottle until, salicylic acid completely dissolves in flexible collodion.

Dispensing: Salicylic acid collodion should be dispensed in small volume (5-10 ml capacity), light resistant, well closed, well filled, container with screw cap, which is fitted with a brush or glass/plastic applicator, should be supplied separately.

Direction: Apply to the affected part with brush, as directed.

Storage: Store in a cool and dark place

Uses: It is used as keratolytic, in the treatment of wrats and in removal of corns, from the toes. It is also used in the treatment of verrucas, condyloma wart and calluses.

> **Note:** Because of high volatile nature of collodion, it should be always kept tightly closed after every use and withdrawing of the preparation should be done, as quickly as possible.

Student's exercise:

1) What is the Latin term for collodions?
2) What is pyroxillin. How it obtained ?
3) Why collodions are used ?
4) What are common ingredients of collodions?
5) How will you apply collodions?
6) Classify the collodions with examples.
7) Give the dispensing technique for collodions.
8) What is the storage condition for collodions? explain with reason.
9) Comment : Collodions is kept moist with industrial methylated spirit.
10) What is the function of alcohol in collodions?
11) What is flexible collodion and colopony?
12) Why castor oil is used in preparation flexible collodion?
13) What is use of salicylic acid collodion ?
14) Write the direction for salicylic acid collodion in Latin.

25 PAINTS

Latin term : Pigmentum

Paints are liquid preparations, applied to the skin or mucous membrane with a soft brush. If paints are applied to the mucous membrane of the throat, then they are called as "Throat paints".

If paints are applied externally to the skin, they are called simply as "paints" (skin paints). Paints should not be used as throat paints.

Paints may contain volatile solvent, that evaporates quickly and leaves a dry or resinous film of the medicament. This resinous film adheres to the affected site and prolongs the action of the medicament. Paint contains medicaments like antiseptics, astringents, analgesics, caustic and resinous substances like benzoin, storex or tolubalsam.

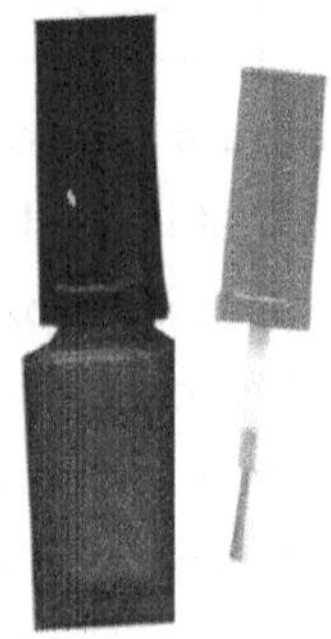

Container for paints

Examples for paints:

1) Crystal violet paint.
2) Coal tar paint
3) Podophyllum paint
4) Mastic paint

Dispensing:

Since paints contain highly volatile solvents, they are dispensed in air tight, amber coloured, narrow mouthed, small glass bottle, closed with the cap, which is fitted with a brush for application. The closure should contain wad and liner, because organic solvents and other ingredients may attack the cork or certain plastic closures.

Direction: Label should contain direction to the patients, about its application.

Example: Applied with brush, as directed.

Storage: Paints should be stored in a cool place. If preparation is very sensitive to the light, then it should be stored in a cool and dark place.

Label: Label of paints should bear necessary requirements of liquid dosage forms. In addition, it should contain auxilliary labels like,

- FOR EXTERNAL USE ONLY.
- STORE IN A COOL AND DARK PLACE.

CRYSTAL VIOLET AND BRILLIANT GREEN PAINT

Synonym : Corn solvent

Rx	
Crystal violet	gr vii ss
Brilliant Green	gr vii ss
Ethanol (90%)	fl. 3 xii ss
Purified water....q.s...	fl. dr xxv
Fiat : Pigmentum	Mitte : fl.oz i
Signa: Cum penicillo parti affectae applicandus, more dicto.	

Conversion :

gr vii ss → 7.5 grains	fl. 3 xii ss → 12.5 fl. drachms
15 grains = 1 g	1 dl. drachm = 4 ml
7.5 grains = 0.5 g	12.5 fl. drachms = 50 ml
	fl. 3 CCL → 250 fl.dr = 1000 ml

Calculation : For fl.oz i → fl.oz 1 = 30 ml

Crystal violet $= \frac{0.5}{100} \times 30 = 0.15$ g

Brilliant Green $= \frac{0.5}{100} \times 30 = 0.15$ g

Ethanol $= \frac{50}{100} \times 30 = 15$ ml

Purified water .....q.s... = 30 ml

Type	Ingredients	Quantity in imperial	Quantity in metric	Quantity taken
Monophasic liquid, for external use.	Crystal violet	7.5 gr	0.5 g	0.15 g
	Brilliant Green	7.5 gr	0.5 g	0.15 g
	Ethanol (90%)	12.5 fl. dr	50 ml	15 ml
	Purified water...q.s....	25 fl. dr	100 ml	30 ml
	Make: Paint	Send: 20 ml		
	Direction: Apply with brush on the affected part, as directed			

Theory:

Crystal violet is also called as Gentian violet, it acts as antiseptic. Brilliant green acts as bacteriostatic. Both are soluble in water and forms a homogenous solution. It is prepared by simple solution method. Alcohol is used to get quick evaporation and cooling sensation, after application to the skin.

Procedure:

1) Accurately weigh crystal violet and brilliant green and transfer, to a previously tared amber coloured bottle.
2) Add measured amount of alcohol (90%). Close the container tightly and dissolve by vigorous shaking, then adjust the final volume with purified water.

Dispensing: This paint contains highly volatile solvent like ethanol (90%) and crystal violet is sensitive to the light, hence it should be dispensed in air tight, amber coloured, narrow mouthed, small glass bottle with the cap, which is fitted with a brush for application. The closure should contain wad liner, because organic solvents and other ingredients may attack the cork or certain plastic closures.

Direction: Apply with brush on the affected part, as directed

Storage: Crystal violet is sensitive to light and temperature. Hence the paint should be stored in a cool and dark place

Auxilliary label:

- FOR EXTERNAL USE ONLY
- STORE IN A COOL AND DARK PLACE

Uses: The paint is used as antiseptic and bacteriostatic, in the treatment of skin diseases.

COMPOUND PODOPHYLLUM PAINT

Rx	
Podophyllum resin	ʒ iii sss
Compound benzoin tincture..q.s..	fl. ʒ xxv
Fiat : Pigmentum	Mitte : fl.oz i
Signa : Parti affeatae bis - ter in die applicandus.	

Conversion :

ʒ iii sss → 3.75 drachms — ʒ xxv → 25 fl. drachms

1 drachm = 4 g — 1 fl. drachm = 4 ml

3.75 drachms = 15 g — 25 fl. drachms = 100 ml

Calculation : For fl.oz i → 1 fl.oz = 30 ml

Podophyllum resin = $\frac{15}{100} \times 30 = 4.5$ g

Compound benzoin tincture ...q.s.. = 30 ml

Type	Ingredients	Quantity in imperial	Quantity in metric	Quantity taken
Monophasic liquid, for external use	Podophyllum resin	3.75 dr	15 g	4.5 g
	Compound benzoin tincture.q.s.	25 fl. dr	100 ml	30 ml
	Make: Paint	Send: 30 ml		
	Direction: Apply on the affected part, two - three times a day.			

Theory:

Podophyllum resin is a powdered mixture of resins, extracted from Podophyllum by percolation with alcohol. It has cytotoxic action, hence used in the treatment of venereal warts. It is also caustic in nature. Compound tincture of benzoin is obtained by maceration of the mixture containing benzoin, prepared Storax, tolubalsum and aloes with alcohol (90%). It acts as protective and antiseptic.

Podophyllum resin is insoluble in water but, soluble in alcohol. compound tincture of benzoin consists of alcohol (90%), which is sufficient to dissolve podophyllum resin. Hence paint is prepared by simple solution method, by mixing podophyllum resin in compound tincture of benzoin.

After application of this paint, alcohol evaporates quickly by leaving a resinous film, which is not easily removed by washing and will be remained adhere, at the site of application, for prolonged period.

Procedure:

1) Accurately weigh podophyllum resin and triturate with small portion of compound tincture of benzoin in a mortar, until to get a smooth paste and then, add little more tincture of benzoin, to make it pourable.

Dispensing: Transfer to a previously tared, amber coloured, narrow mouthed, small volume glass bottle and make up the final volume with sufficient amount of compound tincture of benzoin, close it tightly with plastic screw cap, fitted with brush, and label.

Direction: Apply on the affected part two - three times a day.

Storage: Store in a cool and dark place, away from flame.

Auxilliary label:

- FOR EXTERNAL USE ONLY
- KEEP AWAY FROM CHILDREN
- IT IS VERY IRRITANT TO EYES
- STORE IN A COOL AND DARK PLACE, AWAY FROM FLAME **OR** HEAT

Uses: Compound podophyllum paint is used in the treatment of skin diseases like venereal warts. It is also used as antiseptic and protective.

> **Note:** Podophyllum resin is caustic in nature, hence it is highly irritating to the eyes and mucous membrane. Therefore label should bear the warning (caution) that "It is very irritant to the eyes, do not apply near to the eyes and keep away from children".

Student's exercise:

1) Define paints, Give examples.
2) How paints are differ form throat paints ?
3) For what purpose paints are used?
4) Paints consists what type of medicaments? Give examples.
5) How will you supply the paints and how will you apply ?
6) What are the differences between paints and collodions?
7) What are crystal violet and Brillant green? write their uses.
8) Comment : Alcohol is used as a common ingredient in paints.
9) What is the synonym for crystal violet paint?
10) What is Podophyllum? Why it is used in paints?
11) Define wrats, psoriasis and acne.
12) Define protective, antiseptic, bacteriostatic and bactericidal. Give examples for each.

26 OFFICIAL SOLUTIONS

Solutions are monophasic liquid preparations, which are used for many purposes. They may be sterile or unsterile solutions. Sterile solutions may be parenteral preparations, bladder irrigations, peritoneal dialysis, anticoagulant solutions and dermatological solutions for application to the broken skin. Unsterile solutions are used orally, either alone or as ingredients for medicinal preparations or they are used externally on unbroken surface of the skin.

Each official book (IP, BP, BPC,USP etc...) contains some solutions, which do not fit in to other class of solution. These solutions are called as "official solutions". These solutions are classified as,

A. Solutions for internal administration:

1. Some solutions are used orally either as such or as an ingredient.
   Eg.• Calciferol solution.
   • Aqueous iodine solution.
   • Solution of certain radio pharmaceuticals.
2. Some solutions are used orally, which contain medicaments.
   Eg.• Morphine hydrochloride solution.
   • Aromatic ammonia solution.
   • Strong ammonium acetate solution.
3. Some solutions used as a additives (excipients).
   Eg.• Dye solution for colouring tartrazine solution.
   • Sorbitol solution.
   • Benzoic acid solution.

B. Solutions for external application:

They are used alone or as an ingredient for other pharmaceutical preparations

Eg.• Aluminium acetate solution.
• Lead sub acetate solution.
• Calcium hydroxide solution.
• Coaltar solution.
• Ferric chloride solution.
• Potassium hydroxide solution.
• Sodium chloride solution.

C. Solutions used as antiseptic and disinfectant:

Many antimicrobial agents are represented as solutions.

Eg.• Benzalkonium chloride solution.
• Cresol with soap solution.
• Strong iodine solution.
• Weak iodine solution.
• Chlorhexidine gluconate solution.

- Potassium permanganate solution.
- Hydrogen peroxide solution.
- Formaldehyde solution.
- Cetrimide solution.
- Chlorinated soda solution.
- Chloroxylenol solution.

These solutions are either in concentrated or in dilute form which are suitable for pre- operative preparations of the skin, applications to mucosal membrane, wound and burn treatment, use in obstetrics, cleaning and disinfections of utensils (kichen wares) and general antisepsis in the home.

AQUEOUS IODINE SOLUTIONS I.P.

Rx	
Iodi	ʒ i s
Potassi iodidi	ʒ ii ss
Aquam....q.s.....	fl. ʒ xxv
Fiat : Liquor	Mitte : fl.oz i
Signa : Cochleare amplum, omni nocte sumendum.	

Conversion :

ʒ i s → 1.25 drachms   ʒ ii ss → 2.5 drachms = 10 g

1 drachm = 4 g

1.25 drachms = 5 g   fl. ʒ xxv → 25 fl. drachms = 100 ml

Calculation : For fl.oz i → 1 fl.oz = 30 ml.

Iodine $= \frac{5}{100} \times 30 = 1.5$ g

Potassium iodine $= \frac{10}{100} \times 30 = 3$ g

Purified water.....q.s..... = 30 ml

Type	Ingredients	Quantity in imperial	Quantity in metric	Quantity taken
Solution, for internal use.	Iodine	1.25 dr	5 g	1.5 g
	Potassium iodide	2.5 dr	10 g	3 g
	Purified water......q.s..	25 fl. dr	100 ml	30 ml
	Make: Solution Send: 30ml Direction: One tablespoonful to be taken, at every night.			

Theory :

Iodine is very slightly soluble in water (1:2950 parts). But it is soluble in water in presence of potassium iodide. Because iodine reacts with potassium iodide and forms complex called as "polyiodides". These polyiodides enhance the solubility of iodine and produce a stable aqueous iodine solution.

KI + I_2 ——————> $KI.I_2$ (Potassium mono iodide)

KI + $2I_2$ ——————> $KI.2I_2$ (Potassium di iodide)

KI + $3I_2$ ——————> $KI.3I_2$ (Potassium tri iodide)

Potassium iodide   Iodine   Polyiodides

OR

$$\underset{\text{Potassium iodide}}{KI} + \underset{\text{Iodine}}{nI_2} \longrightarrow \underset{\text{Polyiodides}}{KI.I_2 + KI\ 2I_2 + KI.3I_2 \ldots\ldots\ldots KI.nI_2}$$

Higher polyiodides are more soluble than lower polyiodides. Therefore to get higher polyiodides, the concentrated solution is prepared by dissolving iodine and potassium iodide in small portion of water, then it is diluted with the remaining portion of water, to adjust the final volume.

Procedure:

1) Weigh separately iodine and potassium iodide.
2) Triturate iodine in to fine powder in a glass mortar.
3) In a beaker, dissolve potassium iodide in small portion of water. To this solution, add iodine and dissolve by stirring continuously with glass rod.
4) When iodine dissolves completely, transfer this solution in to a measure, add sufficient quantity of purified water, to produce final volume.

Dispensing: Iodine is sensitive to the light and slowly volatalize at room temperature, hence transfer iodine solution in to an amber coloured (light resistant), narrow mouthed, glass bottle, close tightly with plastic screw cap, polish and label.

Direction: One tablespoonful to be taken, at every night.

Storage: Store in a cool and dark place.

Uses:

1) Internally Aqueous iodine solution is used as source of iodine, in the treatment of simple goiter. (Deficiency of iodine)
2) Externally it is used as antiseptic, because iodine prevents the microbial growth, by the process of oxidation or halogenation of bacterial cell protein.

Note:

1. Iodine stains as brown colour on the skin, cloths, and containers made up of porcelain and metals. Therefore, for the preparation of iodine solution, glass mortar should be used, instead of porcelain.
2. Metal spatula should not be used for handling of iodine and metallic containers should not be used for storing iodine preparations, because iodine being an oxidizing agent, it oxidizes iron and converts in to ferrous iodide.

   $$Fe + I_2 \longrightarrow FeI_2$$

   Hence plastic spoons should be used for handling and containers made up of plastic or glass should be used to store iodine preparations.
3. If necessary, iodine stains can be removed by using Sodium thiosulphate (Hypo solution).

WEAK IODINE SOLUTIONS IP

Synonym: Iodine tincture.

Rx	
Iodi	gr xxx
Potassi iodidi	gr xxxvii ss
Alcoholis (50%)...q.s....	fl. 3 xxv
Fiat : Liquor	Mitte : fl.oz i
Signa : Applicandus cum gossyp, super dolentiparti.	

Conversion :

gr xxx → 30 grains gr xxxvii ss → 37.5 grains

15 grains = 1 g 37.5 grains = 2.5 g

30 grains = 2 g

Calculation : For fl.oz i → 1 fl.oz = 30 ml.

Iodine $= \frac{2}{100} \times 30 = 0.6\,g$

Potassium iodine $= \frac{2.5}{100} \times 30 = 0.75\,g$

Alcohol (50%).....q.s.... = 30 ml

Type	Ingredients	Quantity in imperial	Quantity in metric	Quantity taken
Solution, for external use	Iodine	30 gr	2 g	0.6 g
	Potassium iodide	37.5 gr	2.5 g	0.75 g
	Alcohol (50%)...q.s....	25 fl. dr	100 ml	30 ml
	Make: Solution Send: 30 ml Direction: Apply with cotton (adsorbent), to the affected part.			

Theory :

In weak iodine solution, the concentration of iodine is 20 mg/ml and the percentage of alcohol is also high (50%). Therefore it is used externally as antiseptic, and also called as "Iodine tincture".

Iodine is slightly soluble in water. But it is freely soluble in alcohol. Iodine reacts with potassium iodide and forms complexes - polyiodides. These are highly soluble in water. Higher polyiodides are more soluble than lower polyiodides.

KI	+	I_2 ——————>	$KI.I_2$ (Potassium mono iodide)
KI	+	$2I_2$ ——————>	$KI.2I_2$ (Potassium di iodide)
KI	+	$3I_2$ ——————>	$KI.3I_2$ (Potassium tri iodide)
Potassium iodide		Iodine	Polyiodides

OR

KI	+	nI_2 ——————>	$KI.I_2 + KI\ 2I_2 + KI.3I_2 \ldots\ldots\ldots KI.nI_2$
Potassium iodide		Iodine	Polyiodides

Because of formation of polyiodides, free iodine does not react with ethyl alcohol to form ethyliodide, hydrogen iodide or acetaldehyde. Therefore antibacterial (antiseptic) activity of iodine will be remaining as such.

In this preparation, alcohol (90%) is used as vehicle for following reasons.

1) Alcohol enhances the antiseptic property of the preparation, because alcohol at higher strength (50%) acts as antiseptic.
2) Alcohol acts as permeation enhancer, because it dissolves the skin fats, which increases the pore size. Due to increased pore size, rate of absorption of iodine also increases.
3) Alcohol is volatile in nature. Hence when the tincture is applied on the skin, alcohol evaporates quickly, leaving behind the iodine in very fine particle size. Hence it helps in quicker absorption of iodine through the pores of the skin.
4) Iodine is freely soluble in alcohol. Hence it reduces the requirement of potassium iodide.

Procedure:

1) Accurately weigh iodine and triturate in a glass mortar to get fine powder.
2) In a beaker, dissolve potassium iodide and iodine in ¾ th quantity of alcohol (90%) with stirring.
3) Transfer this content to a measure, and adjust the final volume by adding remaining portion of alcohol.

Dispensing: Iodine is sensitive to the light and slowly volatalize at room temperature, hence transfer tincture of iodine in to an amber colored (light resistant), fluted, narrow mouthed, glass bottle, close tightly with plastic screw cap, polish and label.

Direction: Apply with cotton (adsorbent), to the affected part.

Storage: Store in a cool and dark place.

Auxilliary label: FOR EXTERNAL USE ONLY.

Uses: Weak iodine solution is used as an antiseptic (Tincture).

> **Note:** Due to the presence of high percentage of alcohol (50%), it gives irritating sensation when applied to the wounds or broken skin.

CRESOL WITH SOAP SOLUTION

Synonym: Lysol

Rx	
Cresol	fl. 3 xii ss
Vegetable oil	fl. 3 iv ss
Potassi hydroxidi	3 i
Aquam....q.s.....	fl. 3 xxv
Fiat : Liquor	Mitte : fl.oz ii
Signa : Utendus, more dicto.	

Conversion :

fl. 3 xii ss → 12.5 fl. drachms　　3 i → 1 drachm = 4 g

1 fl. drachm = 4 ml

12.5 fl. drachms = 50 ml　　fl. 3 xxv → 25 fl. dr = 100 ml

fl. 3 iv ss → 4.5 fl.drachms = 18 ml

Calculation : For fl.oz ii → 2 fl.oz = 60 ml.

Cresol $= \frac{50}{100} \times 60 = 3\,\text{ml}$

Vegetable oil $= \frac{18}{100} \times 60 = 10.8\,\text{ml}$

Potassium hydroxide $= \frac{4}{100} \times 60 = 2.4\,\text{g}$

Purified water....q.s...... = 60 ml

Type	Ingredients	Quantity in imperial	Quantity in metric	Quantity taken
Solution for, external use.	Cresol	12.5 fl. dr	50 ml	3 ml
	Vegetable oil	4.5 fl. dr	18 ml	10.8 ml
	Potassium hydroxide	1 dr	4 g	2.4 g
	Purified water.... q.s...	25 fl. dr	100 ml	60 ml
	Make: Solution	Send: 60 ml		
	Direction: To be used, as directed.			

Theory:

Lysol contains 50% v/v of cresol. But cresol has only 2% v/v solubility in water. Therefore the solubility of cresol is increased from 2% v/v to 50% v/v, by using a solubilizing agent – Soap.

Vegetable oils like arachis oil, linseed oil, cotton seed oil consists free fatty acids. These free fatty acids react with alkali like, sodium hydroxide or potassium hydroxide and forms soap. This soap acts as solubilizing agent (surfactant). In this case, soap forms laminar micelle, which takes up more of cresol and enhance the solubility of the cresol from 2% v/v to 50% v/v.

Procedure:

1) Dissolve potassium hydroxide, in ¼ th quantity of purified water.
2) In a small conical flask, take measured quantity of vegetable oil and potassium hydroxide solution, mix well.
3) Heat the mixture on a water bath with occasional stirring, until complete saponification takes place.
4) The completion of saponification reaction is tested by adding one drop of reaction mixture to the test tube containing water and shake well.
    a) If oil globules are not observed in water, it indicates that saponification reaction is completed.
    b) If oil globules are found in water, it indicates saponification is not yet complete. Then continue the heating.
5) After complition of saponification reaction, add measured quantity of cresol to the above mixture with continuous stirring.
6) Add this content to a measure and adjust the final volume with purified water and mix well.

Dispensing: Transfer the solution to a narrow mouthed, coloured, fluted, plastic bottle, close throughly with plastic screw cap, to distinguish it from the preparations meant for internal use, polish and label.

Direction: To be used, as directed.

Storage: Store in a cool place.

Auxilliary label: FOR EXTERNAL USE ONLY.

Uses: Cresol is a mixture of ortho, meta and para cresol. It acts as a disinfectant. Therefore Cresol with soap solution is used as disinfectant.

> **Note:** Cresol is a phenolic compound and hence caustic in nature. Due to its necrotic action to animal tissue, it should be handled carefully and should not be used as antiseptic for human beings.

STRONG AMMONIUM ACETATE SOLUTION I.P.

Rx	
Glacial acetic acid	fl.3 xi s
Ammonium bicarbonatis	3 xi sss
Ammonia strong solution	fl. 3 ii ss
Aquam.....q.s......	fl. 3 xxv
Fiat : Liquor	Mitte : fl.oz ii
Signa : Cochleare amplum, bis in die sumendum.	

Conversion :

fl. 3 xi s → 11.25 fl. drachms   3 xi sss → 11.75 dr = 47 g

1 fl. drachm = 4 ml

11.25 fl. drachms = 45 ml   fl. 3 xxv → 25 fl. drachms = 100 ml

fl. 3 ii ss → 2.5 fl. dr = 10 ml

Calculation : For fl.oz ii → 2 fl.oz = 60 ml.

Glacial acetic acid $= \frac{45}{100} \times 60 = 27$ ml

Ammonium bicarbonate $= \frac{47}{100} \times 60 = 28.2$ g

Ammonia strong solution $= \frac{10}{100} \times 60 = 6$ ml

Purified water....q.s...... = 60 ml

Type	Ingredients	Quantity in imperial	Quantity in metric	Quantity taken
Solution for, internal use.	Glacial acetic acid	11.25 fl. dr	45 ml	27 ml
	Ammonium bicarbonate	11.75 dr	47 g	28.2 g
	Ammonia solution strong	2.5 fl. dr	10 ml	6 ml
	Purified water....q.s......	25 fl. dr	100 ml	60 ml
	Make: Solution	Send: 60 ml		
	Direction: One tablespoonful to be taken, two times a day.			

Theory:

Strong ammonium acetate solution contains 57.5 % v/v of ammonium acetate. It is obtained by neutralization (acid-base) reaction between glacial acetic acid, ammonium bicarbonate and strong ammonia solution.

In this preparation, two alkali substances like, ammonium bicarbonate and strong ammonia solution are used, because only ammonium bicarbonate is not sufficient for complete neutralization of glacial acetic acid, so that at certain point, the reaction between these two substances ceases (stops) and desired product is not produced. Therefore strong ammonia solution is used, to neutralize the remaining glacial acetic acid and to make the preparation alkaline, which is having pH between 7.6 to 8.0.

CH_3COOH	+	NH_4HCO_3	→	$CH_3COONH_4 + H_2O + CO_2\uparrow$
Glacial acetic acid		Ammonium bicarbonate		Ammonium acetate
CH_3COOH	+	NH_4OH	→	$CH_3COONH_4 + H_2O$
Glacial acetic acid		Ammonium hydroxide		Ammonium acetate

For complete neutralization of glacial acetic acid, either ammonium bicarbonate or strong ammonia solution cannot be used in excess quantity. Because,

1) If we use only ammonium bicarbonate, it cannot neutralize the glacial acetic acid completely and also excess of ammonium bicarbonate, will settle at the bottom.
2) If we use strong ammonia solution to neutralize 45 g of glacial acetic acid, 100 ml of ammonia solution is required, which will increase the volume of the preparation.

Therefore, both ammonium bicarbonate and strong ammonia solutions are used in small quantities, for complete neutralization of glacial acetic acid and to make the preparation alkaline, which is having pH between 7.6 to 8.0.

For the adjustment of pH, two indicators such as, Bromothymol blue and Thymol blue are used, because these two indicators produce different colors, at different pH.

a) Bromothymol blue gives:
   Yellow at pH -6 → Green → Blue at pH -7.6
b) Thymol blue gives:
   Yellow at pH -8 → Blue at pH -9.6

Bromothymol blue indicates lower limit pH-7.6 and Thymol blue indicates upper limit pH-8.0. Neutralization point exists between pH 7.6 to 8.0. Therefore pH is maintained between 7.6 (blue with Bromothymol) and 8 (Yellow with Thymol blue).

Procedure:

1) Dilute the glacial acetic acid with ¼th of total volume of water, because ammonium bicarbonate does not reacts in concentrated solution.
2) In a large open vessel (mortar), dissolve ammonium bicarbonate in the dilute glacial acetic acid with continuous stirring, to allow the easy escape of carbon dioxide and avoid spillage of the solution, due to frothing.
3) Measure, strong ammonia solution and add drop by drop with stirring, until one drop of the resulting solution diluted with 10 drops of water gives,
   a) Full blue colour, with a drop of bromothymol blue and
   b) Full yellow colour, with a drop of thymol blue.
4) Then add sufficient amount of purified water, to make up the final volume, mix well.

Dispensing: Ammonium acetate solution dissolves lead salts, therefore transfer the solution to a narrow mouthed, lead free bottle, close it throughly, polish and label.

Direction: One tablespoonful to be taken, two times a day.

Storage: Store in a cool place.

Uses: Strong ammonium acetate solution is used as, diaphoretic (induce sweating) and mild expectorant.

ALUMINIUM SUB ACETATE TOPICAL SOLUTION U.S.P.

Rx	
Aluminii sulphatis	ʒ iii ss
Acetic acid	fl. ʒ ii
Precipitated calci carbonatis	ʒ iv
Aquam....q.s....	fl. ʒ xxv
Fiat : Liquor	Mitte : fl.oz i
Signa : Utendus, more dicto.	

Conversion :

ʒ iii ss → 3.5 drachms

1 drachms = 4 g

3.5 drachms = 14 g

ʒ iv → 4 drachms = 16 g

ʒ ii → 2 fl. drachms = 8 ml

ʒ xxv → 25 fl. drachms = 100 ml

Calculation : For fl.oz i → 1 fl.oz = 30 ml.

Aluminium sulphate $= \frac{14}{100} \times 30 = 4.2\,g$

Acetic acid $= \frac{8}{100} \times 30 = 2.4\,ml$

Precipitated calcium carbonate $= \frac{16}{100} \times 30 = 4.8\,g$

Purified water....q.s...... = 30 ml

Type	Ingredients	Quantity in imperial	Quantity in metric	Quantity taken
Solution for, external use.	Aluminium sulphate	3.5 dr	14 g	4.2 g
	Acetic acid	2 fl. dr	8 ml	2.4 ml
	Precipitated calcium carbonate	4 dr	16 g	4.8 g
	Purified water.......q.s.......	25 fl. dr	100 ml	30 ml
	Make: Solution Direction: To be used, as directed.	Send: 30 ml		

Theory:

Aluminium subacetate solution is obtained by the reaction between aluminium sulphate, acetic acid and precipitated calcium carbonate. In this preparation, the amount of acetic acid used is insufficient to form aluminium acetate, hence it results in the formation of aluminium subacetate.

Calcium carbonate is added, to remove free radicals of sulphate from the solution. Calcium carbonate reacts with sulphate ions of aluminium sulphate and forms insoluble precipitate of calcium sulphate, which is removed by filtration.

$$Al_2SO_4.18H_2O + 3\,CaCO_3 + 4\,CH_3COOH \rightarrow 2(CH_3COO)_2AlOH + 3\,CaSO_4 + CO_2\uparrow + 19H_2O$$

Aluminium sulphate	Calcium carbonate	Acetic acid	Aluminium subacetate	Calcium sulphate

Aluminium sulphate is freely soluble in cold water, than in hot (normal) water. Therefore cold water should be used, to dissolve aluminium sulphate.

Procedure:

1) Separately weigh aluminium sulphate and calcium carbonate.
2) Disperse calcium carbonate in a small portion of water, to make suspension.
3) Dissolve aluminium sulphate in half of the portion of cold water, because it is less soluble in hot water.
4) Filter the solution. To the filtrate, add calcium carbonate suspension with constant stirring.
5) Then slowly add, acetic acid with stirring and keep this mixture aside for 24 hours, to complete the reaction between aluminium sulphate and acetic acid.
6) After 24 hours, filter the product through "Buchner filter (funnel)," by applying vacuum and wash the precipitate with cold water, until the total filtrate measures the required volume.

Dispensing: Transfer the solution to a narrow mouthed, coloured, fluted, plastic or glass bottle, close throughly with plastic screw cap, to distinguish it from preparations meant for internal (oral) use, polish and label.

Direction: To be used, as directed.

Storage: Store in a cool place.

Auxilliary label: FOR EXTERNAL USE ONLY.

Uses: Aluminium subacetate solution is used externally as astringent, as a wash and as wet dressing for skin infections.

CALCIUM HYDROXIDE TOPICAL SOLUTION

Synonym : Lime water

Rx	
Calci hydroxidi	gr vii ss
Aquam (gelidae).....q.s.......	fl. 3 xxv
Fiat : Liquor	Mitte : fl.oz ii
Signa : Parti affectue bis - ter in die applicandus.	

Conversion :

gr vii ss → 7.5 grains	fl. 3 xxv → 25 fl. drachms
15 grains = 1 g	1 fl. drachm = 4 ml
7.5 grains = 0.5 g	25 fl. drachms = 100 ml

Calculation : For fl.oz ii → 2 fl.oz = 60 ml.

Calcium hydroxide $= \frac{0.5}{100} \times 60 = 0.3$ g

Purified water....q.s...... = 60 ml

Type	Ingredients	Quantity in imperial	Quantity in metric	Quantity taken
Solution for, external use.	Calcium hydroxide	7.5 gr	0.5 g	0.3 g
	Purified water(cold)...q.s..	25 fl. dr	100 ml	60 ml
	Make: Solution	Send: 60 ml		
	Direction: To be applied on affeced part, two - three times a day.			

Theory:

Calcium hydroxide is a simple solution, prepared by vigorously agitating calcium hydroxide with cold purified water. The excess amount of calcium hydroxide settles down and the clear supernatent liquid is seperated (decanted) out.

For the preparation of calcium hydroxide solution, temperature is very important. Because the solubility of calcium hydroxide is different, at different temperatures, as given below.

Temperature (°C)	Volume of water required to dissolve 1 g of calcium hydroxide
At 15°C	780 ml
At 25°C	714 ml
At 80°C	3000 ml

Calcium hydroxide has higher solubility at lower temperature. Therefore official calcium hydroxide solution is prepared by using cold water, at room temperature (25 °C).

Hydroxide ions of calcium hydroxide reacts with atmospheric CO_2 and convert into, precipitate of calcium carbonate as follows,

OH	+	CO_2	→	HCO_3^-		
OH	+	HCO_3^-	→	CO_3^-	+	H_2O
CO_3^-	+	Ca^{++}	→	$CaCO_3$		
		Calcium ions		ppt. of Calcium carbonate.		

Hence calcium hydroxide solution should be stored in well filled, airtight container, at temperature not exceeding 25°C.

Therefore for the preparation of any pharmaceutical product, freshly prepared calcium hydroxide solution should be used.

Procedure:

1) Weigh accurately calcium hydroxide.
2) Shake (agitate) calcium hydroxide vigorously, with whole amount of cold water, for about one hour.
3) Allow the solution to stand, for settling of the excess calcium hydroxide.
4) After complete sedimentation of calcium hydroxide, collect the clear supernatant liquid

Dispensing : Hydroxide ions of calcium hydroxide reacts with atmospheric CO_2 and converts into precipitate of calcium carbonate. Therefore immedieatly transfer the solution to a narrow mouthed, fluted, glass or plastic bottle, close tightly with plastic screw cap, polish and label.

Direction: To be applied on affeced part, two or three times a day.

Storage: Store in a cool place.

Auxilliary label: FOR EXTERNAL USE ONLY.

Uses: 1) Internally it is used as antacid.

2) Externally it is used as astringent and it is applied topically, as lotion. It is also used as vehicle, for preparation of lime creams like,
   - Calcium soap emulsion and
   - Oily calamine lotion BP.

CHLOROXYLENOL SOLUTION B.P.C.

Synonym: Roxenol

Rx	
Chloroxylenol	ʒ i s
Olei ricini	fl. ʒ i ss
Potassi hydroxidi	gr xxii ss
Alcoholis	fl. ʒ v
Terpineol	fl. ʒ ii ss
Acidi oleici	M xi s
Aquam........q.s........	fl. ʒ xxv
Fiat : Liquor	Mitte : fl.oz i

Signa : Applicandus cum gossyp, dolentiparti more dicto.

Conversion :

ʒ i s → 1.25 drachms	gr xxii ss → 22.5 grains
1 drachms = 4 g	15 grains = 1 g
1.25 drachms = 5 g	22.5 grains = 1.5 g
fl. ʒ i ss →1.5 fl. drachms = 6 ml	
fl. ʒ v → 5 fl. drachms = 20 ml	M xi s → 11.25 minims
fl. ʒ ii ss → 2.5 fl. drachms = 10 ml	15 minims = 1 ml
fl. ʒ xxv → 25 fl. drachms = 100 ml	11.25 minims = 0.75 ml

Calculation : For fl.oz i → 1 fl.oz = 30 ml.

Chloroxylenol = $\frac{5}{100} \times 30 = 1.5$ g

Castor oil = $\frac{6}{100} \times 30 = 1.8$ ml

Potassium hydroxide = $\frac{1.5}{100} \times 30 = 0.45$ g

Alcohol (95%) = $\frac{20}{100} \times 30 = 6$ ml

Terpeneol = $\frac{10}{100} \times 30 = 3$ ml

Oleic acid = $\frac{0.75}{100} \times 30 = 0.225$ml

Purified water....q.s...... = 30 ml

Type	Ingredients	Quantity in imperial	Quantity in metric	Quantity taken
Solution for, external use.	Chloroxylenol	1.25 dr	5 g	1.5 g
	Castor oil	1.5 fl. dr	6 ml	1.8 ml
	Potassium hydroxide	22.5 gr	1.5 g	0.45 g
	Alcohol (95%)	5 fl. dr	20 ml	6 ml
	Terpineol	2.5 fl. dr	10 ml	3 ml
	Oleic acid	11.25 minims	0.75 ml	0.225 ml
	Purified water...q.s..	25 fl. dr	100 ml	30 ml
	Make: Solution Send: 30 ml Direction: Apply with cotton (adsorbent) to the affected part, as directed.			

Theory:

Roxenol is a clear colloidal solution, in which the chloroxylenol is solubilised by the soap micelles. Chloroxylenol is a chlorinated phenol, acts as a germicide (disinfectant). Terpineol is a volatile oil, used to mask the unpleasant (pungent) phenolic odour of chloroxylenol and prevents separation of chloroxylenol, after dilution.

Both chloroxylenol and terpineol are slightly soluble in water. But they are readily soluble in alcohol 95%. If preparation is done by dissolving chloroxylenol and terpineol in alcohol (95%), the final percentage of the alcohol in this solution will be 20%, which is insufficient to hold, both the ingredients in solution form. Therefore a solubilizing agent is required, which helps in solubilizing both chloroxylenol and terpineol, so as to get a clear colloidal solution.

The free fatty acids of castor oil undergo saponification reaction, with alkali – potassium hydroxide and form soap (potassium recinoleate). This soap acts as a solubilizing agent, which forms micelles and solubilizes chloroxylenol and terpineol and further acts as emulsifying agent, when the solution is diluted with water.

The saponification reaction is fast in presence of alcohol. Therefore alcoholic solution of castor oil is used.

Oleic acid is used to neutralize excess alkali present in the solution, to give optimum pH for bactericidal action of chloroxylenol.

Procedure:

1) Dissolve potassium hydroxide in a small portion of purified water.
2) Separately dissolve castor oil in half of the portion of alcohol.
3) Mix both the solutions with continuous stirring and allow to stand for one hour or until a small portion of the mixture remains clear, when diluted with nineteen times of its volume of purified water then, add oleic acid.

4) First dissolve chloroxylenol in terpineol, which is then mixed with remaining amount of alcohol (95%)
5) Pour this alcoholic solution into soap solution, with stirring and add sufficient amount of water, to produce final volume.

Dispensing: Transfer the solution to a narrow mouthed, fluted, glass or plastic bottle, close tightly with plastic screw cap, polish and label.

Direction: Apply with cotton (adsorbent) to the affected part, as directed.

Auxilliary label: FOR EXTERNAL USE ONLY

Storage: Store at room temperature.

Uses:

1) Chloroxylenol is used as topical antiseptic (germicide)
2) Chloroxylenol is a chlorinated phenol, which is less toxic and more germicidal than phenol or cresol. Therefore its solution is used as topical antiseptic, in the treatment of minor burns, psoriasis, eczema, diaper rash and in the treatment of Athlete's foot.

Note:

1) For preparation of chlorxylenol solution, the industrial methylated spirit may be used, instead of alcohol (95%).
2) Germicidal action of chlorxylenol reduces in alkaline solutions, which may also cause smarting. Therefore oleic acid is used, to neutralize excess alkali present in soap solution.

STRONG LEAD SUBACETATE SOLUTION I.P.

Rx	
Lead acetate	3 vi s
Lead monoxide	3 iv ss
Aquam......q.s.......	fl. 3 xxv
Fiat : Liquor	Mitte : fl.oz i
Signa : Applicandus super dolentiparti S.O.S.	

Conversion :

3 vi s → 6.25 drachms   3 iv ss → 4.5 drachms = 18 g

1 drachm = 4 g

6.25 drachms = 25 g   fl. 3 xxv → 25 fl. dr = 100 ml

Calculation : For fl.oz i → 1 fl.oz = 30 ml.

Lead acetate $= \frac{25}{100} \times 30 = 7.5$ g

Lead monoxide $= \frac{18}{100} \times 30 = 5.4$ g

Purified water....q.s...... = 30 ml

Type	Ingredients	Quantity in imperial	Quantity in metric	Quantity taken
Solution for, external use.	Lead acetate	6.25 dr	25 g	7.5 g
	Lead monoxide	4.5 dr	18 g	5.4 g
	Purified water.....q.s...	25 fl. dr	100 ml	30 ml
	Make: Solution	Send: 30 ml		
	Direction: Apply on the affected part, when ever necessary.			

Theory:

Lead acetate and lead monoxide reacts to form a number of basic lead sub acetates, some of them are soluble and some are insoluble. The principal basic lead subacetate formed is given below.

$$\underset{\text{Lead acetate}}{(CH_3COO)_2Pb} + \underset{\text{Lead monoxide}}{PbO} + H_2O \rightarrow \underset{\text{(Basic) Lead subacetate}}{(CH_3COO)_2Pb.Pb.(OH)_2}$$

This basic lead subacetate $(CH_3COO)_2Pb.Pb.(OH)_2$ is soluble in water. But highly basic lead subacetates are insoluble in nature e.g. $(CH_3COO)_2Pb.5Pb(OH)_2$.

In this preparation, the basic lead acetate reacts with atmospheric CO_2 and precipitates as insoluble basic lead carbonate. Therefore filtration of the solution is done, as quickly as possible directly into a dispensing bottle in such a way that, the filtrate should not expose to atmospheric CO_2 for longer time.

The dissolved CO_2 in water also causes the precipitation of lead acetate, to lead carbonate. Hence adjustment of final volume is made by freshly boiled and cooled water and all the containers used during preparation and dispensing, should be dried before preparation.

Procedure:

1) Dissolve lead acetate in ¾ th of total volume of purified water, in a beaker.
2) To the above solution, add lead monoxide with continuous stirring.
3) Keep this mixture aside for 48 hours with occasional shaking, for complete reaction between lead acetate and lead monoxide.

Dispensing: After 48 hours filter the solution through a filter paper directly to a narrow mouthed, plastic or glass bottle. Immediately adjust the final volume with freshly boiled and cooled water (well filled), close tightly with coloured screw cap, to distinguish it from the preparations, meant for internal use, polish and label.

Direction: Apply on the affected part, when ever necessary.

Auxilliary label: FOR EXTERNAL USE ONLY.

Storage: Store at room temperature.

Uses: Strong lead subacetate solution is used as, soothing astringent.

Student's exercise:

1) Define official solutions and Classify the official solutions with example.
2) What are polyiodides and their use?
3) Comment: Iodine preparations should be dispensed in glass containers
4) What is the synonym for Aqueous iodine solution and Weak iodine solution? How they will differ?
5) How will you dispense Iodine tincture?
6) What is Cresol with soap solution? Why it is used?
7) What is the synonym for Cresol with soap solution?
8) Briefly explain the principle behind the preparation of strong ammonium acetate solution I.P
9) How will you adjust the pH of strong ammonium acetate solution I.P, between 7.6 to 8?
10) What is the use of strong ammonium acetate solution I.P and Aluminium subacetate solution U.S.P?
11) Write the reaction involved in the preparation of Aluminium subacetate solution U.S.P
12) What is the synonym for Calcium hydroxide solution and what is its use?
13) Comment: Calcium hydroxide solution should be stored in well closed container.
14) What is the synonym for Chloroxylenol solution? What is its use?
15) Why oleic acid is used in chloroxylenol solution?
16) How will you dispense chloroxylenol solution?
18) Explain in briefly, the principle behind the preparation of Strong lead subacetate solution I.P

27 AROMATIC WATERS

Synonyms: Medicated Waters; Aquae stillatitiae; Aquae Olei Volatili

Aromatic Waters are vehicles for the mixtures which are saturated solutions (unless otherwise specified) of volatile oils (peppermint, aniseed, caraway, cinnamon, clove, lemon, rose etc.) or other aromatic or volatile substances (camphor, chloroform) in distilled water. They are clear and free from solid impurities.

They are mainly used as flavouring agents but some of them also possess mild therapeutic and/ or preservative properties. They are generally diluted from a concentrated preparation. All aromatic waters are prepared by diluting the concentrated preparation by a 1:40 dilution (i.e. 1 part concentrated preparation and 39 parts of distilled water). Double strength (DS) chloroform water is diluted 1:1 to get chloroform water.

Name of the aromatic water	Concentrated Water (CW)	Dilution	
		CW	Distilled Water
Aniseed water (0.05 % v/v)	Concentrated Aniseed water (2.0 % v/v)	1	39
Camphor water (0.1 % w/v)	Concentrated Camphor water (4.0 % w/v)	1	39
Caraway water	Concentrated Caraway water	1	39
Chloroform water (0.25 % v/v)	Double Strength Chloroform water (0.5% v/v)	1	1
Chloroform water (0.25 % v/v)	Concentrated Chloroform water (10 % v/v)	1	39
Peppermint water (0.05 % v/v)	Concentrated Peppermint water / emulsion (2.0 % v/v)	1	39

Aromatic waters possess an odor similar to the plant or volatile substance from which they are made. They should be protected from strong light and preferably stored in containers which are stoppered with purified cotton to allow access of some air but to exclude dust.

Aromatic Waters can be prepared by any one of the following processes:

1. Distillation :

Place the odoriferous portion of the plant or drug from which the Aromatic water is to be prepared in a suitable still with sufficient water, and distil most of the water, carefully avoiding the development of unpleasant odors through the burning of the substances. Separate any excess of oil, and preserve or use the clear aqueous portion, which should be saturated with the flavoring or aromatic principles of the plant.

It is necessary to observe certain practical rules in conducting the process of distillation. When the substance employed is dry, hard, and fibrous, it should be mechanically divided, and macerated in water for a short time previous to the operation. The quantity of materials should not bear too large a proportion to the capacity of the still, as the water might otherwise boil over into the receiver.

2. Solution :

The Volatile oil, or Other specified volatile substance, 2 ml or 2 g, Distilled Water, a sufficient quantity, to make 1000 ml. Shake the volatile substance with 1000 ml of distilled water in a capacious bottle, and repeat the shaking several times during a period of about fifteen minutes. Set the mixture aside for twelve hours or over night, filter through paper, and pass enough distilled water through the filter to obtain 1000 ml. Sometimes the preparation is not clear, in that case about 50 g of purified talc or a sufficient quantity of purified siliceous earth or pulped filter paper is thoroughly incorporated and mixture is agitated well. The solution is then filtered to get a clear product.

CAMPHOR WATER I.P./ B.P.

Rx	
Camphorae	gr XV
Alcoholis (90%)	M XXX
Aquam .... q. s.....	fl.3 CCL
Fiat: Aquam camphorae	Mitte: fl. oz i
Signa: Cochleare magnum, utendus more dicto.	

Conversion :

gr XV → 15 grains	M XXX → 30 minims
15 grains = 1 g	15 minims = 1 ml
fl.3 CCL → 250 fl.drachms	30 minims= 2 ml
1 fl.drachm = 4 ml	
250 fl.drachms = 1000 ml	

Calculation : For fl.oz i → 1 fl.oz = 30 ml

Camphor $= \frac{1}{1000} \times 30 = 0.03$ g

Alcohol (90%) $= \frac{2}{1000} \times 30 = 0.06$ ml

Purified water q.s. = 30 ml

Type	Ingredients	Quantity in imperial	Quantity in metric	Quantity taken
Monophasic liquid for oral use (Aromatic water)	Camphor	15 gr	1 g	0.03 g
	Alcohol (90%)	30 minims	2 ml	0.06 ml
	Purified water ....q.s....	250 fl.dr	1000 ml	30 ml
	Make: Camphor water Send: 30 ml Direction: One tablespoonful to be taken, as directed.			

Theory:

When applied externally, camphor dilates the vessels of the skin, and is used as a rubefacient and mild counterirritant. Internally, camphor has much the same action as the volatile oils, and is prescribed as a carminative in flatulence and as an antiseptic for the alimentary canal. It mildly excites the circulation, dilating the superficial vessels and slightly increasing the cardiac output. It also directly excites the cerebrum. It is a popular remedy, either taken by the mouth or used as a snuff, for the relief of colds.

Camphor: It is sparingly soluble in water (1 part in 700 parts of water) but is readily soluble in alcohol (1 part in 1 part). Therefore in this preparation, camphor is first dissolved in alcohol and then this alcoholic solution is added drop wise in to water. The small amount of precipitated camphor is re-dissolved by shaking and alcohol in this preparation acts as distributing co-solvent.

Procedure:

1) Weigh the required amount of camphor in a weighing bottle and measure the required quantity of alcohol.
2) Simply mix camphor in alcohol and then add this solution into the purified water in small proportions. Shake vigorously after each addition.
3) After the complete addition, shake occasionally till whole of the camphor gets dissolved.
4) Makeup the final volume with purified water.

Dispensing: Transfer the solution in to a narrow mouth glass container, close tightly with a rubber closure and aluminum cap, polish, label and dispense.

Direction: One tablespoonful to be taken as directed.

Auxiliary label: SHAKE THE BOTTLE WELL BEFORE USE

Storage: Store in tightly closed container at cool place.

Dose: 15 to 30 ml

Uses: It is used as carminative and flavouring agent

Similar Example

Concentrated Camphor Water B. P.

Camphor	40 g
Alcohol (90%)	600 ml
Purified water ....q. s.	1000 ml

Dose: 0.3 – 1.0 ml

This preparation is used as mild analgesic, rubefacient for external applications in liniments and lotions.

CHLOROFORM WATER I.P. / B.P.

Rx	
Chloroformi	M xxxvii ss
Aquam ...... q.s.....	fl. 3 CCL
Fiat : Aquam chloroformi	Mitte : fl.oz ii
Signa : cochleare magnum, utendus more dicto.	

Conversion :

M xxxvii ss → 37.5 minims   fl. 3 CCL → 250 fl.drachms

15 minims = 1 ml   1 fl.drachm = 4 ml

37.5 minims= 2.5 ml   250 fl.drachms = 1000 ml

Calculation : For fl.oz ii → 2 fl.oz   = 60 ml

Chloroform $= \frac{2.5}{1000} \times 60 = 0.15$ ml

Purified water ......q.s. ......   = 60 ml

Type	Ingredients	Quantity in imperial	Quantity in metric	Quantity taken
Monophasic liquid for oral use (Aromatic water)	Chloroform	37.5 minims	2.5 ml	0.15 ml
	Purified water ....q.s....	250 fl.dr	1000 ml	60 ml
	Make: Chloroform water	Send: 60 ml		
	Direction: One tablespoonful to be taken, as directed.			

Theory:

Chloroform is a volatile substance having high vapour pressure. It occurs as a heavy clear, colorless and mobile liquid having characteristic odor and a burning sweet taste. It is but slightly soluble in water (1: 200) but is miscible with alcohol, ether and the fixed and volatile oils. It is a good anesthetic agent when inhaled but when taken orally, small doses are carminative, anodyne and antiseptic, it is therefore used in gastric fermentation and colic. Large doses are sometimes employed as a vermifuge, but are rather dangerous. Excessive doses produce unconsciousness and coma, similarly to the results of its inhalation. It is used as chloroform water B.P. (Single strength chloroform water B.P.), Double strength chloroform water B.P. and Concentrated chloroform water BPC 1959.

Double strength chloroform water (0.5 % v/v) is a good preservative for extracts of vegetative origin and has warm sweet taste. It is widely used as vehicle for mixtures and other liquid preparations for internal use. It is prepared in the same manner as chloroform water by adding 5 ml chloroform to purified water (to 1000 ml). Chloroform water 0.25 % v/v (i.e., single-strength chloroform water) can be prepared by diluting double strength preparation (1:1) with distilled water.

Concentrated chloroform water BPC 1959:

Chloroform	100 ml
Alcohol (90%)	600 ml
Purified water ...... q. s.....	1000 ml

It uses ethanol as a co-solvent to permit the preparation of a solution containing 10 % v/v chloroform. Dose of this preparation is 0.4 – 0.8 ml.

If a preparation equivalent to double strength chloroform water is required (i.e., a solution containing 0.5 % v/v chloroform), one part of the concentrated chloroform water should be diluted with 19 parts of purified water (1 in 20 dilution); this must be further diluted 1:1 to produce a product with a final chloroform content of 0.25 % v/v. To produce a solution having an equivalent strength to chloroform water (i.e., one that contains 0.25% v/v chloroform), one part of concentrated chloroform water should be diluted with 39 parts of purified water (1 in 40 dilution).

Chloroform water prepared from concentrated chloroform water will have a residual ethanol content of about 1.5 % v/v. For the vast majority of patients this level of ethanol will not be a problem. However, it may have implications for patients taking some medicines, and for the use of this preparation in neonates and children.

Procedure:

1) Simply dissolve chloroform into the purified water in small proportions. Shake vigorously after each addition.
2) After the complete addition, makeup the final volume with purified water.

Dispensing: Transfer the solution in to a narrow mouth glass container, close tightly with a rubber closure and aluminum cap, polish, label and dispense.

Auxiliary label: SHAKE THE BOTTLE WELL BEFORE USE

Storage: Store in tightly closed container at cool place.

Dose: 15 to 30 ml

Uses: It is used as preservative, vehicle, flavouring and sweetening agent

CONCENTRATED PEPPERMINT WATER B.P.

Rx	
Olei Mentha piperitae	fl.3 V
Alcoholis (90%)	fl.oz XX
Aquam .... q. s......	fl.3 CCL
Fiat: Aquam mentha piperitae	Mitte: fl. oz i
Signa: Utendus more dicto.	

Conversion:

fl.3 v → 5 fl.drachms   fl.oz i → 1 fl.oz

1 fl.drachm = 4 ml   1 fl.oz = 30 ml

5 fl.drachms = 20 ml   fl.oz XX → 20 fl.oz=600 ml

250 fl.drachms = 1000 ml

Calculation : For fl.oz i → 1 fl.oz = 30 ml

Peppermint oil $= \frac{20}{1000} \times 30 = 0.6$ ml

Alcohol (90%) $= \frac{60}{1000} \times 30 = 18$ ml

Purified water ... q.s..... = 30 ml

Type	Ingredients	Quantity in imperial	Quantity in metric	Quantity taken
Monophasic liquid for oral use (Aromatic Water)	Peppermint oil	5 fl.dr	20 ml	0.6 ml
	Alcohol (90%)	20 fl.oz	600 ml	18 ml
	Purified water.... q.s....	250 fl.dr	1000 ml	30 ml
	Make: Peppermint water Send: 30 ml Direction: To be taken as directed.			

Theory:

Peppermint oil has carminative, antiseptic and flavoring properties and has been included in a range of official and non-official pharmaceutical preparations.

Peppermint water is a saturated solution of peppermint oil (0.05% v/v) in water.

Concentrated peppermint water, like most other aromatic waters, peppermint water is usually prepared by diluting one part of concentrated peppermint water with 39 parts of purified water (1 in 40 dilution), e.g., by diluting 2.5 ml of the concentrated water to 100 ml.

However, to enable concentrated peppermint water to contain 2 % v/v peppermint oil in solution, ethanol has to be included in the formulation as a co-solvent. This concentration of ethanol is also sufficient to act as a preservative for the preparation. Thus, peppermint water prepared by dilution of concentrated peppermint water will contain a residual amount of ethanol, usually about 1.5 % v/v.

Peppermint water is known to support microbial growth and is prone to contamination with Pseudomonas aeruginosa. Neither the peppermint oil nor the residual ethanol in peppermint water is present in sufficiently high concentrations to have effective preservative activity. It has therefore been recommended that peppermint water is prepared under controlled conditions to minimize the risks of contamination and that a limited shelf-life should be assigned to the product.

Antimicrobial preservative systems have been added to peppermint water as a means of extending the shelf-life. They include chloroform (0.25 % v/v) or a combination of methyl hydroxyl-benzoate (0.2 % w/v) and propyl hydroxyl-benzoate (0.02 % w/v).

Procedure:

1) Dissolve the measured amount of peppermint oil in alcohol (90%) and add this (in small proportions) to sufficient amount of purified water, shaking vigorously after each addition.
2) Add 50 g of purified talc to the preparation and shake well to disperse.
3) Allow the preparation to stand for twelve hours or overnight with occasional shaking.
4) Filter the preparation and pass sufficient amount of purified water through the filter to make up the required volume.

Dispensing: Transfer the solution in to a narrow mouth glass container, close tightly with a rubber closure and aluminium cap, polish, label and dispense.

Direction: To be taken as directed.

Auxiliary label: SHAKE THE BOTTLE WELL BEFORE USE

Storage: Store in tightly closed container at cool place.

Dose: 0.25 to 1 ml

Uses: It is used as mild carminative and flavouring agent.

OTHER PREPARATIONS

1) CONCENTRATED ANISEED WATER B.P.

Rx

Anise oil	20 ml
Alcohol (90%)	700 ml
Purified water ..... q. s	1000 ml

Uses: It is used mainly as a pleasant vehicle for the administration of milk of magnesia, and such cathartics as jalap, rhubarb, and senna, to modify their griping action. It is useful as a carminative to expel flatus in indigestion accompanied with gaseous accumulations. The dose is from 8 ml to 30 ml.

2) CARAWAY WATER U.S.P.

Rx

Oil of Carum	2 ml
Purified water ..... q. s	1000 ml

3) CINNAMON WATER U.S.P.

Rx

Oil of cinnamon	2 ml
Purified water .... q. s	1000 ml

Uses: Cinnamon water is useful in passive hemorrhage from the lungs, stomach, kidneys, or uterus, in chronic diarrhoea and dysentery, and in flatulency. It is frequently employed to cover the unpleasant taste of other remedies, especially opiates, and will often allay vomiting. Its dose is from 8 ml to 60 ml. It should not be used when fever or inflammation is present.

4) FENNEL WATER U.S.P.

Rx

Oil of fennel	2 ml
Purified water .... q. s	1000 ml

Uses: Fennel water is a pleasant aromatic, stimulant and carminative.

28 SPIRITS

Spirits are the alcoholic or hydro-alcoholic solutions of volatile substances. The volatile substances used may be in the form of solid, liquid or gas. Spirits are also called as Essences.

They generally contain higher percentage of alcohol than that in Tinctures and Aromatic waters and they usually contain 50 to 90% of alcohol.

Eg: The range of alcoholic content among the current official preparations being from a low of 62-68% required for Aromatic spirit of Ammonia USP, to a high of 79-85% required for Peppermint spirit USP. The high alcoholic contents maintain water-insoluble oils in solution. If water is added to a spirit the oil gets separated.

Eg: Chloroform spirits, Peppermint spirit, Lemon spirit, Compound orange spirit, Benzaldehyde spirit, Aromatic spirit of ammonia, Soft soap spirit, Surgical spirit, Spirit of ether.

Methods of preparation of spirits

Spirits can be prepared by any of the following methods:

1. Simple solution
2. Solution with maceration
3. Chemical reaction
4. Distillation

1) Simple solution Method:

Most of the spirits are made by solution method. This method involves simple dissolution of volatile substance or materials in alcohol. The solution may be filtered to obtain a sparkling clear liquid. Some times talc is added and filtered to get clear solution.

E.g. Spirits prepared by this method include chloroform spirit, peppermint spirit, spirit of ether etc.

2) Solution with maceration:

In this method, crude drug containing volatile substance is macerated with purified water to extract water soluble constituents. The marc is pressed and expressed liquid is mixed with the extract. Then to the marc, sufficient quantity of alcohol is added and liquid is colleted and filtered. The filtered liquid is mixed with the extract.

The spirits prepared by this method possesses green colour due to the presence of soluble chlorophyll.

E.g. Official peppermint spirit is made by this process but Peppermint spirit B.P.C, which is prepared by dissolving peppermint oil in alcohol.

3) Chemical reaction

No official spirits are prepared by this process, but in the preparation of Ethyl nitrite spirit, this method is employed using sodium nitrite with the mixture of alcohol and sulphuric acid in cold.

4) Distillation

Aromatic spirit of ammonia I.P is prepared by this method. The distilled spirits are prepared from aromatic vegetable substances, the essential oils of which rise with the vapor of alcohol and condense with it in the receiver.

Some of the oils, however, will not rise at the temperature of boiling alcohol, but may be distilled with water. In this case, it is necessary to employ diluted alcohol or proof spirit, with the water of which the oil comes over in the latter part of the process.

The aromatic substance should be macerated for some days with the alcohol before the distillation, as the oil being thus dissolved, rises more readily with the spirituous vapor than when confined in the tissue.

Sufficient water must, therefore, be added to cover the vegetable matter after the alcohol shall have been distilled, and as a rule, the heat should be applied by means of a water bath, or of steam.

In preparing the spirits, care should be taken to avoid the color and flavor arising from the decomposition of the vegetable matter by heat.

As the proof spirit of commerce is often impregnated with foreign matter, which gives it an unpleasant flavor, it is better to use alcohol which has been carefully rectified, and to dilute it with the que proportion of water, as directed by the U.S. Pharmacopoeia.

Incompatibility

Spirits may show incompatibility when mixed with water or with an aqueous preparation; the volatile substances present in spirits generally evaporate from solution and form a milky preparation and causes turbidity.

Some times dilution of spirit causes precipitation of the volatile constituent resulting turbid product. In certain cases salts present in the formulation precipitate due to high percentage of alcohol in spirit. Hence while preparing spirits, contact with water must be avoided and all glassware and utensils must either be dried or final rinsed with alcohol rather than with water.

If a spirit is to be filtered, filter it through a dry filter paper or one moistened with a small portion of alcohol. Denatured spirit is prepared by diluting 19 volumes of alcohol with 1 volume of approved wood naphtha.

Storage

Spirits must be stored in tightly closed containers to avoid the loss of alcohol or volatile principle by evaporation. Light energy decomposes the volatile constituents with the loss of flavour. Hence the container should also be light resistant.

Spirits should be kept in cool place (20°C) and they should be protected from flame or fire.

Uses

They are used internally as well as externally by inhalation for their medicinal value while a large number of them are used as flavouring agents. When used for medicinal purposes, they may be taken orally or applied externally, or used by inhalation depending upon the type of preparation.

Some spirits are used as flavoring agents called as aromatic spirits e.g. Lemon spirit, Compound orange spirit, Cardamom spirit etc. and some spirits are used as medicinal agents e.g. aromatic ammonia spirit.

Spirits may be used in the formulation of aromatic waters or other pharmaceuticals in which flavor is required.

The aromatic spirits are used to impart a pleasant odor and taste to mixtures, and to correct the nauseating and griping effects of other medicines. They also serve as carminatives in flatulent colic, and as agreeable stimulants in debility of the stomach.

PEPPERMINT/SPIRIT

Rx	
Olei manthae piperitae	fl.3 ii ss
Alcoholis (90%) .....q.s....	fl.3 xxv
Fiat : Spiritus	Mitte : fl. oz. ii
Signa : Utendus more dicto.	

Conversion :

fl. 3 ii ss → 2.5 fl.dr	fl. 3 xxv → 25 fl.dr
1 fl. drachm = 4 ml	1 fl. drachm = 4 ml
2.5 fl. drachms = 10 ml	25 fl. drachms = 100 ml

Calculation : For fl.oz ii → 2 fl.oz = 60 ml

Peppermint oil $= \frac{10}{100} \times 60 = 6$ ml

Alcohol (90%) ..... q.s..... = 60 ml

Type	Ingredients	Quantity in imperial	Quantity in metric	Quantity taken
Monophasic liquid	Peppermint oil	2.5 fl.dr	10 ml	6 ml
	Alcohol (90%).... q.s....	25 fl.dr	100 ml	60 ml
	Make: Spirit	Send: 60 ml		
	Direction: To be used, as directed.			

Theory:

Peppermint oil is obtained by distillation from the fresh flowering tops of Mentha piperita. It is a colorless or pale yellow liquid having a strong penetrating odour of peppermint and a pungent taste, followed by a sensation of cold when air is drawn into the mouth. The odor of fresh peppermint is due to the presence of about 2.0% of a volatile oil, most of which is lost due to drying off.

Peppermint spirit B.P.C. is prepared by solution method in which peppermint oil is dissolved in alcohol. But Official peppermint spirit (USP) is prepared by solution with maceration process.

Procedure:

1) Dissolve peppermint oil in a small amount of alcohol. If the solution is not clear, shake it with purified talc (5% w/v) and set aside for sometime and then filter to get the clear liquid.
2) Add sufficient amount of ethanol to make up the volume.

Dispensing: Transfer to a amber coloured glass bottle (light resistant container) and close tightly to avoid the loss of alcohol or volatile principle by evaporation and decomposition of the volatile constituents with the loss of flavor by light.

Storage: Peppermint oil and alcohol are volatile in nature; therefore, the preparation is stored in cool place (20ºC) and they should be protected from flame or fire.

Auxiliary label: KEEP AWAY FROM DIRECT FLAME OR FIRE.

Uses: Peppermint spirit is used as flavoring agent and carminative in flatulence and nausea. It is also used as an antiseptic and local anesthetic.

It is also used as a flavoring agent in pharmaceutical preparations and in certain candies, chewing gum, etc.

Similar example

1) **Peppermint spirit U.S.P.**

Rx

Peppermint oil	100 ml
Peppermint, in coarse powder	10 g
Alcohol ......q.s.......	1000 ml

Uses: It is used as flavouring agent.

CHLOROFORM SPIRIT

Rx	
Chloroformi	fl. 3 i s
Alcoholis (90%) .....q.s.	fl. 3 xxv
Fiat : Spiritus	Mitte : fl. oz. i
Signa : Utendus more dicto.	

Conversion :

fl. 3 i s →1.25 fl.dr — fl. 3 xxv → 25 fl.dr

1 fl. drachm = 4 ml — 1 fl. drachm = 4 ml

1.25 fl. drachms = 5 ml — 25 fl. drachms = 100 ml

Calculation : For fl.oz i → 1 fl.oz = 30 ml

Peppermint oil $= \frac{5}{100} \times 30 = 1.5\,\text{ml}$

Alcohol (90%) ...... q.s..... = 30 ml

Type	Ingredients	Quantity in imperial	Quantity in metric	Quantity taken
Monophasic liquid	Peppermint oil	1.25 fl.dr	5 ml	1.5 ml
	Alcohol (90%).... q.s....	25 fl.dr	100 ml	30 ml
	Make: Spirit	Send: 30 ml		
	Direction: To be used, as directed.			

Theory:

When chloroform is exposed to light or air, oxidation takes place. If the alcohol is added in small proportion it retards the oxidation. Hence chloroform is most of the times used as spirit.

Procedure:

1) Mix chloroform with ethanol (90% v/v) and shake it.
2) Add sufficient ethanol to produce the required volume of spirit and mix it well.

Dispensing: Transfer to a amber coloured glass bottle (light resistant container) and close tightly to avoid the loss of alcohol or volatile principle by evaporation and decomposition of the volatile constituents with the loss of flavours by light.

Storage: It should be stored in a well-closed, completely filled container in a cool place to prevent the volatilisation of volatile ingredients and to retard the oxidation.

Auxiliary label: KEEP AWAY FROM DIRECT FLAME OR FIRE.

Uses: Chloroform spirit is used as sweetening agent, carminative and preservative. It is one of the main ingredients of carminative mixtures.

Chloroform is also used as analgesic, anesthetic and muscle relaxant.

> **Note:** It is less as anesthetic as some times it is poisonous due to formation of phosgene gas during the storage in the presence of light.

BENZALDEHYDE SPIRIT

Rx	
Benzaldehyde	M xv
Alcoholis	fl. 3 xx
Aquam ..... q.s.	fl. 3 xxv
Fiat : Spiritus	Mitte : fl. oz. ii
Signa : Utendus more dicto.	

Conversion :

M xv → 15 minims

15 minims = 1 ml

fl. 3 xx → 20 fl.dr

1 fl. drachm = 4 ml

20 fl. drachms = 80 ml

fl.3 xxv → 25 fl.drachms = 100 ml

Calculation : For fl.oz ii → 2 fl.oz = 60 ml

Benzaldehyde $= \frac{1}{100} \times 60 = 0.6\,\text{ml}$

Alcohol $= \frac{80}{100} \times 60 = 48\,\text{ml}$

Water ...... q.s..... = 60 ml

Type	Ingredients	Quantity in imperial	Quantity in metric	Quantity taken
Monophasic liquid	Benzaldehyde	15 minims	1 ml	0.6 ml
	Alcohol	20 fl.dr	80 ml	48 ml
	Water .... q.s....	25 fl. dr	100 ml	60 ml
	Make: Spirit	Send: 60 ml		
	Direction: To be used, as directed			

Theory:

Benzaldehyde is also known as artificial essential almond oil. It is a colorless, strongly refractive liquid and has an odour resembling that of bitter almond oil with a burning aromatic taste.

Benzaldehyde is used in place of bitter almond oil for flavoring purposes. It is much safer than almond oil as it contains no hydrocyanic acid. It is also used in perfumery and in manufacturing of dyestuffs and many other organic compounds.

Procedure:

1) Dissolve measured amount of benzaldehyde in the required volume of ethanol (90%).
2) Add sufficient purified water to make up the volume and mix properly by shaking.

Dispensing: Transfer to a amber coloured glass bottle and close tightly to avoid the loss of alcohol or volatile principle by evaporation and decomposition of the volatile constituents with the loss of flavours by light.

Auxiliary label: KEEP AWAY FROM NAKED FLAME OR FIRE.

Storage: Benzaldehyde spirit should be protected from light and stored in cool place (20ºC).

Uses: Benzaldehyde spirit is used as flavoring agent.

AROMATIC SPIRIT OF AMMONIA

Synonym: Spirit of Sal volatile

Rx	
Ammonii bicarbonatis	3 vi s
Liquoris ammoniae	fl. 3 xvii ss
Olei lemonis	fl. 3 i s
Olei natmeg	M VL
Alcoholis (90%)	fl. oz xxv
Aquam ..... q.s.	fl. 3 CCL
Fiat : Spiritus	Mitte : fl.oz. ii
Signa : Utendus more dicto.	

Conversion :

3 vi s → 6.25 drachms
1 drachm = 4 g
6.25 drachms = 25 gm

M V L → 45 minims
15 minims = 1 ml
45 minims = 3 ml

fl.3 xvii ss → 17.5 fl.dr
1 fl. drachms = 4 ml
17.5 fl. drachms = 70 ml
fl. 3 i s → 1.25 fl.dr = 5 ml

fl. oz xxv → 25 fl.oz
1 fl. oz = 30 ml
25 fl. oz → 750 ml
fl. 3 CCL = 250 fl.dr = 1000 ml

Calculation : For fl.oz ii → 2 fl.oz = 60 ml

Ammonium bicarbonate $= \frac{25}{1000} \times 60 = 1.5$ g

Ammnia solution $= \frac{70}{1000} \times 60 = 4.2$ ml

Lemon oil $= \frac{5}{1000} \times 60 = 0.3$ ml

Nutmeg oil $= \frac{3}{1000} \times 60 = 0.18$ ml

Alcohol (90%) $= \frac{750}{1000} \times 60 = 45$ ml

Water ...... q.s..... = 60 ml

Type	Ingredients	Quantity in imperial	Quantity in metric	Quantity taken
Monophasic liquid	Ammonium bicarbonate	6.25 dr	25 gm	1.5 g
	Ammnia solution	17.5 fl.dr	70 ml	4.2 ml
	Lemon oil	1.25 fl.dr	5 ml	0.3 ml
	Nutmeg oil	45 minims	3 ml	0.18 ml
	Alcohol (90%)	25 fl.oz	750 ml	45 ml
	Water .... q.s....	250 fl.dr	1000 ml	60 ml
	Make: Spirit Send: 60 ml Direction: To be used, as directed.			

Theory:

Generally the spirits are prepared by solution method but aromatic spirit of ammonia is prepared by distillation method, because the oil of Nutmeg contains non-volatile resinous matter, due to which the preparation changes to dark color on storage. Here the distillate is collected in two portions. They are different in their characteristic form.

First portion is water in alcohol type i.e. first part of distillate contains a major part of alcohol, volatile oils and a small proportion of water. This part contains volatile oils; hence this part can not be subjected to heat.

The second portion is alcohol in water i.e. the second portion of distillate contains a major part of water, a little quantity of alcohol and volatile oil. Second portion of distillate is heated with ammonium bicarbonate and ammonia to coverts it into ammonium carbonate.

Ammonia and ammonium bicarbonate when dissolved are converted into normal carbonate (ammonium carbonate).

$$NH_4HCO_3 + NH_3 \rightarrow (NH_4)_2\ CO_3$$

The conversion of ammonium bicarbonate to ammonium carbonate is necessary before mixing it with alcoholic portion of the distillate, because ammonium bicarbonate is almost insoluble in alcohol. Complete process is performed in a closed vessel to prevent the escape of carbon dioxide which is produced during heating.

Freshly prepared ammonium carbonate is used because ammonium carbonate on storage partially changes into ammonium bicarbonate. Due to this reason the bottles are well filled and due to the presence of volatile ingredients it is stored in a cool placed in well-closed containers.

Procedure :

1) Place nutmeg oil, lemon oil and alcohol, 90 % with 350 ml of purified water in a distillation flask.
2) Collect first 75 ml of the distillate in a separate container and keep it aside.
3) Collect the second distillate of about 35 ml and place it in a separate flask. Add the ammonium bicarbonate and strong ammonia solution in to second distillate and heat on a water-bath at 60°C with frequent shaking till the salt dissolves. Cool it and filter through cotton wool. Mix this filtrate gradually with the first distillate.

4. Finally, add sufficient water to make the volume. Keep the product in a wall filled well closed container in a cool place.

Dispensing: Transfer to a amber coloured glass bottle and close tightly to avoid the loss of alcohol or volatile principle by evaporation and decomposition of the volatile constituents with the loss of flavours by light.

Auxiliary label: KEEP AWAY FROM NAKED FLAME OR FIRE.

Storage: It should be stored in cool place (20°C) and protected from sun light.

Uses: Aromatic spirit of ammonia is used as stimulant, diuretic and diaphoretic.

It is dispensed in bulk in suitable tight, light resistant containers or as a single-dose glass vial wrapped in a soft cotton envelope. The vial is broken easily, the cotton acts as a sponge for spirit.

Similar examples

1) Spirit of ether

Anaesthetic ether	33.0 ml
Ethanol (90%) ......q.s......	100.0 ml

Uses: Ether when administered by inhalation produced anesthesia. When administered by oral route it gives narcotic action similar to that to alcohol. It has a carminative action and its spirit is used in various pharmaceutical preparations.

In the preparation of spirit of ether, anesthetic ether acts as an active medicament, whereas alcohol plays the role of solvent and finely distributes ether.

Anesthetic ether is also known as Diethyl-ether. It is highly inflammable; therefore, it should be kept away from an open flame and stored in an air tight container.

2) Surgical Spirit:

Methyl salicylate	5 ml
Diethyl phthalate	20 ml
Castor oil	25 ml
Industrial methylated spirit .....q.s...	100 ml

Uses: It is used as surgical dressing

Auxiliary label: This preparation is inflammable. Keep away from a naked flame. FOR EXTERNAL USE ONLY.

3) Soap spirit

Soft soap	65.0 g
Ethanol (90%) .....q.s.....	100.0 ml

Uses: For external use, as a detergent.

LEMON SPIRIT

Rx	
Terpeneless Lemon oil	fl. 3 ii ss
Alcoholis (90%) .... q.s....	fl. 3 xxv
Fiat : Spiritus	Mitte : fl. oz. i
Signa : Utendus more dicto.	

Conversion :

fl. 3 ii s → 2.5 fl. drachms	fl. 3 xxv = 25 fl. drachms
1 fl. drachm = 4 ml	1 fl.drachm = 4 ml
2.5 fl. drachms = 10 ml	25 fl. drachms = 100 ml

Calculation : For fl.oz i → 1 fl.oz = 30 ml

Terpeneless lemon oil $= \frac{10}{100} \times 30 = 3$ ml

Alcohol (90%) .... q.s.... = 30 ml

Type	Ingredients	Quantity in imperial	Quantity in metric	Quantity taken
Monophasic liquid	Terpeneless Lemon oil	2.5 fl.dr.	10 ml	3 ml
	Alcohol .. q.s....	25 fl.dr.	100 ml	30 ml
	Make: Spirit Direction: To be used, as directed.	Send: 30 ml		

Theory:

Terpeneless lemon oil is obtained from the fresh peel of fruit of *Citrus lemon*. It is pale yellow to deep yellow or greenish yellow liquid with the characteristic odor and taste.

For pharmaceutical preparations, terpeneless lemon oil is preferred, because due to the presence of terpenes, simple lemon oil readily undergoes deterioration by oxidation and gets terebenthine odour.

Procedure:

1) Mix measured amount of terpeneless lemon oil with ethanol (90%).
2) Add remaining volume of ethanol and make up the volume.

Dispensing: Transfer to a amber coloured glass bottle and close tightly to avoid the loss of alcohol or volatile principle by evaporation and decomposition of the volatile constituents with the loss of flavours by Light energy.

Auxiliary label: KEEP AWAY FROM DIRECT FLAME OR FIRE.

Storage: Lemon spirit should be kept in a well-filled container and protected from light.

Uses: It is used a flavoring agent in pharmaceutical preparations and in certain candies and foods.

Similar example

1) **Compound orange spirit**

Rx

Terpeneless lemon oil	1.3 ml
Terpeneless orange oil	2.5 ml
Anise oil	4.25 ml
Coriander oil	6.25 ml
Ethanol (90%), sufficient to produce ...q.s...	1000.0 ml

Uses: Flavoring agent and carminative.

2) **Surgical Spirits**

Rx

Methyl Salicylate	5 ml
Diethyl ether	20 ml
Castor oil	25 ml
Industrial methylated spirit...... q.s.....	1000 ml

Use: To be used, as directed.

29 TINCTURES

Tinctures are alcoholic or hydro-alcoholic solutions usually containing comparatively low concentration of the active principles of vegetable drugs or animal drugs.

When only one drug is used for making a tincture, it is simply designated as 'Tincture' but when more then one vegetable or animal drug is used; the preparation is known as 'Compound Tincture'.

According to international protocol, the chemical substances dissolved in alcohol should not be named as tinctures. But they should be designated as solutions i.e Weak iodine solution or Strong iodine solution, etc.

Tinctures vary widely in their method of preparation, the strength their active ingredients, their alcohol content, and their intended use in medicine and pharmaceutical field.

Eg: Some tinctures are used externally as protectants (e.g. Compound Tincture of Benzoin)

Some are used internally as cardiotonics (e.g. Tincture of Digitalis),

As anticholinergics (e.g. Tincture of Digitalis), and

For pharmaceutical purposes as flavouring agents (e.g. Tincture of Sweet Orange Peel U.S.P. or Orange tincture I.P.)

In recent years, increasing use of pure drugs isolated form animals, plants, or prepared by synthetic processes have reduced the use of plant or animal extracts. However, tinctures are still in use where comparatively low potency and large dosages are recommended.

Tinctures are very stable preparations and can be stored for long period without loss of potency, decomposition or degradation.

Tinctures differ from spirits that, the tinctures contain low concentration of active principles of vegetable drugs whereas spirits contain volatile substances only.

Eg.
- Orange tincture
- Lemon tincture
- Belladonna tincture
- Compound benzoin tincture
- Compound cardamom tincture
- Aromatic cardamom tincture
- Capsicum tincture
- Nux Vomica tincture.
- Opium tincture
- Strong Ginger tincture

Alcohol is widely used as a solvent for tinctures because of following reasons:

1. The medicinally active ingredients of many drugs are soluble alcohol.
2. Alcoholic preparations remain stable for a long period of time without degradation, decomposition or loss of potency. It also prevents Microbial growth

3. Alcohol precipitates gums and aluminous matter; therefore alcoholic preparations can be filtered to obtain a clear liquid.

Strength of Alcohol in Tinctures

Tinctures contain alcohol ranging form15 to 80% v/v. The alcoholic strength also varies form one tincture to another.

Eg.

Orange tincture consist of 73-78 %

Opium tincture consist of 41-46 %

Camphorated Opium tincture consist of 56-60 %

It is necessary to keep the alcoholic strength of tinctures within limits, so that the solute remains in solution. If the desired balance of alcohol and water is disturbed i.e mixing the tincture with other very diverse liquids having different solvent power, may increase the instability of the preparation. This happens because; some of the solute may be precipitated out.

Eg: Tincture of Balsam of Tolu is prepared with alcohol as a menstruum and if this tincture is mixed with aqueous solutions, the alcohol-soluble principles will be actually precipitated out of solution.

It is not essential that the alcohol employed shall be strong (90 %) in order to secure this effect. In most cases the permanency of tincture can be secured by the use of a 45 % alcohol.

A diluted alcohol, however, has in some degree the properties of both alcohol and water, and alcohols of 45, 60, 70, and 90 % strengths are employed in the preparation of the tinctures. The more dilute the alcohol the more closely do its properties approximate to those of water, and of course, the more economical is the manufacture of the tincture.

Dehydrated alcohol is not preferred for making tinctures. Diluted alcohol or proof spirit is often preferable to official alcohol, as it is capable of extracting a larger proportion of those active principles of plants which require an aqueous menstruum, while at the same time it is strong enough to prevent spontaneous decomposition, and has the advantages of being cheaper and less stimulating.

Alcohol or rectified spirit, is preferred as a solvent when the substance to be extracted or dissolved is nearly or quite insoluble in water, as in the instances of resins, camphor, and the essential oils.

Diluted alcohol, or proof spirit, is employed when the substance is a soluble both in alcohol and in water; or when one or more of the ingredients are soluble in the one fluid and one or more in the other, as in the case of vegetable bodies which contain extractive or tannin, or the natural salts of the alkaloids, or gum united with resin or volatile oil.

In the preparation of the tinctures, the drug should be dry and properly comminuted by being sliced, or pulverized. It is usually better in a moderately fine than in a very fine powder; the proper degree depends, however, upon the ease with which the menstruum extracts the soluble principles.

Eg. Some examples include :

- Tincture of Cannabis sativa
- Ticture of Benzoin
- Tincture of cantharides
- Tincture of opium
- Camphorated opium tincture (paregoric)

Before completion of the final product, many tinctures have to be assayed, either chemically or biologically, and based on the result of the determination; the potency is adjusted according to the prescribed standards in the Pharmacopoeia.

In tinctures prepared by percolation process, there often occurs a deposit of some of the extractives on standing, however, it is found that the deposit consists mainly of inert material and, therefore, potency of the finished product is not affected. The deposit can be filtered out in most dispensing pharmacies. The pharmacist is often able to dispense the clear portion of the tincture by simply decanting carefully, i. e. without stirring or agitating the sediment.

A few tinctures when prepared with weak alcoholic menstruum undergo some deterioration with time, as a result of acetous fermentation taking place in the alcoholic fluid. The best preventive is to keep them in full and well-closed bottles, at a low temperature.

Preparation of tinctures

Generally tinctures are prepared by the following processes:

1) Maceration process 2) Percolation process

1) Maceration process

A. Maceration process for tinctures made form organized drugs.

Organized drugs are those which have well defined cell structure. Maceration is the extraction process, in which the solid drug is placed in contact with whole amount of the menstruum in a closed vessel for 2-7 days with occasional stirring.

The liquid is strained and marc is pressed, adding the expressed liquid to the strained liquid. 'The combined liquids are clarified by decantation or filtration. Final volume is not adjusted. Here the volume is not adjusted to obtain uniformity of strength of the finished product. If the volume will be adjusted then the product would vary in strength with the apparatus used for expression.

Eg: Tinctures prepared by this method includes

- Tinctures of orange
- Tincture of capsicum,
- Tincture of lemon
- Tincture of gentian etc.

B. Maceration process for tincture made form unorganised drugs

Unorganized drugs are the plant exudates. Eg: Resins or Oleo-gum resins.

For the preparation of tinctures from unorganized drugs the ordinary maceration process described above is used with certain modifications. Such as,

1) The marc is not pressed.
2) The product is adjusted to volume.
3) The time period of maceration is reduced in certain cases.

Drugs suitable for maceration process:

1) Drugs which can not be powdered or which are difficult to be powdered owing of their hygroscopic character Eg: squill
2) Drugs which are not having relatively important therapeutic value.
3) Unorganized drug, i.e. gum resins, because these drugs would block the percolator.
4) Drugs which are relatively very cheap.

Eg: Preparations made by this process include,
Compound tincture of benzoin,
Tincture of myrrh,
Tincture of tolu etc.

2) Percolation process

Percolation is another method of extraction of active constituents form the drugs used in the preparation of tinctures and liquid extracts.

1) The solid ingredient(s) are moistened by keeping them with a sufficient quantity of the solvent in an air tight vessel for 4 hours and packed firmly in a suitable percolator and sufficient solvent is added to saturate the mass, and the top of the percolator is closed.
2) When the liquid is about to drip, the lower outlet of the percolator is closed, sufficient solvent is added to give a shallow layer above the mass, and the mixture is allowed to macerate in the closed percolator for 24 hours.
3) The percolation is then allowed to proceed slowly until the percolate slowly until the percolate measures about three quarters of the required volume of the finished tincture.
4) The marc is pressed. The expressed liquid is mixed with the percolate, and sufficient solvent is added to produce the required volume.
5) The combined liquids are mixed and clarified by filtration or by allowing them to stand and decanting.

Drugs suitable for percolation process are,

1) Drugs having cellular structure i. e. organized drug.
2) Drugs in powdered form, varying from coarse to moderately fine.
3) Drug having medicinally active constituents.

4) Drugs which are relatively expensive.

Tinctures prepared by percolation process include tincture of belladonna, compound tincture of cardamom, strong tincture of ginger etc.

Storage

Tinctures should be kept in tightly-closed containers to prevent loss of alcohol by evaporation, resulting in change of concentration of active principles.

Hydro-alcoholic menstruum being a fractionating menstruum, there is likelihood of microbial growth if the strength of alcohol is reduced very low. Hence, tinctures are directed to be stored in tightly closed containers and not exposed to excessive temperatures.

Many of the constituents of tinctures being light-sensitive undergo photochemical changes on exposure to light, hence tinctures should be stored in light-resistant containers and protected from sunlight.

If the active principle of the tincture deteriorates with time (on storage) it should be discarded after one year,

Eg: Aconite tincture, Belladonna tincture and Hyoscyamus tincture.

ORANGE TINCTURE

Rx	
Fresh Orange peal	3 vi s
Alcoholis (90%)...q.s..	fl. 3 XXV
Fiat : Tincturae	Mitte : fl. oz. i
Signa : Utendus more dicto.	

Conversion :

3 vi s → 6.25 dr — fl.3 xxv → 25 fl.drachms

1 drachms = 4 g — 1 fl.drachms = 4 ml

6.25 drachms = 25 g — 2.5 fl.drachms = 100 ml

Calculation : For fl.oz i → 1 fl.oz = 30 ml

Orange peal = $\frac{25}{100} \times 30 = 7.5$ g

Alchol (90%) .... q.s.... = 30 ml

Type	Ingredients	Quantity in imperial	Quantity in metric	Quantity taken
Monophasic liquid	Fresh orange peal	6.25 dr	25 g	7.5 g
	Alcohol (90%).....q.s.....	25 fl.dr	100 ml	30 ml
	Make: Tincture	Send: 30 ml		
	Direction: To be used, as directed.			

Theory :

Fresh orange peel is the fresh outer part of the pericarp of the ripe or nearly ripe fruit of Citrus uranium, family Rutaceae. Fresh orange peel is used for extraction because it contains more volatile oil than the dry peel. The inner white portion of the peel is excluded because it gives bitter taste to the preparation. The peel is thinly sliced to expose the oil glands embodied therein and to expose more surface area to the action of solvent.

Generally, alcohol in a concentration of 70 % or more is required to solubilize the volatile oils but since fresh orange peel contains a large proportion of water, it dilutes alcohol and therefore, 90 % alcohol is used which is diluted to 73-78 % v/v.

During maceration process occasional stirring is necessary to displace the saturated layers of menstruum around the drug. This leads to more effective extraction. Filtration is necessary to remove insoluble cell contents which are introduced due to pressing of marc. Adjustment of final volume is not done to keep uniformity of the strength of the finished product.

Procedure :

1) Take fresh orange peel and cut into thin slices. Weigh the required quantity of thin slices and macerate it with whole quantity of alcohol in a covered vessel.
2) Allow to macerate for 7 days with occasional stirring. Strain the liquid, press the marc and mix the expressed liquid to the strained liquid. Clarify the combined liquids by filtration.

Dispensing: Transfer to a amber coloured glass bottle (light resistant container) and close tightly to avoid the loss of alcohol or volatile principle by evaporation and decomposition (photochemical changes) of the volatile constituents with the loss of flavor by light.

Direction : To be used, as directed.

Storage: It should be stored in a well-closed light-resistant container and in a cool place to prevent the volatilization and deterioration of active constituents.

Uses: Orange tincture is used as flavouring agent.

BENZOIN TINCTURE

Rx	
Benzoin crushed	3 XXV
Alcoholos (90%) ... q.s....	fl. 3 CCL
Fiat : Tincturae	Milte fl.oz.ii
Signa : Utendus more dicto.	

Conversion :

3 xxv → 25 drachms — fl.3 CCL → 250 fl.drachms

1 drachm = 4 g — 1 fl.drachm = 4 ml

25 drachms = 100 g — 250 fl.drachms = 1000 ml

Calculation : For fl.oz ii → 2 fl.oz = 60 ml

Benzoin crushed $= \frac{100}{1000} \times 60 = 6\ g$

Alchol (90%) ....q.s.... = 60 ml

Type	Ingredients	Quantity in imperial	Quantity in metric	Quantity taken
Monophasic liquid	Benzoin crushed	25 dr	100 g	6 g
	Alcohol (90%)....q.s....	250 fl.dr	1000 ml	60 ml
	Make: Tincture	Send: 60 ml		
	Direction: To be used, as directed.			

Theory :

Benzoin is a balsamic resin obtained from Styrax benzoin, known as Sumatra benzoin. It contains benzoic and cinnamic acid esters of the alcohol benzoresinol; free benzoic and cinnamic acid.

Crushed benzoin is used to expose a large surface area to the solvent action of the menstruum and thus ensure complete extraction of the constituent. Alcohol (90%) is used to dissolve the volatile oils and resins. The alcohol strength in the final preparation is reduced due to dissolved oil and resin, and not due to dilution with water.

In the beginning 80% of the menstruum is used because the oil and resin which pass into solution occupy a variable volume. This is adequately covered by adding remaining amount of menstruum to the preparation. The liquid is filtered to separate the alcoholic layer from the gummy matter. Sufficient menstruum is passed through the filter to wash any adherent alcoholic liquid from the gummy matter.

Procedure :

Macerate the benzoin (crushed) in 800 ml of alcohol for one hour with frequent agitation, filter and pass sufficient alcohol through the filter to produce the required volume.

Dispensing: Transfer to a amber coloured glass bottle (light resistant container) and close tightly to avoid the loss of alcohol or volatile principle by evaporation and decomposition (photochemical changes) of the volatile constituents with the loss of flavor by light.

Storage: It should be stored in a well-closed light-resistant container and in a cool place to prevent the volatilization and deterioration of active constituents.

Uses :

Tincture of benzoin has two main medicinal uses, as a treatment for damaged skin, and as an inhalant.

1. It is used as an inhalation in the treatment of upper respiratory tract infections, including bronchitis and colds. For this purpose about 5 ml of the preparation is added to warm water and the vapors are inhaled.
2. When it is mixed with glycerine and water, it can be used as an antiseptic. Hence the tincture may be applied locally for cutaneous ulcers, bedsores, cracked nipples, and fissures of the lips and anus.
3. It is often applied to skin before applying tape or other adhesive bandages. To some degree, it protects the skin from allergy to the adhesive in the tape or bandage, but mostly it makes the tape or bandages adhere much longer.
4. It is also used by athletes for its reputation of toughening skin exposed to the tincture.

COMPOUND CARDAMOM TINCTURE

Rx	
Cardmom Seeds	3 iii ss
Caraway	3 iii ss
Cinnamon	gr XL ii
Amaranth	3 i s
Glycerin	fl. xii sss
Alcoholis (45%) .... q.s.....	fl. 3 CCL
Fiat : Tincturae	Milte fl.oz.i
Signa : Utendus more dicto.	

Conversion :

3 iii ss → 3.5 drachms
1 drachm = 4 g
3.5 drachms = 14 g

3 i s → 1.25 drachms
1 drachm = 4 g
1.25 drachms = 5 g

gr XL ii → 42 grains
15 grains = 1 g
42 grains = 2.8 g

fl.3 xii ss →12.5 fl.dr
1 fl.drachm = 4 ml
12.5 fl.dr = 50 ml
fl. 3 CCC = 250 fl.dr = 1000 ml

Calculation : For fl.oz i → 1 fl.oz = 30 ml

Cordamom Seeds $= \frac{14}{1000} \times 30 = 0.42$ g

Caraway $= \frac{14}{1000} \times 30 = 0.42$ g

Cinnamon $= \frac{2.8}{1000} \times 30 = 0.084$ g

Amaranth $= \frac{5}{1000} \times 30 = 0.15$ g

Glycerin $= \frac{50}{1000} \times 30 = 1.5$ ml

Alcohol (45%) .... q.s.... = 30 ml

Type	Ingredients	Quantity in imperial	Quantity in metric	Quantity taken
Monophasic liquid	Cardamon	3.5 dr	14 g	0.42 g
	Caraway (Mod..)	3.5 dr	14 g	0.42 g
	Cinnamon	42 grains	2.8 g	0.084 g
	Amaranth	1.25 grains	5 g	0.15 g
	Glycerin	12.75 fl.dr	50 ml	1.5 ml
	Alcohol (40%) ...q.s....	250 fl.dr	1000 ml	30 ml
	Make: Tincture Direction: To be used, as directed.	Send: 30 ml		

Theory:

As the preparation contains more than one ingredient for extraction, it is termed as compound tincture. Glycerine prevents the precipitation of tannins and hence increases the stability of the product. Amarnth imparts colour to the tincture.

This tincture is prepared by percolation process. Cardamom seeds recently removed from the capsules should be used for powdering because it contains the required volatile constituents. Already removed or stored seeds will contain less amount of volatile ingredients.

Moderately coarse powders are used to expose an adequately large surface to the solvent action of the menstruum, moreover in case of non-reduction the menstruum will trickle down from spaces without penetrating the drug tissues. Imbibation is done to swell the drug before packing in the percolator. If dry drug is packed there will be air entrapment through which the menstruum will flow and may disturb the packing of the drug in the percolator thus obstructing smooth percolation.

Moistened plug of cotton wool is placed over the perforated disc so as to prevent the falling of the drug particles in the tap of percolator thus blocking the tap. Moistening of cotton wool is done to prevent the fibres to fall in the tap. Packing of the moistened drug should be uniform. It should neither be too tight nor loose. Tight packing will not allow the menstruum to pass freely which will led to slow extraction rate. Similarly loose packing will allow the menstruum to pass through quickly resulting in incomplete contact with the drug, hence less dissolution of active constituents.

After packing the material in the percolator a piece of filter paper is placed over top layer of the packed material. On the filter paper a small quantity of washed sand is placed to prevent disturbance of the packed materials. After packing the column, sufficient menstruum is added to saturate the material and allowed to set aside to 24 hours so that during this period much of the soluble matter passes into solution. Under no circumstances the column is allowed to become dry otherwise cracks will appear in the packed column resulting in inefficient percolation.

Procedure

1) Mix the weighed amounts of Cardamom, Caraway and Cinnamon powders and moisten them with a sufficient quantity of alcohol. Pack the moistened drug in the percolator. Pour sufficient menstruum onto the drug so as to saturate the column of drug throughout its length and also form a layer above it. Set aside for 24 hours.
2) Collect the extract.
3) Separately dissolve amaranth in small amount of alcohol. To this add glycerine. Incorporate this solution to the collected extract.
4) Add more of alcohol to produce the required volume. Filter, if necessary.

Dispensing: Transfer to a amber coloured glass bottle (light resistant container) and close tightly to avoid the loss of alcohol or volatile principle by evaporation and decomposition (photochemical changes) of the volatile constituents with the loss of flavor by light.

Direction : To be used, as directed.

Storage: It should be stored in a well-closed light-resistant container and in a cool place to prevent the volatilization and deterioration of active constituents.

Uses: It is used as carminative and flavouring agent.

Similar example

1) **Aromatic cardamom tincture**

Rx

Cardamom oil	0.3 ml
Cinnamon oil	1.0 ml
Caraway oil	1.0 ml
Clove oil	1.0 ml
Strong ginger tincture	6.0 ml
Ethanol (90%), ...q.s...	100.0 ml

Uses: This is a very agreeable aromatic tincture, used as a carminative, but more frequently as an additive to mixtures, infusions, etc., to make them pleasant to taste.

STRONG GINGER TINCTURE

Rx	
Ginger in moderately coarse powder	3 CXXV
Alcoholis (90%) .....q.s.....	fl. 3 CCL
Fiat : Tincturae	Mitte : fl.oz.ii
Signa : Utendus more dicto.	

Conversion :

3 CXXV = 125 drachms fl.3 **CCL** = 250 fl.drachms

1 drachm = 4 g 1 fl.drachms = 4 ml

125 drachms = 500 gm 250 fl.drachms = 1000 ml

Calculation : For fl.oz ii → 2 fl.oz = 60 ml

Ginger powder $= \frac{500}{1000} \times 60 = 30$ g

Alchol (90%) ....q.s.... = 60 ml

Type	Ingredients	Quantity in imperial	Quantity in metric	Quantity taken
Monophasic liquid	Ginger (mod...)	125 dr	500 g	30g
	Alcohol (90%) .....q.s.....	250 fl.dr	1000 ml	60 ml
	Make: Tincture	Send: 60 ml		
	Direction: To be used, as directed.			

Theory:

Ginger consists of the rhizome of Zingiber officinale, family Zingibracae. The oleo-resins present in the ginger are not soluble in water or dilute alcohol hence, a strong alcohol must be used to effect extraction. Weak tincture is prepared by diluting the strong tincture in 1:5 proportion with alcohol 90 %.

It is prepared by percolation process. Ginger, in moderately coarse powder, is used to expose an adequately large surface to the solvent action of the menstruum. Before packing the drug into the percolator, moistening is done to swell the drug otherwise if the swelling takes place in the percolator it will lead to tight packing of the drug and percolation would not take place.

After packing the moistened drug in the percolator, sufficient menstruum is poured and allowed to set aside for 24 hours so that during this period much of the soluble matter passes into solution. The marc is pressed to recover the menstruum to the maximum. Filtration is done to remove the cell debris expelled by expression of the marc.

Procedure :

1) Moisten the drug with a portion of the menstruum and set aside for 4-6 hours. Pack the moistened drug in the percolator. Pour sufficient menstruum onto the drug so as to saturate the column of drug throughout its length and also form a layer above it. Set aside for 24 hours.
2) Commence the percolation and collect the percolate in a vessel. Continue percolation until 3/4 of volume of the finished product is obtained. Test the percolate for complete exhaustion of the drug. Press the marc and add the expressed liquid to the already collected percolate. The total volume should be about 80-90% of the final volume.
3) Add more of menstruum to produce the required volume. Allow the liquid to stand to settle the suspended particles. Decant or clarify the liquid by filtration.

Dispensing: Transfer to an amber colored glass bottle (light resistant container) and close tightly to avoid the loss of alcohol or volatile principle by evaporation and decomposition (photochemical changes) of the volatile constituents with the loss of flavor by light.

Storage: It should be stored in a well-closed light-resistant container and in a cool place to prevent the volatilization and deterioration of active constituents.

Uses: It is used as carminative and flavouring agent.

Similar examples

1) Compound Benzoin tincture

Synonyms: Friars' Balsam

Aloes	2.0 g
Tolu balsam	2.5 g
Prepared styrex	7.5 g
Benzoin, crushed	10.0 g
Ethanol (90%), ...q.s....	100.0 ml

Uses: The tincture is used to protect and toughen skin in the treatment of bedsores, ulcers, cracked nipples, and fissures of the lips and anus and as an inhalant in bronchitis and respiratory conditions.

2) Tincture of Nux Vomica

Nux Vomica, coarse power	100 g
Alcohol (45 %), ...q.s......	1000 ml

Uses: Bitter tonic in gastric atony.

3) Capsicum tincture

Capsicum, moderately coarse powder	50 g
Alcohol (60%) ....q.s.....	1000 ml

Use: As carminative, stomachic and local counter irritant.

4) Belladonna Tincture

Belladonna Herb (Moderately coarse powder) 100 g

Alcohol (70 %) ....q.s..... 1000 ml

Uses: It is used as parasympatholytic and spasmolytic in the cases of intestinal spasms.

5) Datura Tincture

Datura liquid extract 100 ml

Alcohol (45 %) ....q.s..... 1000 ml

Uses: As parasympatholytic

6) Opium Tincture

Opium, sliced capsule 10 g

Alcohol (90 %) ....q.s..... 100 ml

Uses: In I.P. it is categorised as hypnotic and sedative, depending on the dose. In U.S.P. it is categorised as an antiperistaltic, used in diarrhea.

Students Exercise:

1. What are Tinctures?
2. What are the processes for making tinctures?
3. How to prepare tincture?
4. How to preserve tinctures?
5. Why is alcohol used as a menstruum and what should be the strength of alcohol used as a menstruum for extracting vegetable drugs?
6. Define: Maceration, Percolation.
7. Why marc is pressed in case of organised drug and not is unorganised drug?
8. Why is the final volume not adjusted in case of organized drugs and adjusted in unorganized drugs?
9. What are the several distinct operations required in the extraction of drugs by percolation?
10. Which types of drug is suitable / unsuitable for extraction by the method of percolation?
11. What is the difference between tincture and extraction?
12. What is the use of cardamom tincture?
13. What is the use of orange tincture?
14. Give pharmaceutical application of tinctures.
15. What is percolation?

30 SUSPENSIONS

Suspensions are bi-phasic liquid dosage forms or dispersion systems, in which the finely divided, insoluble solid particles are suspended or dispersed in a liquid.

The size of the dispersed solids ranges from 0.1 to 1000 μ.

a) Solid particles constitute as : Dispersed phase (Internal phase)

b) Liquid medium constitute as : Continuous phase (External or Dispersion phase)

Pharmaceutical suspensions may be used for,

Internal (Oral) use	:	Eg. Antacids
External use	:	Eg. Lotions (Calamine lotion)
Parenteral use	:	Eg. Procaine penicillin G injection
Opthalmic use	:	Eg. Eye drops.

Significance (advantages or importance) of suspensions :

1) **Stability:** Some drugs are unstable, when they are formulated in solution form. Hence such drugs are converted into insoluble form and formulated as suspensions, to improve their stability.

   Ex. Procaine penicillin G injection: in which penicillin G is soluble in water, but this solution form is unstable. Hence penicillin G is converted into insoluble form as, Procaine penicillin G and formulated as suspension for parenteral use.

2) **To mask the taste:** The disagreeable (bitter) taste of some drugs in solution form is masked, by converting such drugs into insoluble form as a suspension. Eg. Insoluble Chloroamphenicol palmitate is used in the form of suspension, to reduce the bitter taste of soluble chloramphenicol.

3) **Prolonged action:** Prolonged (Controlled release) action of drug can be obtained, by converting the drugs into complex form or insoluble form and administered as suspensions.

   Ex. Insulin is complexed with Zinc and converted into protamine - Zinc insulin to get prolonged action, in the form of parenteral suspension (Depot therapy.) (Hence parenteral suspensions are used in "Depot therapy". This is based on the slow release of drug, from the suspension for extended action.)

4) **Bio-availability:** Drugs in the form of suspensions have higher (more) bio-availability, compared to the tablets and capsules.

   Ex. Antacid suspensions have quick action, compared to the same antacid tablets.

5) **Choice of solvent:** If drug is not soluble in water and other solvents are not suitable for that drugs and for administration, then drug is formulated in the form of suspension.

   Ex. Cortico-steroids are used as suspensions (injections), by dispersing insoluble corticosteroids in water.

6) **Route of administration:** Another important reason for using drug in suspension form is, their applicability in different routes like oral, parenteral, external and ophthalmic routes.

Disadvantages of suspensions : The suspensions also have some disadvantages such as :

1) Sedimentation may give the problem in measuring of accurate dose and uniform distribution of drug, throughout the system.
2) Compared to the unit dosage forms, dose of drug in suspensions is not accurate. Hence potent drugs cannot be administered in suspension form.
3) Since suspensions are liquid dosage forms, microbial growth takes place easily. Therefore suspensions should be properly preserved, by using preservatives.
4) Suspensions being liquid dosage forms, may require sufficient care during handling and transportation compared to the solid dosage form.
5) In case of accidental breakage, the container of suspension may result in loss of whole of the dosage form.
6) Suspensions require additional additives like :
   Suspending agents
   Flocculating agents
   Viscosity increasing agents
   Wetting agents
7) The drug in suspension is liable to undergo oxidation and hydrolysis. Hence chemical stability is a problem, so needs proper attention (care).

Ideal properties of suspensions:

A well formulated pharmaceutical suspension, should have the following ideal characteristics (properties) such as,

1) The solid particles should have size that, they do not settle rapidly (size range should be 0.1 to 1000 µ (microns))
2) The dispersed particles should not settle rapidly. Even though particles settles down, they should be easily redispersed after shaking.
3) Sediment should not form a hard cake, because it is difficult to redisperse even after shaking.
4) The particles should be uniformly distributed (dispersed) through out the external phase.
5) Suspensions should be elegant in appearance (good looking).
6) Suspensions should be physically, chemically and micro-biologically stable.
7) Suspensions should have suitable viscosity, so that they can be easily poured from container, for measurement of dose.
8) The suspensions meant for internal (oral) use, should be palatable (have good taste and odour).
9) Suspensions used for external (topical) use, should spread easily and leave a film of medicament at the site of application.
10) Suspensions meant for ophthalmic use, should be free from irritation.

11) Suspensions meant for parenteral use, should not loose their efficacy during sterilization.
12) Suspensions meant for parenteral use should have proper particle size and viscosity, so that it can be easily pass through the needle of a syringe.

Classification of suspensions: Suspensions are classified into different types,

I. **Classification of suspensions based on route of administration;**

1) Oral suspensions
2) Topical suspensions
3) Parenteral suspensions
4) Opthalmic suspensions

II. **Classification of suspensions based on, their method of preparation:** (i.e. depending on the nature of substance to be dispersed) as,

1) Suspensions containing diffusible solids.
2) Suspensions containing indiffisuble solids
3) Suspensions containing poorly wettable solids.
4) Suspensions containing precipitate forming liquid
5) Dispersions of oil in inhalation
6) Suspensions produced by chemical reaction.

III. **Classification of suspensions based on, the nature of suspending particles:**

1) Flocculated suspensions
2) Deflocculated suspensions.

1) Flocculated suspensions:

In a flocculated suspension, the individual particles of suspended phase are in contact with one another and form a loose network like structure, called as "floccules" or "aggregates".

- These floccules are light, fluffy and held together by weak Vander Wall's forces of attraction. This flocculation (aggregation) is also achieved, by adding flocculating agents.
- The floccules settle down rapidly within short period of time, due to gravity and density of floccules and form a loosly packed sediment. Hence this sediment will be re-dispersed easily after small shaking of the container, so it gives homogenous (uniform) suspension.

Advantages:

1) The formation of hard cake can be reduced by converting the drug into floccules.
2) The controlled release (prolonged action) of drug can be obtained by converting the drug in the form of floccules.
3) Even though sedimentation rate is fast, the formed sediment can be easily re-dispersed, on moderate shaking.

Disadvantages:

1) Compared to the deflocculated suspensions, flocculated suspensions are not elegant in appearance (i.e. not having good appearance) because after removing the suspension from bottle, floccules remain sticking to the walls of the container and hence gives the non-elegant appearance.
2) Compared to the deflocculated suspensions, the bio-availability of drugs in flocculated suspensions is less. Because, the drug absorption is slow, due to the formation of network like floccules (i.e. due to bigger size of drug particles first floccules should break down into small and individual particles and they undergo dissolution and absorption).

2) De-flocculated (non-flocculated) suspensions:

In deflocculated suspensions, each suspended particle exists as a separate entity. Therefore in this system, the rate of sedimentation is slow, but after sedimentation it forms a hard compact cake. This hard cake is very difficult to re-disperse, to get a homogenous suspension after moderate shaking.

Advantages:

1) Deflocculated suspensions are elegant in appearance, because individual particles do not stick to the container.
2) Sedimentation rate is slow.
3) Bio-availability in deflocculated suspensions is high, because each individual drug particles will be quickly absorbed.

Disadvantages:

In deflocculated suspensions after sedimentation, "hard cake" will be formed. It is very difficult to re-disperse even after shaking. This will lead to the non-uniform distribution of drug and dose.

Difference between Flocculated and Deflocculated suspensions:

Sr.no	Flocculated suspensions	Deflocculated suspensions
1)	In these suspensions, solid particles exist as loose network like structure called as floccules.	In these suspensions, particles exist as separate entities.
2)	Rate of sedimentation is fast (high), due to high density of floccules.	Rate of sedimentation is slow, due to less density of individual particles.
3)	Sediment is loosely packed.	Sediment formed is hard compact cake.
4)	Loosely packed sediment can be easily re-dispersed, by moderate shaking.	Hard cake is difficult to redisperse, by moderate shaking.
5)	The Bio-availability in flocculated suspension is less (slow).	The Bio-availability in deflocculated suspension is high (fast).

6)	These have non-elegant appearance, because floccules stick to the walls of the container.	These are elegant (pleasant) in appearance, because after sedimentation particles will not stick to the wells of the container.
7)	Sediment volume is high.	Sediment volume is small.
8)	The supernatant liquid becomes clear, because floccules settle down rapidly.	The supernatant liquid remains cloudly for a longer time, because small particles take very long time to settle.

Formulation (preparation) of suspensions : For the formulation of suspensions, along with medicament and vehicle other additives are also used, as shown in the table.

S.n.	Type	Example for additives	
1.	Flocculating agents	a. Surfactants	Tweens Spans
		b. Electrolytes	Aluminium chloride Potassium phosphate
		c. Hydrophilic polymers	Hydro-colloids, Bentonite, Alginates, Carbowaxes, Silicates.
2.	Suspending and Thickening agents	a. Natural polysaccharides	Gum acacia Gum tragacanth Guar gum Sodium alginate Starch Xanthan gum
		b. Semi synthetic Polysaccharides	Methyl cellulose Sodium carboxy methyl cellulose Hydroxy cellulose Hydroxy propyl cellulose Hydroxy propyl methyl cellulose Micro crystalline cellulose
		c. Inorganic agents	Clays, Bentonite Aluminium hydroxide
		d. Synthetic agents	Colloidal silicon dioxide Carbomer (Carboxy vinyl polymer)
3.	Wetting agents	——	Alcohol, Glycerin, Polysorbate, Tragacanth mucilage, Sodium alginate, Bentonite dispersion, Surfactants having HLB value between 7 to 9, Sodium lauryl sulphate,

4.	Preservatives	——	Benzoic acid, Chloroform, Sodium benzoate, Methyl paraben, Propyl paraben,
5.	Colouring agents	——	Amaranth Tartrazine (Pink & Yellow) Sunset yellow Quninie yellow Brillient green Erithrosine
6.	Flavouring agents	——	Lemon oil, Orange oil, Pineapple flavour.
7.	Sweetening agents	——	Sucrose, Saccharin.
8.	Stabilizers	——	Sodium citrate

Dispensing :

1. **Suspensions meant for oral use:** These suspensions are dispensed in narrow mouthed clear or amber coloured glass bottle, closed with metallic screw cap. These containers should have adequate air space above the liquid, to permit adequate shaking, before use.
2. **Suspension meant for external application :** Suspensions which are less viscous in nature should be dispensed in coloured fluted, narrow mouthed, plastic containers closed with coloured, plastic screw cap or hinged lids to differentiate from the preparations, which are meant for internal use.
   Ex. Calamine lotion
   Sulphur lotion.

Storage:

1. Since viscosity is inversely proportional to the temperature, at higher temperature, viscosity of suspension will decreases.
2. Suspension should not be stored at freezing temperature (in refrigerator), because very low temperature leads to aggregation of suspended particles.
   Therefore suspensions should be stored in a cool place or at a room temperature, not exceeding 25 ºC.

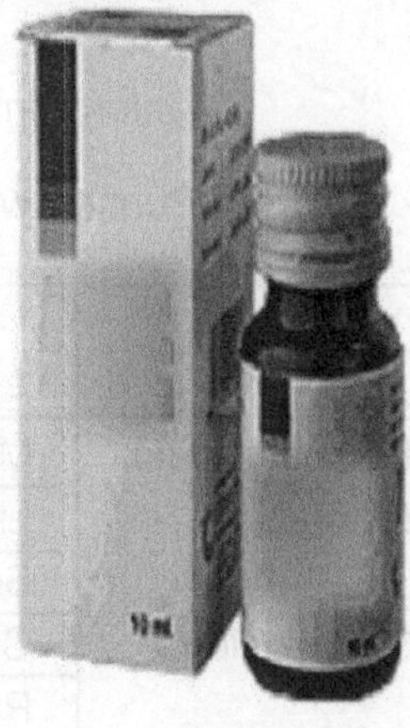
Container for suspension

Label : Along with general requirements of label, suspensions should bear auxilliary label like,

- SHAKE WELL BEFORE USE.

If suspension is meant for external use it should bear, auxilliary label as

- FOR EXTERNAL USE ONLY,
- SHAKE WELL BEFORE USE.

MAGNESIUM HYDROXIDE MIXTURE B.P.

Synonyms : Milk of magnesia or Cream of magnesia or Magnesium hydroxide oral suspension

Rx	
Magnesii sulphatis	3 xii
Light magnelsic oxidi	3 xiii s
Sodii hydroxidi	3 iii sss
Chloroformi	fl. 3 sss
Aquam .... q.s...	fl. 3 CCL
Fiat : Suspension	Mitte: 1 fl.oz
Signa : Duo cochleare minimum b.i.d sumendum.	

Conversion :

3 xii → 12 dr
1 dr = 4 g
12 dr = 48 g
3 Xiii s → 13.25 dr = 53 g
3 iii ss → 3.75 dr = 15 g

fl 3 sss → 0.75 fl. dr
1 fl.dr = 4 ml
0.75 dr = 3 ml
fl.3 CCL → 250 fl.dr = 1000 ml

Calculation: For 1 fl.oz → 30 ml

Magnesium sulphate $= \frac{48}{1000} \times 30 = 1.44$ g

Light magnesium oxide $= \frac{53}{1000} \times 30 = 1.59$ g

Sodium hydroxide $= \frac{15}{1000} \times 30 = 0.45$ g

Chloroform $= \frac{3}{1000} \times 30 = 0.09$ ml

Purified water...q.s... 30 ml

Type	Ingredients	Quantity in imperial	Quantity in metric	Quantity taken
Biphasic liquid	Magnesium sulphate	12 dr	48 g	1.44 g
for oral use.	Light magnesium oxide	13.25 dr	53 g	1.59 g
	Sodium hydroxide	3.75 dr	15 g	0.45 g
Suspension	Chloroform	0.75 fl. dr	3 ml	0.09 ml
	Purified water ...q.s...	250 fl. dr	1000 ml	30 ml
Mixture	Make : Suspension Send : 30 ml Direction : Two teaspoonful to be taken two times a day.			

Theory : • Milk of Magnesia is an aqueous colloidal dispersion of magnesium hydroxide. Magnesium hydroxide is prepared by :

(1) Hydration of magnesium oxide and

(2) Precipitation (double decomposition) of magnesium sulphate and sodium hydroxide. As shown in the reaction,

$$1)\ MgO + H_2O \xrightarrow{(Hydration)} Mg(OH)_2$$

$$2)\ MgSO_4 + 2NaOH \xrightarrow{(precipitation)} Mg(OH)_2 + Na_2SO_4$$

• Magnesium hydroxide mixture cannot be prepared directly by suspending (dispersing) the magnesium hydroxide powder in water, because it absorbs carbon dioxide and moisture from atmosphere. Therefore, magnesium hydroxide should be prepared "insitu" by the reaction between magnesium oxide, magnesium sulphate and sodium hydroxide.

• In this preparation, both magnesium oxide and magnesium sulphate are used, because

(a) If the mixture is prepared only by using magnesium oxide (hydration reaction), mixture becomes very viscous and unpourable after storage.

(b) If the mixture is prepared only by using magnesium sulphate (precipitate reaction), the particles of magnesium hydroxide sediment quickly and, hence does not remain uniformly suspended.

Therefore, Magnesium hydroxide mixture is prepared by using both magnesium oxide and magnesium sulphate (i.e. using both the reactions) so that, particles remain suspended uniformly and the preparation does not become too viscous and easily pourable.

• The pH of the mixture (preparation) is about 10, hence it attacks the soda lime glass containers, which leads to leaching of the alkali from the glass and imparts a bitter taste to the preparation.

• To minimize this problem 0.1% of citric acid can be added to the preparation. It also enhances the palatability, because it gives acidic taste to the preparation.

• In this preparation, a large volume of water is used to get the particles of smaller (desired) size. After getting magnesium hydroxide mixture, it should be filtered and precipitate of magnesium hydroxide should be repeatedly washed with water, to remove sulphate (SO_4^{-2}) ions of sodium sulphate, because sulphate ions gives purgative effect to this mixture.

• To determine the absence or presence of sulphate ions, the testing can be done by "Sulphate test" using Barium chloride solution.

• To improve the palatability of the mixture, flavouring agent up to 0.05% can also incorporated. Chloroform is used as a preservative.

Procedure : In this preparation, a large volume of water is required to get the particles of smaller (desired) size.

1) Hence, separately dissolve magnesium sulphate in a 200 ml of purified water.
2) Dissolve the weighed amount of sodium hydroxide in a little portion of purified water (i.e. 10-15% of the total volume of the mixture) in a mortar.
3) To the sodium hydroxide solution, add light magnesium oxide and triturate to form a smooth cream. After getting smooth cream, add sufficient purified water to produce 200-250 ml.
4) To the magnesium sulphate solution, pour the dispersion of sodium hydroxide and magnesium oxide in a thin stream, into a solution with continuous stirring.
5) After complete mixing, precipitate of magnesium hydroxide will be formed. Allow this precipitate to settle down, after settling, decant (remove) the clear supernatant liquid and transfer the residue to a calico strainer.
6) Wash the precipitate with purified water several times, until the precipitate should be free from sulphate ions. The presence or absence of sulphate ions in the filtrate is confirmed by conducting "sulphate test" using Barium chloride solution.
7) If filtrate passes the sulphate test, then mix the washed precipitate with purified water and add chloroform and mix uniformly.
8) Transfer the mixture (dispersion) to a measure, add required amount of citric acid and adjust the final volume with water.

Dispensing: The magnesium hydroxide mixture should be dispensed in a well filled and well closed, glass or plastic bottle, to protect it from atmospheric carbon dioxide, because carbon dioxide reacts with hydroxide ion (OH-) of magnesium hydroxide and converts into magnesium carbonate, which is indiffusible in nature.

If glass containers are used for supplying the milk of magnesia, 0.1% citric acid should used to prevent the leaching of alkali from the glass, made up of soda lime. If plastic containers are used, there is no need of adding citric acid. Generally blue coloured glass bottle is used to enhance the white appearance of the milk of magnesia.

The tannins of the cork can change the colour of the mixture, therefore the cork should be used after dipping in melted paraffin

Therefore transfer the dispersion to a narrow mouthed, blue coloured glass bottle, close it thoroughly with metallic screw cap, polish and label.

Direction : Two teaspoonful to be taken two times a day.

Storage : Milk of magnesia should not be stored at freezing temperature (refrigerator), because freezing leads to the co-arsening (aggregation)of the dispersed particles. Hence the colloidal size of the particles increases (alters). Temperature above the 35°C decreases the gel structure of the mixture

Therefore, store the magnesium hydroxide mixture at cool temperature (or at room temperature not exceeding 25°C.)

Auxilliary label : SHAKE WELL BEFORE USE.
DO NOT STORE IN REFRIGERATOR (COLD PLACE).

Uses : Milk of magnesia is used as an antacid of choice, because it has the advantage over carbonates and bicarbonates, as there is no liberation of CO_2 and it does not produce alkalosis. It also has laxative action at higher doses. But most of the time it is used as antacid at lower doses 5-10 ml.

Note : Other examples for suspensions, which are already discussed in other categories (classification).

Sr. no	Type of Preparation	Example	P.no.
1)	Suspensions containing diffusible solids. (Mixture)	a) Magnesium sulphate mixture	39
		b) Light kaolin and magnesium carbonate mixture	40
		c) Magnesium trisilicate mixture	42
2)	Suspensions containing indiffusible solids (Mixture)	a) Mixture of Prepared chalk	45
		b) Phenacetin and caffeine mixture	47
		c) Sulphadiamadine mixture	51
		d) Bismuth carbonate mixture	53
3)	Suspensions containing precipitate forming liquid (Mixture)	a) Mixture of Ethereal tincture of Lobelia	56
		b) Mixture of tincture of Myrrh and potassium iodide	58
4)	Lotions (Suspensions produced by chemical reaction)	a) Sulphurated potash lotion	221
		b) White Lotion NF (Sulphide lotion)	223
		c) Calamine lotion IP	216
5)	Inhalation (Dispersion of oils in Inhanlations)	a) Menthol-Eucalyptus oil Inhalation	191

Other examples for suspensions :

(1) Amoxycillin trihydrate suspension :

Amoxycilling trihydrate	:	4 g
Sodium carboxy methyl cellulose	:	1.8 g
Sodium benzoate	:	0.45 g
Sugar	:	90 g
Tartrazine colour	:	0.02 g
Pineapple flavour	:	1 g
Purified water....q.s...	:	100 ml

Uses : This suspension is used as, antibacterial.

(2) Cortisone acetate suspension :

Cortisone acetate	:	2.5 g
Sodium CMC	:	0.5 g
Sodium chloride	:	0.9 g
Polysorbate-80	:	0.4 ml
Benzyl alcohol	:	0.9 ml
Purified water ...q.s...	:	100 ml

Uses : This suspension is used as, adreno-cortical hormone.

(3) Mixture of Aluminium hydroxide (Synonyms : Antacid suspension)

Aluminium hydroxide gel	:	36 g
Sorbitol	:	7 g
Methyl paraben	:	0.2 g
Propyl paragal	:	0.2 g
Peppermint oil	:	0.005 ml
Alcohol	:	1 ml
Purified water....q.s...	:	100 ml

Uses : This suspension is used as, antacid.

31 EMULSIONS

Latin term : Emulsio

The word 'Emulsion' originates from the Latin word "emulgere", which means milk. Since milk is a natural emulsion, all the products having similar nature to milk, are called as emulsions.

An emulsion is defined as, "biphasic or heterogenous liquid preparation containing two immiscible liquids, one of which is dispersed as minute globules in another liquid". The diameter of dispersed globules ranges from 0.1 to 100 μ (microns).

The liquid, which is converted into minute globules, is called as "dispersed phase" or "internal phase" and the liquid in which the globules are dispersed is called as "continuous phase" or "external phase" or "dispersion medium".

Emulsion posses a minimum thermodynamic stability, because two immiscible liquids cannot be remain dispersed for a longer period, droplets of dispersed phase quickly coalesce and the two liquids get separated. Therefore emulsifying agent is added, to increase the stability of emulsion. It forms a film around the globules and keeps the globules of dispersed phase separately, from other globules and prevent coalescence.

Classification of emulsions: Emulsions are classified mainly into two types,

1. Oil in water (o/w) type emulsions: In this type of emulsions, oil is dispersed as minute globules in the water. These emulsions are prepared by using emulsifying agents like gum acacia, tragacanth, methyl cellulose, soaps formed from monovalent bases like Na^+, K^+ and NH_4^+.

(o/w) type emulsions are mainly used for internal (oral) use because, the unpleasant taste and odour is masked by emulsification and oil being in a finely dispersed state, it is more quickly absorbed in GIT.

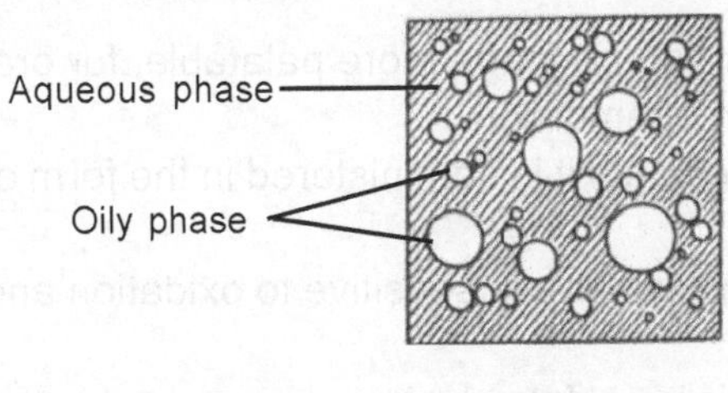

O/W type emulsion

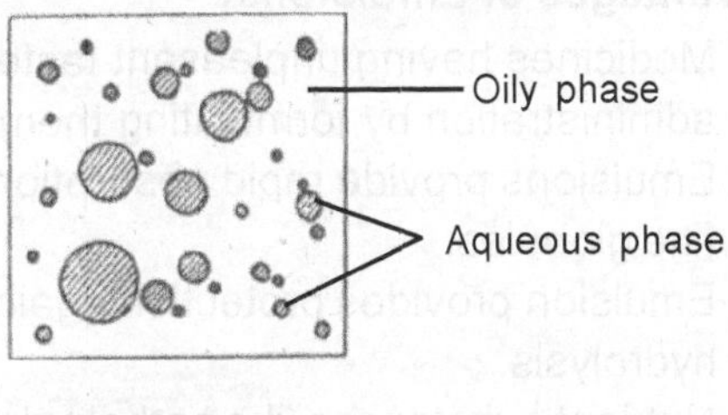

W/O type emulsion

2. Water in oil (w/o) type emulsions: In this type of emulsions, water is dispersed as minute globules in the oil. These emulsions are prepared by using emulsifying agents like bees wax, wool fat, resins, synthetic compounds, and soaps formed from divalent bases like Ca^{++}, Mg^{++} and Zn^{++}. These emulsions are mainly used for external purpose as lotions, liniments, creams, and emulsified ointments.

Special type of emulsions (Depending on the globule size):

1. **Micro-emulsions:**

Micro emulsions are emulsions, which contain globules of size less than 0.1μ (microns). Droplets of such dimensions cannot reflect light, hence globules are invisible to the naked eyes. Therefore micro-emulsions appear, as transparent solutions.

These emulsions are physically more stable, compared to conventional emulsions. Micro emulsions are used for preparation of both internal and external purpose and they show increased bioavailability of drug compared to conventional emulsions, hence now-a-days they are becoming more popular.

Eg: • Etoposide emulsion • Methotrexate emulsion

Multiple emulsions (Double emulsion):

Multiple emulsions are complex type of emulsions. These are also called as 'emulsion – within – emulsion'. Multiple emulsions are represented (designated) as,

1) o/w/o type emulsion 2) w/o/w type emulsion

o/w/o emulsions: In this type of emulsion, (o/w) type of emulsion is re-dispersed in the oil phase.

w/o/w emulsions: In this type of emulsion, (w/o) type of emulsion is re-dispersed in the aqueous phase.

These types of emulsions can be prepared by proper selection of emulsifying agents, depending on H.L.B. scale.

Applications: In multiple emulsions, the drug is entrapped (incorporated) in the inner most phase. Hence the drug must cross two phase boundaries, before getting absorbed. Hence this mechanism is used in the preparation of controlled (sustained) release emulsions (formulations), meant for the both,

1) Internal or oral use.
2) In 'Depot therapy', as intramuscular injections.

Advantages of Emulsions:

1) Medicines having unpleasant taste and odour can be made more palatable, for oral administration by formulating them in the form of emulsion.
2) Emulsions provide rapid absorption of drug, because it is administered in the form of fine globules.
3) Emulsion provides protection against the drugs, which are sensitive to oxidation and hydrolysis.
4) Nutrient substances like carbohydrates, vitamins and fats can be administered to the patients, who are unable to swallow them orally. Therefore these substances are formulated as sterile and stable intravenous emulsions.
5) Dermatological preparations like lotions, creams, foam aerosols and certain ointments can be formulated in the form of emulsion.
6) Radio-opaque emulsions are used as diagnostic agents, in X-Ray examination.
7) Multiple emulsions are used in depot therapy, for sustained release of drugs.
8) Emulsions are economically cheap because, water is used as one of its phase.

Disadvantages of emulsions:

1) Improper emulsification may cause breaking of emulsion on storage.
2) Sometimes emulsions are difficult to prepare, because special processing parameters are required.
3) Because of their instability, emulsions have short shelf life.
4) Since emulsions are liquid dosage forms, packing, handling and storage is difficult compared to solid dosage forms.

Formulation of emulsions:

I. Emulsifying agents / Emulsifiers / Emulgents:

Emulsifying agent is a substance, which reduces the interfacial tension between oily phase and aqueous phase and forms a film around the dispersed globules, hence prevents the coalescence of droplets and thus makes them, miscible with each other to get a stable emulsion. Therefore an ideal emulsifying agent, must possess the following ideal properties:

1) It should be capable of reducing the interfacial tension, between the two immiscible liquids.
2) It should form complete and coherent film, around dispersed globules, so as to prevent their coalescence.
3) It should be compatible with other ingredients of the preparation.
4) It should be non-toxic and chemically stable.
5) It should be capable of producing and maintaining the required consistency (viscosity) of the emulsion.

Emulsifying agents are classified as:

1)	Natural emulsifying agents	a. From vegetable source	Gum acacia, Karaya gum, Tragacanth gum, Agar, Pectin, Starch, Irish moss, Alginate, Gaur gum, Soyabean.
		b. From animal source	Gelatin, Egg yolk, Casein, Wool fat, Serum albumin.
2)	Semi-synthetic polysaccharides		Methyl cellulose, Carboxy methyl cellulose, Sodium carboxy methyl cellulose, Hydroxy propyl methyl cellulose, Micro crystalline cellu lose.
3)	Synthetic subtances	a. Anionic	Sodium lauryl sulphate, Polypeptide condensates, Trioleyl phosphate, Sarcosinates,
		b. Cationic	Alkoxyalkylamines, Benzalkonium chloride, Cetrimide, Benzethonium chloride.
		c. Non-ionic	Polyoxyethylene, polyoxyethylene alkyl ethers,Polyoxypropylene, Sorbitan ester,Glyceryl ester, Sucrose esters,Polyoxyethylene fatty acids ester.

4)	Inorganic subtances	—	Magnesium oxide, Milk of magnesia, Magnesium trisilicate, Magnesium aluminium silicate, Bentonite.
5)	Alcoholic substances	—	Polyethylene glycols (Carbowaxes), Cholesterol, Lauryl alcohol, Lecthins.

Note: When the vehicle is having medicinal value, eg. cinnamon water, mucilage of tragacanth should not be used as it may displace some amount of the vehicle and hence reduce its dose and its medicinal action.

II. Preservatives:

Emulsions are prepared by using different emulsifying agents like carbohydrates, proteins, non-ionic surfactants, which may leads to the growth of bacteria, fungi and moulds in presence of water. This leads to the contamination and breakdown (cracking) of emulsions.

To prevent this problem, preservatives should be incorporated.

Eg.
- Benzoic acid (0.1-0.2%),
- Chloroform (0.25%),
- Methyl paraben (0.1-0.2%),
- Propyl paraben (0.1-0.2%),
- Chlorocresol (0.1%)
- Cetrimide (0.002-0.01%)
- Sodium benzoate

III. Anti-oxidants:

During storage of emulsions, many oil and animal fats may undergo oxidation by atmospheric oxygen and leads to rancidity. To avoid these undesirable changes, suitable anti-oxidants are used, which have high affinity for oxygen and compete for it, with liable substances in the formulation.

Eg.
- Tocopherol,
- Ascorbic acid,
- Citric acid,
- Catechol,
- Gallic acid,
- Propyl gallate,
- Ethyl gallate,
- Pyrogallon.

IV. Flavouring agents:

To prevent the unpleasant taste of some emulsifying agents and fixed oils, flavouring agents like vanillin, benzaldehyde spirit and aromatic waters like chloroform water, cinnamon water, peppermint water are used. A combination of flavouring and sweetening agent, provides greater palatability to the emulsion.

Preparation of emulsions :

For small scale, emulsions are prepared by using mortar and pestle. For large scale homogenizer or colloid mill is used.

Emulsions are classified as,

1) Emulsions for internal use and

2) Emulsions for external use.

These emulsions are once again classified in to different groups, depending on the nature of emulsifying agents used, as shown in the table.

1) Classification of emulsions meant for internal use:

Sr.no	Types of emulsion	Examples
1)	Acacia emulsions.	Castor oil emulsion, Arachis oil emulsion, Olive oil emulsion, Codliver oil emulsion, Turpentine oil emulsion.
2)	Methyl cellulose emulsions.	Liquid paraffin oral emulsion.
3)	Emulsions containing oil or Water insoluble substances.	Liquid paraffin and Phenolphthalein emulsion.
4)	Emulsions containing a small proportion of oil.	Calciferol emulsion.
5)	Emulsion containing resinous tinctures	Terbene emulsion.
6)	Emulsions containing more than one oil	Liquid paraffin and castor oil emulsion.
7)	Irish moss emulsion	Cod liver oil emulsion with mucilage of irish moss
8)	Tragacanth emulsions (Emulsions containing combination of emulsifying agents or secondary emulsifying agent)	Shark liver oil emulsion. Liquid paraffin emulsion with acacia and tragacanth. Liquid paraffin emulsion with agar and acacia.
9)	Emulsions containing salts of alginic acid	Liquid paraffin emulsion with sodium alginate.
10)	Emulsions prepared with egg yolk.	Olive oil emulsion with egg yolk.

2) Classification of emulsions meant for external use:

w/o type of emulsions are used for external purpose or application. These may be used as lotions, liniments, applications, creams or as ointments. Their consistency may vary from liquid, semi-solid to solid.

Sr.no	Types of emulsions	Examples
(A)	**Soap emulsions:**	
1)	Alkali soap type	Turpentine liniment BP.
2)	Ammonium soap type	Ammonium soap emulsion. (White liniment BPC)

3)	Lime cream type	Lime cream (Calcium soap emulsion). Lime cream type lotion.
(B)	**Anionic emulsifying wax emulsions :**	Benzyl benzoate application BP.
(C)	**Semi solid emulsions:** 1) Wool fat emulsions 2) Wool alcohol emulsions 3) Lime cream emulsion 4) Borax creams	 Proflavine cream BPC, Oily cream BP. Barrier cream. Zinc cream BP (Lime cream). Zinc cream BP (Oily calamine cream) Cold cream.
D)	**Anionic emulsifying wax creams**	Aqueous cream BP, Buffered cream BPC.
E)	**Cationic emulsifying wax creams**	Cetrimide lotion BPC, Dimethicone cream,
F)	**Starch emulsion**	Castor oil enema.
G)	**Creams emulsified with non-ionic surfactants**	Cetomacrol cream BPC, Ichthamol cream, Chlorohexidine cream BPC.

> **Note :** Emulsions meant for external use are discussed in detail, which are coming under different categories like lotions, liniments, creams and ointments. Students are required to refer under particular categories.

The emulsions meant for internal use are usually prepared with acacia gum. To stabilize the acacia emulsions, other emulsifying agents like tragacanth and agar are used in the combination with acacia. These emulsions are prepared by using mortar and pestle.

Before preparing these emulsions, proportions of oil, water and gum (emulsifying agent) should be selected according to primary emulsion ratio, depending on the nature of oil used. The following table gives the proportion of oil, water, gum, required for different types of oils, for preparing primary emulsion.

Sr. No.	Type of the oil	Examples	Ratio of Oil: Water: Gum
1)	Fixed oils	Castor oil Cod liver oil Almond oil Arachis oil Olive oil Halaibut liver oil Calciferol oil (Vit.D)	4:2:1

2)	Volatile oil	Turpentine oil Sandal wood oil Cinnamon oil Peppermint oil Terbene oil Oil of cubebs	2:2:1
3)	Mineral oil	Liquid paraffin Balsam of peru	3:2:1
4)	Oleo-resin	Extract of male fern.	1:2:1

Primary emulsion : Primary emulsion is an initial thick emulsion, which is obtained by trituration of oil, water and gum, either by dry gum or wet gum method, where globules of internal phase of emulsion is reduced to their minimum size. The formation of primary emulsion is indicated by getting a white or nearly white (product) cream and a clicking or cracking or chit-chat sound is produced. Once the primary emulsion is formed, it is then diluted with the vehicle up to final volume by light trituration.

When an emulsion consists of more than one oil, the quantity of each oil is calculated separately and sum of these quantities is considered for preparing primary emulsion.

I. Dry gum method: In this method, oil is first triturated with gum and then water is added, to make a primary emulsion.

Procedure:

1) Calculate the quantities of oil, water and gum required for primary emulsion, depending on the nature of oil. For this method always use dry measure, mortar and pestle.
2) Take measured quantity of oil and gum in a mortar and mix them gently with pestle just, to disperse the gum in oil uniformly.
3) Add a measured quantity of water at once and triturate vigourously in a single direction without stopping, until a clicking sound is produced and product becomes thick white or nearly white, due to the internal light reflection. At this stage, product is called as primary emulsion.
4) The primary emulsion is then diluted, with remaining amount of aqueous vehicle (water), to make it pourable.
5) Transfer the content to a measure, and make up the final volume with water.

II. Wet gum method:

This method is used, only when the emulsifying agents are available in mucilage form themselves or they are required to be used in their mucilage forms. In this method, gum is first triturated with water, to form mucilage and then triturated with oil to make primary emulsion.

Procedure:

1) Calculate the quantities of oil, water and gum for primary emulsion, depending on nature of the oil.
2) Take a measured quantity of gum and water in a mortar and triturate, to form a mucilage.
3) To the mucilage, add oil in small portions with light trituration in a single direction.
4) When whole amount of oil has been added, triturate vigorously until a thick, white or nearly white product is formed and clicking sound is produced. (Until a thick primary emulsion is formed.)
5) To the primary emulsion, incorporate water in small portions with trituration, to make it pourable.
6) Transfer the content to a measure and make up the final volume with water.

> **Note :** Wet gum method has not become much popular compared to dry gum method because,
>
> 1) It does not gives stable emulsion (more chances of breaking of emulsion).
> 2) This method is slower process than dry gum method.

III Bottle method:

It is a modified method of dry gum method. Bottle method is used for the preparation of emulsions of volatile oils and other non-viscous oils. The proportions for primary emulsion ratio is, oil: water: gum is 2:2:1.

1) Measure the required quantity of the oil and transfer into a large bottle. Add the required amount of powdered gum acacia, close it thoroughly with the cap.
2) Shake the bottle vigorously, until the oil and gum are mixed thoroughly.
3) Add measured quantity of water and shake until, an uniform emulsion is formed.

Stability of emulsions

Stability of emulsion means, a formulated emulsion should retain its original characters, throughout its self life i.e. the dispersed globules should be uniformly distributed throughout the dispersion medium, during its storage.

Emulsion should be chemically stable, and they should not allow any bacterial growth to takes place. Instability in emulsion occurs during the storage, due to following three reasons.

1) Creaming
2) Cracking
3) Phase inversion.

1) **Creaming:** Creaming of emulsions is the upward movement of dispersed globules, to form a layer at the surface of the emulsion depending on its density. But creaming is a revesible process (i.e. cream can be re-dispersed by shaking or stirring, to get homogenous emulsion).

The creaming of dispersed phase can be minimized by utilizing Stoke's Law :

$$V = \frac{d^2 (\delta_1 - \delta_2) g}{18\eta}$$

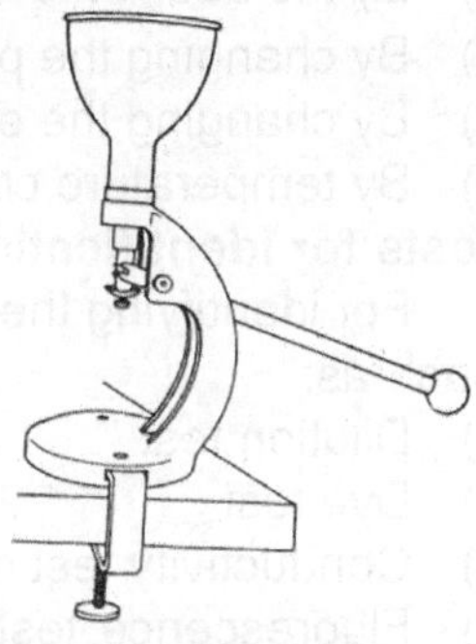
Hand homogeniser

Where V = Rate of creaming
d = Diameter of globules
δ_1 = Density of dispersed phase
δ_2 = Density of continuous phase
η = Viscosity of the continuous phase
g = Gravitational constant.

Creaming can be reduced :

a) By reducing the size of the globules, by passing the emulsion through homogenizer.

b) By reducing the difference in the density between two phases, by adding oil soluble substances to oily phase like α-bromo napthlene, bromoform. But it is not therapeutically desirable.

c) By increasing the viscosity of continuous phase, by adding thickening agents like tragacanth or methyl cellulose.

2) Cracking or Coalescence: Cracking means, coalescence of the globules of dispersed phase due to which, the separation of layers of dispersed and continuous phase occurs. Cracking is a irreversible process (i.e. it cannot be redispersed by shaking).

This may occur due to :

a) Decomposition or precipitation of emulsifying agent.
Eg : Alkali soaps are decomposed by acids.

b) Addition of an emulsifying agent, of opposite type.
Eg : Monovalent metal soap produces o/w emulsions while soap of divalent metal soap produces w/o emulsions.

c) By addition of common solvent.
Eg : Addition of a liquid in which, both disperse and continuous phase are soluble, which forms one phase system and destroys the emulsions.

d) Microbial contamination.

e) Changes in temperature.

f) Incorporation of excess dispersed phase.

3) Phase inversion:

Phase inversion in emulsions means, reversal of phases – i.e. the change of one type of emulsion into another type. Eg : o/w type emulsion changes into w/o type emulsion and vice versa.

Phase inversion occurs due to following reasons,

a) By the addition of an electrolyte.
b) By changing the phase – volume ratio.
c) By changing the emulsifying agents.
d) By temperature change.

Tests for identification of type of an emulsion:

For identifying the type of an emulsion mainly four tests are used. Such as,

1) Dilution test
2) Dye test
3) Conductivity test or Electrical conductivity test
4) Fluorescence test

Other evaluation tests for emulsions,

1) Particle size or globule size analysis by microscopic method.
2) Rate of phase separation by centrifugation.
3) Viscosity by viscometer.
4) Electophoretic properties.
5) Measurement of dielectric constant.

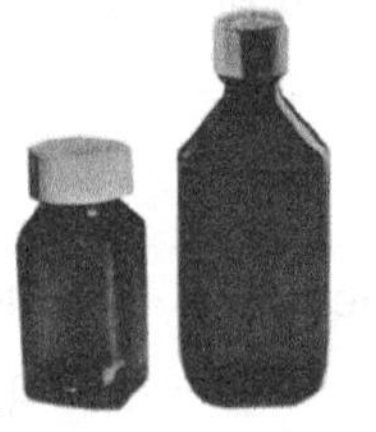

Narrow mouthed - amber coloured glass bottles

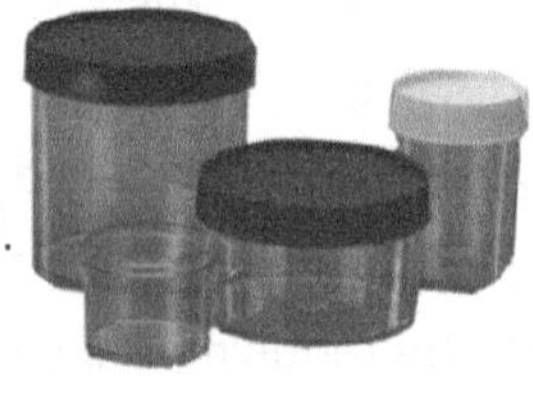

Small plastic wide mouthed containers

Dispensing of emulsions:

1) Emulsions meant for (oral) internal administration should be dispensed in narrow mouthed, plain or amber coloured glass bottle, closed with metallic screw cap. These containers should be airtight and having a sufficient air space above the emulsion, so as to permit adequate shaking before it's use.

Label: Label should bear all necessary requirements of liquid dosage forms for internal use, in addition it should contain auxilliary label like,
- SHAKE WELL BEFORE USE',
- STORE IN COOL PLACE.

2) Emulsions, which are meant for external use, should be dispensed in narrow mouthed, fluted, coloured plastic bottle. If emulsion has semisolid consistency, then it should be dispensed in small, wide mouthed glass or plastic bottle, so as to remove it easily from the container, closed with coloured plastic screw cap to differentiate it from the preparations meant for internal use.

Label: Label should bear all necessary requirements of liquid dosage forms, in addition it should contain auxilliary label like, 'FOR EXTERNAL USE ONLY',
'SHAKE WELL BEFORE USE',
'STORE IN A COOL PLACE'.

Storage: Emulsions should be protected from light, freezing and excess heat, because freezing temperature leads to the cracking of emulsion, higher temperature leads to the decrease in viscosity of dispersion medium, which finally leads to downward creaming. Hence they should be stored in a cool place.

Direction: Emulsions meant for external use should bear the direction on the label, about how to apply, how much to apply and how many times to apply.

Note : Emulsions meant for external use are discussed in detail, which are coming under different categories like lotions, liniments, creams and ointments. Students are required to refer under particular categories.

FERRIC AMMONIUM CITRATE EMULSION

Rx	
Olei morrhuae	fl. ʒ iv
Syrupi	fl. ʒ ii
Ferri ammonii citratis	gr xviii
Aquam cinnamoni....q.s...	fl.oz ii
Fiat : Emulsio	Mitte : fl.oz i
Signa : Cochleare parvum, bis in die capiendus.	

Conversion :

ʒ iv → 4 fluid drachms	gr xviii → 18 grains
1 fluid drachm = 4 ml	15 grains = 1 g
4 fluid drachms = 16 ml	18 grains = 1.2 g
fl. ʒ ii → 2 fl. dr = 8 ml	
fl.oz ii → 2 fl.oz = 60 ml	

Calculation : For fl.oz i → 1 fl.oz = 30 ml

Cod liver oil = $\frac{16}{60} \times 30 = 8$ ml

Syrup = $\frac{8}{60} \times 30 = 4$ ml

Ferric ammonium citrate = $\frac{1.2}{60} \times 30 = 0.6$ g

Cinnamon water....q.s........... = 30 ml

Primary emulsion: Since Cod liver oil is fixed oil, the primary emulsion ratio for,

oil : water : gum = 4 : 2 : 1

Cod liver oil = $\frac{8 \times 4}{4} = 8$ ml

Cinnamon water = $\frac{8 \times 2}{4} = 4$ ml

Acacia = $\frac{8 \times 1}{4} = 2$ g

Revised formula for primary emulsion:

Cod liver oil	---	8 ml
Cinnamon water	---	4 ml
Acacia	---	2 g
		----------
		14 ml

Revised formula for finished emulsion:

Primary emulsion --- 14 ml
Cinnamon water --- 16 ml
----
30 ml

Type	Ingredients	Quantity in imperial	Quantity in metric	Quantity taken
O/W type of emulsion containing fixed oil, emulsified with acacia gum	Cod liver oil	4 fl.dr	16 ml	8 ml
	Syrup	2 fl.dr	8 ml	4 ml
	Ferric ammonium citrate	18 gr	1.2 g	0.6 g
	Cinnamon water....q.s...	2 fl.oz	60 ml	30 ml
	Make: Emulsion	Send: 30 ml		
	Direction: One teaspoonful to be taken, two times a day.			

Theory:

This is an emulsion containing fixed oil. Cod liver oil is a valuable source of vitamin D and a readily digestible fat. Because of its vitamin D content, cod liver oil ensures optimum absorption of calcium and phosphorus, from the gut and prevents the rickets. Therefore it is used as a dietary supplement for infants and children as anti-rachitic agent.

Cod liver oil is insoluble in water and also posses unpleasant odour and taste, hence it causes nausea. Therefore it is formulated in the form of o/w type of emulsion, to mask its unpleasant taste and odour, using acacia as emulsifying agent.

Ferric ammonium citrate is water soluble substance and acts as haematinic. Syrup is used as sweetening agent. Cinnamon water constitutes as continuous phase and also acts as carminative. Since cod liver oil is a fixed oil, the primary emulsion ratio will be oil: water: gum acacia (4:2:1).

Procedure: (By dry gum method)

1) Measure cod liver oil in a dry measure and transfer to a dry mortar.
2) Weigh required amount of acacia and place on the oil. Mix them gently to disperse.
3) Add about 4 ml of cinnamon water, triturate lightly and continuously in a single direction, until mixture is thickened. Continue the trituration until product becomes white or nearly white and clicking sound is produced (primary emulsion).
4) Dissolve ferric ammonium citrate in few ml of cinnamon water. To this solution, add syrup and mix well. Gradually add this mixture to the mortar with continuous trituration.
5) Transfer the content to a measure and adjust the final volume with cinnamon water and mix well.

Dispensing: Transfer the emulsion to a narrow mouthed glass bottle, close it thoroughly with metallic screw cap, polish and label.

Direction: One teaspoonful to be taken, two times a day.

Storage: Store in a cool place.

Auxilliary label: SHAKE WELL BEFORE USE.

Use: This emulsion is used as anti-rachitic and haematinic.

CASTOR OIL - EMULSION

Rx	
Olei ricini	fl. 3 ii ss
Aquam cinnamoni...q.s...	fl. 3 vi s
Fiat : Emulsio	Mitte : fl.oz i
Signa : Cochleare amplum, hora somni utendus.	

Conversion :

fl. 3 ii ss → 2.5 fluid drachms   fl. 3 vi s → 6.25 fluid drachms = 25 ml

1 fluid drachm = 4 ml

2.5 fluid drachms = 10 ml

Calculation : For fl.oz i → 1 fl.oz = 30 ml

Castor oil = $\frac{10}{25} \times 30 = 12$ ml

Cinnamon water....q.s... = 30 ml

Primary emulsion: Since Castor oil is a fixed oil, primary emulsion ratio,

4 : 2 : 1 = oil : water : gum.

Castor oil = $\frac{12 \times 4}{4} = 12$ ml

Cinnamon water = $\frac{12 \times 2}{4} = 6$ ml

Acacia = $\frac{12 \times 1}{4} = 3$ g

Revised formula for primary emulsion:

Castor oil	---	12 ml
Cinnamon water	---	6 ml
Acacia	---	3 g
		21 ml

Revised formula for finished emulsion:

Primary emulsion	---	21 ml
Cinnamon water	---	9 ml
		30 ml

<table>
<tr><th>Type</th><th>Ingredients</th><th>Quantity in imperial</th><th>Quantity in metric</th><th>Quantity taken</th></tr>
<tr><td rowspan="4">O/W type of emulsion, containing fixed oil, emulsified with acacia gum.</td><td>Castor oil</td><td>2.5 fl. dr</td><td>10 ml</td><td>12 ml</td></tr>
<tr><td>Cinnamon water…q.s..</td><td>6.25 fl. dr</td><td>25 ml</td><td>30 ml</td></tr>
<tr><td>Make: Emulsion</td><td colspan="3">Send:30 ml</td></tr>
<tr><td colspan="4">Direction: One table spoonful to be taken, at bed time.</td></tr>
</table>

Theory:

This is an emulsion containing fixed oil. Castor oil, is a fixed oil obtained from castor seeds of Ricinus communis. Castor oil gets hydrolysed in the intestine, by pancreatic lipase and liberates as ricinoleic acid (ricino-oleate), which is irritant in nature and hence produces a purgative effect.

Castor oil is insoluble in water, possesses unpleasant odour and blunt taste, hence it causes nausea. Therefore to mask its unpleasant odour, it is formulated in the form of o/w type of emulsion, using acacia as emulsifying agent.

In this preparation, cinnamon water is used as continuous phase and also acts as carminative and flavouring agent.

Since castor oil is a fixed oil, the primary emulsion ratio for oil: water: gum is (4:2:1).

Procedure: (By wet gum method)

1) Weigh gum acacia and transfer to a mortar, to this add few ml of cinnamon water and triturate to form mucilage.
2) Add castor oil in small quantities with constant and rapid trituration in a single direction to produce a thick cream, continue the trituration until, product becomes white or nearly white and clicking sound is produced (primary emulsion).
3) To the primary emulsion, gradually add cinnamon water, with continuous trituration and transfer to a measure.
4) Rinse the pestle and mortar with cinnamon water and transfer to the measure.
5) Adjust the final volume with the cinnamon water and mix well.

Dispensing: Transfer the emulsion to a narrow mouthed glass bottle, close it thoroughly with metallic screw cap, polish and label.

Direction: One table spoonful to be taken, at bed time.

Storage: Store in a cool place.

Auxilliary label: SHAKE WELL BEFORE USE.

Uses: Castor oil emulsion is used as laxative, when patients are undergoing gastrointestinal surgeries, colon X-ray and endoscopic examinations, to empty the gastrointestinal tract.

ARACHIS OIL EMULSION

Synonym: Groundnut oil emulsion, Peanut oil emulsion

Rx	
Olei arachis	fl. 3 xii ss
Menthae piperitae emulsio (conc)	fl. 3 i s
Aquam chloroformi	fl. 3 xxv
Aquam.........q.s...	fl. 3 L
Fiat : Emulsio	Mitte : fl.oz i
Signa : Cochleare parvum, semel in die, anti cibos sumendum.	

Conversion :

fl. 3 xii ss → 12.5 fluid drachms　　fl. 3 i s → 1.25 fl. dr = 5 ml

1 fl. drachm = 4 ml　　fl. 3 xxv → 25 fl. dr = 100 ml

12.5 fl. drachms = 50 ml　　fl. 3 L → 50 fl. dr = 200 ml

Calculation : For fl.oz i → 1 fl.oz = 30 ml

Arachis oil $= \frac{50}{200} \times 30 = 7.5$ ml

Peppermint emulsion conc. $= \frac{5}{200} \times 30 = 0.75$ ml

Chloroform water $= \frac{100}{200} \times 30 = 15$ ml

Water....q.s................ = 30 ml

Primary emulsion: Since Arachis oil is a fixed oil, primary emulsion ratio for,

oil : water : gum = 4 : 2 : 1 .

Arachis oil $= \frac{7.5 \times 4}{4} = 7.5$ ml

Water $= \frac{7.5 \times 2}{4} = 3.75$ ml

Acacia $= \frac{7.5 \times 1}{4} = 1.875$ g

Revised formula for primary emulsion:

Arachis oil --- 7.5 ml

Water --- 3.75 ml

Acacia --- 1.875 g

13.125 ml

Revised formula for finished emulsion:

Primary emulsion	---	13.125 ml
Peppermint emulsion	---	0.75 ml
Chloroform water	---	15 ml
Water	---	1.125 ml
		------------
		30 ml

Type	Ingredients	Quantity in imperial	Quantity in metric	Quantity taken
O/W type of emulsion containing fixed oil, emulsified with acacia gum.	Arachis oil	12.5 fl. dr	50 ml	7.5 ml
	Peppermint emulsion concentrated	1.25 fl. dr	5 ml	0.75 ml
	Chloroform water double strength	25 fl. dr	100 ml	15 ml
	Water.....q.s.....	50 fl. dr	200 ml	30 ml
	Make: Emulsion	Send: 30 ml		
	Direction: One teaspoonful to be taken, once a day, before meals.			

Theory:

This is an emulsion containing fixed oil like arachis oil. Arachis oil is mainly used as food article (nutrient), demulcent and also as lubricant, but it can not be taken orally as such, because of its unpleasant taste and odour. Hence this taste is masked by formulating it in the form of emulsion, using acacia as a emulsifying agent, which produces o/w type of emulsion.

Peppermint emulsion concentrated is used as flavouring agent, to give an acceptable odour to the emulsion and chloroform water is used as continuous phase, which also acts as preservative.

Since arachis oil is a fixed oil, the ratio for primary emulsion will be (4:2:1).

Procedure: (By dry gum method)

1) Accurately measure arachis oil in a dry measure and transfer to a dry mortar.
2) Weigh accurately gum acacia and place on the oil, mix gently to disperse. Immediately add water at once. Triturate lightly and continuously in single direction, until product becomes white or nearly white and clicking sound is produced (primary emulsion).
3) Mix peppermint emulsion concentrated with the chloroform water double strength and gradually add to the mortar, with continuous trituration.
4) Transfer to a measure and adjust the volume with water, stir well.

Dispensing: Transfer the emulsion to a narrow mouthed clear or amber coloured glass bottle, close it thoroughly with metallic screw cap, polish and label.

Direction: One teaspoonful to be taken, once a day, before meals.

Storage: Store in a cool place.

Auxilliary label: SHAKE WELL BEFORE USE.

Use: This emulsion is used as nutrient and laxative.

TURPENTINE OIL EMULSION

Rx	
Olei turbinthinae	fl. 3 ii
Aquam cinnamoni....q.s...	fl. 3 x
Fiat : Emulsio	Mitte : fl.oz i
Signa : Sumendum hastus, semel.	

Conversion :

fl. 3 ii → 2 fluid drachms   fl. 3 x → 10 fluid dr = 40 ml

1 fluid drachm = 4 ml

2 fluid drachms = 8 ml

Calculation : For fl.oz i → 1 fl.oz = 30 ml

Turpentine oil $= \frac{8}{40} \times 30 = 6$ ml

Cinnamon water....q.s........ = 30 ml

Primary emulsion: Since Turpentine oil is a volatile oil, Primary emulsion ratio for

oil : water : gum = 2 : 2 : 1

Turpentine oil $= \frac{6 \times 2}{2} = 6$ ml

Cinnamon water $= \frac{6 \times 2}{2} = 6$ ml

Acacia $= \frac{6 \times 1}{2} = 3$ g

Revised formula for primary emulsion:

Turpentine oil --- 6 ml
Cinnamon water --- 6 ml
Acacia --- 3 g
----
15 ml

Revised formula for finished emulsion:

Primary emulsion --- 15 ml
Cinnamon water --- 15 ml
----
30 ml

Type	Ingredients	Quantity in imperial	Quantity in metric	Quantity taken
O/W type of emulsion, containing volatile oil, emulsified with acacia gum.	Turpentine oil	2 fl. dr	8 ml	6 ml
	Cinnamon water…q.s..	10 fl. dr	40 ml	30 ml
	Make: Emulsion Send: 30 ml Direction: To be taken as drought, at once.			

Theory:

It is an internal emulsion, containing volatile oil like turpentine oil, which acts as expectorant hence mainly used in the treatment of chronic bronchitis. Cinnamon water constitutes as continuous phase, which acts as, flavouring agent and carminative.

Turpentine oil is a volatile oil, therefore to prevent its volatilization it is prepared by bottle method, as oil in water (o/w) type emulsion, using acacia as emulsifying agent.

Since turpentine oil is volatile oil, the primary emulsion ratio will be, oil: water: gum (2:2:1).

Procedure (By bottle method):

1) Accurately measure turpentine oil in a dry measure and transfer to a previously tared calibrated bottle.
2) Add the required amount of powdered gum acacia, close it throughly with metallic screw cap.
3) Shake the bottle vigarously, until oil and gum should mix completly.
4) Add measured quantity of cinnamon water and shake well. After getting a good emulsion, polish and label.

Direction: To be taken as drought, at once.

Storage: Store in a cool place.

Auxilliary label: SHAKE WELL BEFORE USE.

Use: This emulsion is used as expectorant, in the treatment of chronic bronchitis.

LIQUID PARAFFIN – CASTOR OIL EMULSION

Rx	
Liquidi paraffini	fl. 3 ii ss
Olei ricini	fl. 3 ii ss
Syrupi	fl. 3 vii ss
Aquam .....q.s...	fl. 3 xxv
Fiat : Emulsio	Mitte : fl.oz ii
Signa : Sumendum, hastus semel.	

Conversion :

fl. 3 ii ss → 2.5 fl. drachms

1 fl. drachm = 4 ml

2.5 fl. drachms = 10 ml

fl. 3 vii ss → 7.5 fl. dr = 30 ml

fl. 3 xxv → 25 fl. dr = 100 ml

Calculation : For fl.oz ii → 2 fl.oz = 60 ml

Liquid paraffin = $\frac{10}{100} \times 60 = 6$ ml

Castor oil = $\frac{10}{100} \times 60 = 6$ ml

Simlpe syrup = $\frac{30}{100} \times 60 = 18$ ml

Water....q.s........ = 30 ml

Primary emulsion: Since Liquid paraffin is a mineral oil, the primary emulsion ratio for, oil : water : gum = 3 : 2 : 1.

Liquid paraffin = $\frac{6 \times 3}{3} = 6$ ml

Water = $\frac{6 \times 2}{3} = 4$ ml

Acacia = $\frac{6 \times 1}{3} = 2$ g

Since Castor oil is a fixed oil, the primary emulsion ratio for, oil : water : gum = 4 : 2 : 1.

Castor oil = $\frac{6 \times 4}{4} = 6$ ml

Water = $\frac{6 \times 2}{4} = 3$ ml

Acacia = $\frac{6 \times 1}{4} = 1.5$ g

Revised formula for primary emulsion:

Liquid paraffin	---	6 ml
Castor oil	---	6 ml
Water	---	3 + 4 = 7 ml
Acacia	---	1.5 + 2 = 3.5 g

		22.5 ml

Revised formula for finished emulsion:

Primary emulsion	---	22.5 ml
Simple syrup	---	18.0 ml
Water	---	19.5 ml
		------------
		60 ml

Type	Ingredients	Quantity in imperial	Quantity in metric	Quantity taken
Internal emulsion, containing more than one oil	Liquid paraffin	2.5 fl. dr	10 ml	6 ml
	Castor oil	2.5 fl.dr	10 ml	6 ml
	Simple syrup	7.5 fl.dr	30 ml	18 ml
	Water.....q.s.....	25 fl.dr	100 ml	60 ml
	Make: Emulsion	Send: 60 ml		
	Direction: To be taken as drought, at once.			

Theory:

This is an emulsion containing more than one oil i.e it consists a combination of mineral oil (liquid paraffin) and a fixed oil (castor oil). Liquid paraffin, when taken orally, it keeps the stools soft and therefore particularly useful, in the treatment of chronic constipation and in the presence of painful conditions of the anus and rectum, such as haemorrhoids and anal fissure and fistula.

Castor oil acts as mild purgative (laxative), its action being exerted as a result of saponification in the small intestine, with formation of the irritant alkali.

This emulsion is prepared as o/w type emulsion, by dry gum method using o/w type of emulsifying agent – Acacia. In which both liquid paraffin and castor oil constitutes as dispersed phase and water constitutes as dispersion (continuous) phase.

For preparation of primary emulsion, the quantities of both acacia and water should be calculated for each oil, separately. Since liquid paraffin is a mineral oil, its primary emulsion ratio is 3:2:1 and castor oil is a fixed oil its primary emulsion ratio is 4:2:1. The total quantities of acacia and water together with both the oils, should be used for preparing primary emulsion.

Simple syrup is used as sweetening agent, to give an acceptable odour to the emulsion, because castor oil has unpleasant blunt taste. Simple syrup also acts as a preservative.

Procedure: (By dry gum method)

1) Measure liquid paraffin, transfer into a dry mortar and add half quantity of weighed acacia, mix well by trituration.
2) To the above mixture, add castor oil and remaining amount of acacia, triturate well.
3) Add calculated amount of water at once. Triturate lightly and continuously in single direction, until the mixture becomes white or nearly white and clicking sound is produced (primary emulsion).
4) Dilute the syrup with half quantity of water. Gradually add to the mortar with continuous trituration.
5) Transfer the content to a measure and adjust the final volume with water and mix well.

Dispensing: Transfer the emulsion to a narrow mouthed glass bottle, close it thoroughly with metallic screw cap, polish and label.

Directions: To be taken as drought, at once.

Storage: Store in a cool place.

Auxilliary label: SHAKE WELL BEFORE USE.

Uses: The liquid paraffin-castor oil emulsion is used, as mild purgative (laxative)

- In the treatment of haemorrhoids,
- For emptying the bowel before delivery or any surgery,
- For emptying the bowel in diarrhoea, due to food poisoning.

LIQUID PARAFFIN ORAL EMULSION B.P.

Synonym: Liquid paraffin emulsion

Rx	
Liquidi paraffini	fl. 3 xii ss
Methyl cellulose	gr xxx
Acidi benzoici	M xxx
Chloroformi	M iii sss
Vanillin	gr i
Sodii sacchari	... q.s..(5 mg)
Aquam.....q.s....	fl. 3 xxv
Fiat : Emulsio	Mitte : fl.oz ii
Signa : Cochleare magnum, bis in die sumendum.	

Conversion :

fl. 3 xii ss → 12.5 fluid dr	gr xxx → 30 grains
1 fl. drachm = 4 ml	15 grains = 1 g
12.5 fl. dr = 50 ml	30 grains = 2 g
fl. 3 xxv → 25 fl. dr = 100 ml	gr i → 1 grain = 60 mg
	M iii sss → 3.75 minims
	15 minims = 1 ml
	3.75 minims = 0.25 ml
	M xxx → 30 minims = 2 ml

Calculation : For fl.oz ii → 2 fl.oz = 60 ml

Liquid paraffin = $\frac{50}{100} \times 60 = 30$ ml

Methyl cellulose = $\frac{2}{100} \times 60 = 1.2$ g

Benzoic acid solution = $\frac{2}{100} \times 60 = 1.2$ ml

Chloroform = $\frac{0.25}{100} \times 60 = 0.15$ ml

Vanillin = $\frac{60}{100} \times 60 = 36$ mg

Sodium saccharin = $\frac{5}{100} \times 60 = 3$ mg

Water....q.s........ = 60 ml

Preparation of sodium saccharin solution:

Sodium saccharin : 100 mg

Water : 100 ml

Dissolve sodium saccharin in water, 3 ml of this dilution contains 3 mg of sodium saccharin

Type	Ingredients	Quantity in imperial	Quantity in metric	Quantity taken
O/w type emulsion, emulsified by Methyl cellulose	Liquid paraffin	12.5 fl.dr	50 ml	30 ml
	Methyl cellulose	30 gr	2 g	1.2 g
	Benzoic acid solution	30 minims	2 ml	1.2 ml
	Chloroform	3.75 minims	0.25 ml	0.15 ml
	Vanillin	1 gr	60 mg	36 mg
	sodium saccharin	..q.s..	5 mg	5 ml
	Water…q.s…	25 fl.dr	100 ml	60 ml
	Make: Emulsion Send: 60 ml Direction: One table spoonful to be taken, twice a day.			

Theory:

This is an internal emulsion containing mineral oil like liquid paraffin, which is emulsified with methyl cellulose. Liquid paraffin is a mineral oil, obtained by distillation of petroleum, which get emulsified in the gastro-intestinal tract and holds water. Hence it keeps the stools soft and do not allow feacal matter to become dry. This helps in easy evacuation of bowel. Hence liquid paraffin is useful, in the treatment of chronic constipation.

In this preparation, methyl cellulose -20 is used as emulsifying agent, at a concentration of 2%. Benzoic acid and chloroform water are used as preservatives. Sodium saccharin is used as sweetening agent and vanillin is used to give an pleasant flavour, to the liquid paraffin emulsion.

Procedure: Preparation of liquid paraffin emulsion involves two stages such as:

(A) preparation of Mucilage of methyl cellulose

1) Mix methyl cellulose-20 with about six times its weight of boiling water and allow it to hydrate (swell) for about 30 minutes.
2) Add an equal weight (about 15 g) of ice and stir mechanically, until the mucilage becomes homogenous.

(B) preparation of emulsion using Mucilage of methyl cellulose :

3) Since vanillin is a volatile substance, it is more soluble in organic solvents than in water, dissolve it in a mixture of benzoic acid solution and chloroform. Add this solution to the mucilage and stir for 5 minutes.
4) Make a suitable dilution of small quantity of sodium saccharin with water. From this dilution, add required quantity of sodium saccharin solution, to the mucilage.

5) Make up the volume of the mucilage up to 30 ml by stirring, (care should be taken to ensure that, there is no entrapment of air in the mucilage).
6) Make the emulsion by adding (mixing), eqaul volume of liquid paraffin and mucilage of methyl cellulose (i.e. 30 ml of liquid paraffin and 30 ml of Mucilage of methyl cellulose) with constant stirring.
7) Usually liquid paraffin emulsion is very coarse in nature, hence for further reducing of the globule's size and to get a stable and whitner emulsion, final emulsion should be passed through Homogeniser.

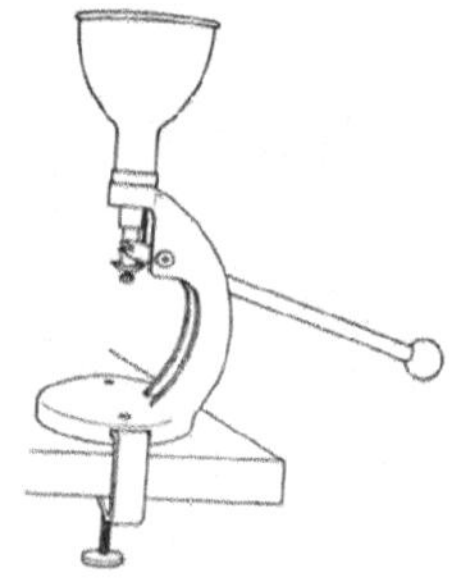

Hand homogeniser

Dispensing: Transfer the liquid paraffin emulsion in to a amber coloured, narrow mouthed glass bottle, close throughly with a child resistant closure, polish and label.

Direction: One table spoonful to be taken, twice a day.

Advice for patients while dispensing:

This emulsion should not be taken, within 30 minutes of meal time and preferably on empty stomach (Patients are also advised about the importance of fibre and fluid intake, in the diet should be emphasized).

Storage: Store in a cool place but do not allow to freeze.

Note: This is an official preparation with effective preservative system, hence it remains stable for longer period (on storage).

Auxilliary label: SHAKE WELL BEFORE USE.

Uses: Liquid paraffin oral emulsion is used as a laxative, in the treatment of constipation.

LIQUID PARAFFIN AND PHENOLPHTHALEIN EMULSION

Rx	
Liquidi paraffini	fl.oz ii
Phenolphthalein	gr xxx
Agar	gr xx
Acacia	3 iii sss
Syrupi	fl.oz ½
Aquam cinnamoni...q.s...	fl.oz vi
Fiat : Emulsio	Mitte : fl.oz i
Signa : Duo cochleare minimum, nocte sumendum.	

Conversion :

fl.oz ii → 2 fl.oz	gr xxx → 30 grains = 2 g
1 fl.oz = 30 ml	gr xx → 20 grains = 1.35 g
2 fl.oz = 60 ml	
½ fl.oz = 15 ml	3 iii sss → 3.75 drachms
fl.oz vi → 6 fl.oz = 180 ml	1 drachm = 4 g
	3.75 drachms = 15 g

Calculation : For fl.oz i → 1 fl.oz = 30 ml

Liquid paraffin $= \frac{60}{180} \times 30 = 10$ ml

Phenolphthalein $= \frac{2}{180} \times 30 = 0.33$ g

Agar $= \frac{1.35}{180} \times 30 = 0.225$g

Acacia $= \frac{15}{180} \times 30 = 2.5$ g

Syrup $= \frac{15}{180} \times 30 = 2.5$ ml

Cinnamon water....q.s.... = 30 ml

Type	Ingredients	Quantity in imperial	Quantity in metric	Quantity taken
O/w type emulsion,	Liquid paraffin	2 fl.oz	60 ml	10 ml
containing water	Phenolphthalein	30 gr	2 g	0.33 g
and oil insoluble	Agar	20 gr	1.35 g	0.225 g
substance.	Acacia	3.75 dr	15 g	2.5 g
Emulsified by	Syrup	½ fl.oz	15 ml	2.5 ml
combination of	Cinnamon water…q.s.…	6 fl.oz	180 ml	30 ml
emulsifying agents	Make: Emulsion	Send: 30 ml		
	Direction: Two teaspoonful to be taken, at night.			

Theory : This is an emulsion of a mineral oil like liquid paraffin, with a water and oil insoluble substance Phenolphthalein, which acts as cathartic. Liquid paraffin acts as laxative by lubricating the stool.

Since phenolphthalein is insoluble in both liquid paraffin and water, it is suspended in liquid paraffin emulsion. Therefore it is finely powdered (micronised) and triturated with gum acacia, before adding liquid paraffin or chloroform water, to prepare primary emulsion.

It is prepared as o/w type emulsion, using gum acacia as a emulsifying agent by dry gum method, because of its low viscosity, a stable emulsion cannot be produced. Hence to increase the viscosity of emulsion, agar is used as secondary emulsifying agent (i.e. as emulsion stabilizer). Agar should be used only in small proportions (less than 1%) along with primary emulsifier, because more than 1% of agar, will produce a solid or semi solid preparation.

In this preparation, cinnamon water is used as continuous phase, which also acts as flavouring agent. Syrup is used as sweetening agent and acacia acts as o/w type emulsifying agent.

Since liquid paraffin is a mineral oil, primary emulsion ratio will be 3:2:1.

Procedure: The preparation of emulsion involves two steps,

A) Preparation of agar solution:

1) In a tared dish, dissolve accurately weighed agar in about 30 ml of water by gentle heating, while hot itself, adjust the volume to 30 ml, to compensate the loss of water during heating due to evaporation.
2) To this, add syrup and cinnamon water and stir well to get a homogenous mass (mixture).

B) Preparation of emulsion (By dry gum method):

1) Accurately weigh phenolphthalein and acacia.
2) Finely powder the phenolphthalein and place in a hot mortar and mix with acacia by trituration. To this, add liquid paraffin and triturate well.
3) To this triturate, incorporate cinnamon water required for primary emulsion, little at a time with constant trituration, until a clicking sound is produced and a white cream is formed (i.e. a primary emulsion is formed.)
4) Gradually add the hot solution of agar to the primary emulsion with constant trituration, until a uniform product is obtained.
5) Transfer the emulsion to a measuring cylinder and adjust the final volume, by rinsing out the mortar with cinnamon water.
6) Usually liquid paraffin emulsion is very coarse in nature, hence for further reducing of the globule's size and to get a stable and whitner emulsion, final emulsion should be passed through Homogeniser.

Dispensing: Transfer this emulsion to a narrow mouthed, amber coloured glass bottle close with child resistant closure and label.

Direction: Two teaspoonful to be taken, at night.

Storage: Store in a cool place.

Auxilliary label: SHAKE WELL BEFORE USE.

Uses: Phenolphthalein acts as a cathartic, which exerts its action directly on the intestinal mucous membrane and causes copious water secretion. It produces loose motion in 4 to 6 hours after administration. Hence it is usually given at night to act in the morning. It is administered along with other purgatives like liquid paraffin, which enhance its action.

Liquid paraffin acts as purgative by lubricating the stools and make them soft. Therefore this emulsion is used as a laxative (purgative) in the treatment of chronic constipation and in the painful conditions of anus and rectum like haemorrhoids and anal fissure.

CALCIFEROL EMULSION

Rx	
Liquoris calciferolis	M xxii ss
Glyerini	M VL
Aquam....q.s...	fl. 3 xii ss
Fiat : Emulsio	Mitte : fl.oz i
Signa : Cochleare minimum, nocte sumendum.	

Conversion :

fl. 3 xii ss → 12.5 fl. dr	M xxii ss → 22.5 minims
1 fl. dracham = 4 ml	15 minims = 1 ml
12.5 fl. dr = 50 ml	22.5 minims = 1.5 ml
	M VL → 45 minims = 3 ml

Calculation : For fl.oz i → 1 fl.oz = 30 ml

Calciferol solution = $\frac{1.5}{50} \times 30 = 0.9$ ml

Glycerin = $\frac{3}{50} \times 30 = 1.8$ ml

Purified water .....q.s.... = 30 ml

The percentage of calciferol (oil) is very less (i.e 3 %), which is less than 20 %. This percentage is raised to 20 % by the addition of a bland oil like, Arachis oil.

i.e..0.9 ml of calciferol solution should be raised to 20 % = $\frac{20}{100} \times 30 = 6$ ml

Volume of Arachis oil required = 6 ml - 0.9 ml = 5.1 ml

Primary emulsion: Since, Calciferol and Arachis oil are fixed oils, the primary emulsion ratio for oil : water : gum = 4 : 2 : 1.

Calciferol solution + Arachis oil = 0.9 + 5.1 = 6 ml

Water = $\frac{6 \times 2}{4} = 3$ ml

Acacia = $\frac{6 \times 1}{4} = 1.5$ g

Revised formula for primary emulsion:

Calciferol solution	---	0.9 ml
Arachis oil	---	5.1 ml
Water	---	3 ml
Acacia	---	1.5 g

		10.5 ml

Revised formula for finished emulsion:

Primary emulsion --- 10.5 ml
Glycerin --- 1.8 ml
Water --- 17.7 ml
----
30 ml

Type	Ingredients	Quantity in imperial	Quantity in metric	Quantity taken
O/w acacia emulsion, containing a small quantity of oily substance.	Calciferol solution	22.5 minims	1.5 ml	0.9 ml
	Glycerin	45 minims	3 ml	1.8 ml
	Purified water...q.s...	12.5 fl.dr	50 ml	30 ml
	Make: Emulsion, for a 1 year old child. Send: 30 ml			
	Direction: One teaspoonful to be taken, at night.			

Theory: It is an o/w type emulsion – emulsified with acacia, containing small volume of oily substance. In this prescription, calciferol solution constitutes as oily phase, which is prescribed in very low concentration (3%).

In case of acacia emulsion, if oil phase is less than 20%, it leads to the instability of emulsion due to creaming. Therefore to prevent the creaming, the percentage of oily phase should be increased from 3% to 20% of the total volume, using a fixed (bland) oil like arachis oil.

Calciferol solution and arachis oil are fixed oils, hence primary emulsion ratio will be 4:2:1. For primary emulsion, total quantity of both calciferol solution and arachis oil should be considered.

Glycerin is used as a sweetening agent, to mask the unpleasant blunt taste of arachis oil. It also increases the viscosity of the preparation.

Procedure: (By dry gum method)

1) Accurately measure calciferol solution and arachis oil, according to primary emulsion ratio and transfer to a dry mortar, mix well.
2) Add weighed amount of acacia and mix thoroughly by trituration, to disperse uniformly.
3) Add a small portion of water (about 5 ml) at once, triturate gently and continuously in a single direction, until a white or creamy product and clicking sound is produced (primary emulsion).
4) Dilute the glycerin with little portion of water and add gradually, to the primary emulsion with continuous trituration.
5) Transfer the content to a measure, rinse the mortar and pestle with water and transfer to the measure. Make up to the final volume, with remaining amount of water.

Dispensing: Transfer the emulsion to a narrow mouthed, amber coloured glass bottle, close it thoroughly, with metallic screw cap, polish and label.

Direction: One teaspoonful to be taken, at night.

Storage: Store in a cool place.

Auxilliary label: SHAKE WELL BEFORE USE.

Uses: Calciferol emulsion is used as source of Vitamin 'D' for the prevention of rickets and osteomalacia, in infants and children.

COD LIVER OIL EMULSION

Rx	
Olei morrhuae	fl. 3 xii ss
Acacia	3 iii s
Tragacanth	gr xi s
Benzaldehyde spirit	M iii sss
Chloroformi	M iii sss
Sodii sacchari	...q.s...
Aquam....q.s...	fl. 3 xxv
Fiat : Emulsio	Mitte : fl.oz i
Signa : Cochleare minimum, omni nocte sumendum.	

Conversion :

fl. 3 xii ss → 12.5 fl. drachams

1 fl. dracham = 4 ml

12.5 fl. drachams = 50 ml

M iii sss → 3.75 minims

15 minims = 1 ml

3.75 minims = 0.25 ml

fl. 3 xxv → 25 fl. drachams = 100 ml

3 iii s → 3.25 drachams = 13 g

gr xi s → 11.25 grains

15 grains = 1 g

11.25 grains = 0.75 g

Calculation : For fl.oz i → 1 fl.oz = 30 ml

Cod liver oil = $\frac{50}{100} \times 30 = 15$ ml

Acacia = $\frac{13}{100} \times 30 = 3.9$ g

Tragacanth = $\frac{0.75}{100} \times 30 = 0.225$ g

Benzaldehyde spirit = $\frac{0.25}{100} \times 30 = 0.075$ ml

Chloroform = $\frac{0.25}{100} \times 30 = 0.075$ ml

Sodium saccharin .... = ...q.s...

Purified water .....q.s.... = 30 ml

Preparation of sodium saccharin solution:

Sodium saccharin ---- 100 mg

Water ---- 100 ml

Dissolve sodium saccharin in water, 5 ml of this dilution contains 5 mg of sodium saccharin.

Type	Ingredients	Quantity in imperial	Quantity in Metric	Quantity Taken
Internal emulsion containing a fixed oil, emulsified with combination of emulsifying agents acacia and tragacanth	Cod liver oil	12.5 fl.dr	50 ml	15 ml
	Acacia powder	3.25 dr	13 g	3.9 g
	Tragacanth powder	11.25 gr	0.75 g	0.225 g
	Benzaldehyde spirit	3.75 minims	0.25 ml	0.075 ml
	Chloroform	3.75 minims	0.25 ml	0.075 ml
	Saccharin sodium	5 mg (q.s)	5 mg	5 ml
	Purified water ...q.s....	25 fl.dr	100 ml	30 ml
	Make: Emulsion, for 2 years old child Send: 30 ml. Direction: One teaspoonful to be taken, at every night.			

Theory:

It is an o/w type (internal) emulsion, containing a fixed oil like cod liver oil, which is emulsified by combination of emulsifying agents like acacia and tragacanth.

In this preparation, if acacia is used alone, it produces low viscosity in the emulsion, which leads to the downward creaming. Therefore viscosity of acacia emulsion is increased by adding thickening agents like tragacanth, agar or sodium alginate as stabilizers.

In this preparation, tragacanth is included as an emulsion stabilizer. The emulsifying ability of tragacanth is mainly due to the high viscosity of its mucilage.

Benzaldehyde spirit and chloroform are used as preservatives. Sodium saccharin is used as sweetening agent, to mask the blunt taste of cod-liver oil.

Procedure: (By dry gum method)

1) Weigh calculated quantities of acacia and tragacanth, mix them uniformly in a dry mortar.
2) Add cod-liver oil and triturate lightly to disperse gum in the oil. Add calculated amount of water at once and triturate vigorously, in a single direction, until to form a primary emulsion.
3) Dilute the primary emulsion, by adding more amount of water gradually in small portions with constant trituration.
4) Add sodium saccharin solution, chloroform and triturate well. Add benzaldehyde spirit drop by drop to the centre of the emulsion with continuous trituration, to prevent the precipitation of the emulsifying agent (acacia) by alcohol.
5) Transfer the content to a measure and make up the final volume with water.

Dispensing: Transfer the emulsion to a narrow mouthed, amber coloured glass bottle, close it thoroughly with metallic screw cap, polish and label.

Direction: One teaspoonful to be taken, at every night.

Storage: Store in a cool place.

Auxilliary label: SHAKE WELL BEFORE USE.

Uses: Cod liver oil is a fixed oil, which consists Vitamin 'D', hence this emulsion is used as source of Vitamin 'D', as antirachitic in infants and children.

BENZYL BENZOATE APPLICATION B.P.

Rx	
Benzyl benzoate	fl. 3 vi s
Emulsifying wax	gr xxx
Aquam.....q.s....	fl. 3 xxv
Fiat : Application	Mitte : fl.oz i
Signa : Applicandus cum gossyp, super dolentiparti, more dicto.	

Conversion :

fl. 3 vi s → 6.25 fl. drachms	gr xxx → 30 grains
1 fl. drachm = 4 ml	15 grains = 1 g
6.25 fl. drachms = 25 ml	30 grains = 2 g
fl. 3 xxv → 25 fl. dr = 100 ml	

Calculation : For fl.oz i → 1 fl.oz = 30 ml

Benzyl benzoate = $\frac{25}{100} \times 30 = 7.5$ ml

Emulsifying wax = $\frac{2}{100} \times 30 = 0.6$ g

Water ......q.s.... = 30 ml

Type	Ingredients	Quantity in imperial	Quantity in Metric	Quantity Taken
Emulsion meant for external use. Emulsified by, emulsifying wax	Benzyl benzoate	6.25 fl. dr	25 ml	7.5 ml
	Emulsifying wax	30 gr	2 g	0.6 g
	Purified water (freshly boiled and cooled)	25 fl.dr	100 ml	30 ml
	Make : Application Send: 30 ml Direction: Apply with cotton (adsorbent), on the affected part, as directed.			

Theory:

It is an emulsion, prepared by using anionic emulsifying agent like, emulsifying wax, which is used for external purpose as an application. Emulsifying wax, acts as emulsifying agent.

Benzyl benzoate exists in liquid form, which acts as scabicide and constitutes as dispersed phase. It is emulsified by, anionic emulsifying wax.

Application is prepared by fusion method. i.e. emulsifying wax and benzyl benzoate are fused together by melting them and cooled to 60 °C. The aqueous phase is also warmed to same temperature and added to oily mixture with constant stirring, which is continued until the preparation becomes cold.

Procedure: (By fusion method)

1) For the preparation of this emulsion, previously warmed bottle is used, because melted wax will be solidified in to a solid mass, at room temperature. Therefore calibrate the bottle (jar) to the prescribed volume and put on a water bath to warm.
2) Accurately weigh benzyl benzoate and emulsifying wax in a china dish and melt them together. Allow this mixture to cool to about 60 ºC to 70 ºC.
3) Warm the water to 60 ºC to 70 ºC.
4) Transfer the oily mixture to the calibrated and warmed bottle and add warm water once at a time, upto the mark.

> **Note:**
> 1) Preparation froths after shaking, hence water should be added at once up to the mark, instead of adding water in small portions.
> 2) For cooling the preparation, it should not be put on a cold surface, because it may cause separation of emulsifying wax.
> 3) To get a fine emulsion, use an electric stirrer.

Dispensing: The preparation becomes thick, after cooling to room temperature. Therefore transfer benzyl benzoate application to a wide mouthed, amber coloured jar or bottle, to facilitate easy removal, stir until it becomes cool. Close it thoroughly with plastic screw cap, polish and label.

Direction: Apply with cotton (adsorbent), on the affected part, as directed.

Auxilliary label:
- FOR EXTERNAL USE ONLY.
- SHAKE WELL BEFORE USE.

Storage: Store in a cool place.

Uses: This application is used, as scabicide.

LIME CREAMS

Lime creams are w/o type emulsions of fixed oils, which are emulsified with liquid alkali like calcium hydroxide (Lime water).

Certain fixed oils (Eg. Olive oil), consists sufficient free fatty acids. These free fatty acids reacts with alkali – calcium hydroxide and undergoes saponification reaction and produces enough calcium soap (calcium oleate). This calcium soap is a divalent soap, which acts as emulsifying agent and hence produces w/o type emulsions.

Therefore generally creams, lotions or applications, prepared by emulsification (saponification) of fixed oils with lime water (calcium hydroxide) are considered as "Lime creams".

But certain fixed oils like arachis oil does not contain sufficient fatty acids, to form enough soap, for the complete emulsification. Therefore addition of little free fatty acids (like Oleic acid) is necessary, to obtain a satisfactory emulsion.

Examples for Lime creams,

1) Calcium soap emulsion (Lime cream or Calamine-zinc oxide lime cream).
2) Oily calamine lotion B.P. (Calamine soap emulsion).

A) CALCIUM SOAP EMULSION

Synonym: Lime cream or Calamine-zinc oxide lime cream.

Rx	
Calamine	gr xv
Zinci oxidi	gr xv
Olive oil	fl. ʒ iii sss
Lime water	fl. ʒ iii sss
Fiat : Emulsio	Mitte : fl.oz ½
Signa : Applicandus cum gossyp, super dolentiparti, more dicto.	

Conversion :

gr xv → 15 grains	fl. ʒ iii sss → 3.75 fl.dr
15 grains = 1 g	1 fl.dr = 4 ml
	3.75 fl.dr = 15 ml

Calculation : For fl.oz ½ = 15 ml

Calamine $= \frac{1}{30} \times 15 = 0.5$ g

Zinc oxide $= \frac{1}{30} \times 15 = 0.5$ g

Olive oil $= \frac{15}{30} \times 15 = 7.5$ ml

Lime water $= \frac{15}{30} \times 15 = 7.5$ ml

Type	Ingredients	Quantity in imperial	Quantity in metric	Quantity taken
w/o emulsion, for external use.	Calamine	15 gr	1 g	0.5 g
	Zinc oxide	15 gr	1 g	0.5 g
	Olive oil	3.75 fl.dr	15 ml	7.5 ml
	Lime water….q.s…..	3.75 fl.dr	15 ml	7.5 ml
	Make: Emulsion	Send: 15 ml		
	Direction: Apply with cotton (adsorbent) on the affected part, as directed.			

Theory:

It is a divalent (w/o) type soap emulsion, prepared by using lime water (calcium hydroxide solution). Olive oil is a fixed oil consists sufficient free fatty acids, which undergo saponification reaction with alkali-calcium hydroxide solution and produces calcium soap (calcium oleate). The calcium soap is a divalent soap, and acts as (w/o) type emulsifying agent, hence produces a (w/o) type emulsion. Therefore this emulsion is called as "calcium soap emulsion" or as "Lime cream". In this preparation, lime water constitutes as dispersed phase and olive oil constitutes as continuous phase.

$$\underset{\text{Oleic acid}}{2CH_3(CH_2)_7 - CH = CH\,(CH_2)_7\,COOH} + \underset{\text{Lime water}}{Ca(OH)_2} \xrightarrow{(Saponification)}$$

$$\underset{\text{Calcium soap (Calcium oleate)}}{[CH_3(CH_2)_7 - CH = CH\,(CH_2)_7\,COO]_2{:}Ca} + 2H_2O$$

Calcium hydroxide solution absorbs atmospheric carbon dioxide and precipitates out as calcium carbonate, as shown in the reaction,

$$OH^- + CO_2 \rightarrow HCO_3^-$$

$$OH^- + HCO_3 \rightarrow CO_3^- + H_2O$$

$$Ca^{++} + CO_3^- \rightarrow CaCO_3$$

Therefore for the preparation of lime cream, freshly prepared saturated calcium hydroxide (lime water) solution should be used.

Calamine and zinc oxide are insoluble in calcium hydroxide solution, hence they are dispersed in the emulsion.

Procedure:

A) Preparation of calcium hydroxide solution (Lime water): Lime water is a simple solution prepared by dissolving calcium hydroxide in water. (Note: Procedure for preparation of calcium hydroxide solution is given in detail in Calcium hydroxide solution I.P See page no 261)

B) Preparation of Lime cream:

1) Weigh accurately calamine and zinc oxide and transfer to a mortar and mix well by trituration.
2) Transfer olive oil into mortar and triturate well to get a paste.
3) Add lime water at once and triturate briskly, until cream is formed.

Dispensing: Transfer to a narrow mouthed glass or plastic bottle, close it thoroughly with plastic screw cap, polish and label.

Direction: Apply with cotton (adsorbent) on the affected part, as directed.

Storage: Store in a cool place.

Auxilliary label:
- FOR EXTERNAL USE ONLY.
- SHAKE WELL BEFORE USE.

Uses: This emulsion is used as astringent and soothing agent, in the treatment of dermatitis and eczema.

B) OILY CALAMINE LOTION B.P.

Synonym: Calamine soap emulsion

Rx	
Calamine	ʒ i s
Olei arachisi	fl. ʒ xii ss
Acidi oleici	M vii ss
Adipis lanae	gr xv
Lime water....q.s	fl. ʒ xxv
Fiat : Emulsio (lotio)	Mitte : fl.oz i
Signa : Applicandus cum linteum, super dolentiparti, more dicto.	

Conversion :

ʒ i s → 1.25 drachms	fl. ʒ xii ss → 12.5 fl.dr
1 drachm = 4 g	1 fl.dr = 4 ml
1.25 drachms = 5 g	12.5 fl.dr = 50 ml
M vii ss → 7.5 minims	fl. ʒ xxv → 25 fl. dr = 100 ml
15 minims = 1 ml	
7.5 minims = 0.5 ml	gr xv → 15 grains = 1 g

Calculation : For fl.oz i → 1 fl.oz = 30 ml

Calamine $= \frac{5}{100} \times 30 = 1.5$ g

Arachis oil $= \frac{50}{100} \times 30 = 15$ ml

Oleic acid $= \frac{0.5}{100} \times 30 = 0.15$ ml

Wool fat $= \frac{1}{100} \times 30 = 0.3$ g

Lime water ......q.s.... = 30 ml

Type	Ingredients	Quantity in imperial	Quantity in metric	Quantity taken
W/O Calcium	Calamine	1.25 dr	5 g	1.5 g
soap emulsion.	Arachis oil	12.5 fl.dr	50 ml	15 ml
	Oleic acid	7.5 minims	0.5 ml	0.15 ml
Biphasic liquid for	Wool fat	15 gr	1 g	0.3 g
external use.	Lime water	25 fl.dr	100 ml	30 ml
	Make: Emulsion (lotion)	Send: 30 ml		
Lime cream.	Direction: Apply with lint, on affected part as directed.			

Theory : This is a 'Lime cream' type of lotion. Arachis oil is a fixed oil, which does not contain sufficient free fatty acids, to form enough soap with lime water. Hence oleic acid is used in addition to arachis oil. Oleic acid provides sufficient free fatty acids, necessary to obtain satisfactory emulsion i.e. free fatty acids of oleic acid and 50% of arachis oil undergoes saponification reaction with alkali – calcium hydroxide and produce divalent calcium (lime) soap. This soap acts a emulsifying agent, which is used to emulsify the remaining 50% of arachis oil, to prepare w/o type emulsion.

Wool fat is used to stabilize this emulsion. In this emulsion, arachis oil constitutes as continuous phase and calcium hydroxide solution constitutes as internal or dispersed phase. Calamine is insoluble either in arachis oil or calcium hydroxide solution. Hence it is suspended in emulsion, by levigation method.

Procedure:

1) Place wool fat, oleic acid and arachis oil together in a china dish and heat on a water bath, until they melt and mix well.
2) Finely sift the calamine, sieve and place an accurately weighed calamine on a warmed tile. Add a little of the oily mixture and rub (levigate) with ointment spatula, until a smooth cream is produced.
3) Dilute the cream, until it becomes fluid and pourable, stir with glass pestle (rod) to distribute the suspension evenly.
4) Pour this content to a calibrated bottle, which is previously warmed slightly on the water bath, because melted wax get solidified at room temperature of the bottle. Add the lime water in small amounts, shake vigorously after each addition. Repeat the shaking until oil disperses as fine globules.

Dispensing: Transfer the emulsion to a narrow mouthed, coloured, fluted, plastic bottle, close it thoroughly with a coloured plastic screw cap, to distinguish it from the preparations meant for external use.

Direction: Apply with lint, on affected part, as directed.

Storage: Store in a cool place.

Auxilliary label:
- FOR EXTERNAL USE ONLY.
- SHAKE WELL BEFORE USE.

Uses: Calamine acts as mild astringent and protective. Therefore, oily calamine lotion is used as soothing lotion, for the treatment of eczema and for releaving the pain and swelling or for sun burn and astringent.

Other examples of Emulsions

1) Halibut liver oil emulsion (Fixed oil / Dry gum method)

Rx

Halibut liver oil	-	2 ml
Glycerin	-	2 ml
Cinnamon water	-	30 ml

Uses : This emulsion is used as a good source of Vitamin 'A' and 'D'.

2) **Cod liver oil – Egg yolk emulsion** (Fixed oil)

Rx

Cod liver oil	-	30 ml
Egg Yolk	-	4 ml
Purified water	-	60 ml

Uses: This emulsion is used as anti rachitic agent.

3) **Almond oil emulsion** (Dry gum method containing two oils – fixed oil and volatile oil)

Rx

Almond oil	-	16 ml
Turpentine oil	-	6 ml
Tincture Tolu	-	8 ml
Tincture Ipecac	-	8 ml
Water ...q.s..	-	180 ml

Uses: This emulsion is used as expectorant.

4) **Ammonium chloride emulsion** (o/w ammonium soap emulsion for external use)

Rx

Ammonium chloride	-	12.5 g
Dilute ammonium solution	-	45 ml
Oleic acid	-	85 ml
Turpentine oil	-	250 ml
Water	-	625 ml

Uses: This emulsion is acts as rubifacient and counter irritant.

5) **Triethanolamine - Oleic acid emulsion** (o/w organic soap emulsion for external use)

Rx

Triethanolamine	-	1 ml
Oleic acid	-	4 ml
Benzyl benzoate	-	25 ml
Water….q.s…..	-	100 ml.

Uses: This emulsion is contain benzyl benzoate as a dispersed phase, which acts as scabicide.

Student's exercise:

1) Define emulsions and classify.
2) What are emulgents? Give examples for each class.
3) What types of emulsifiers are used for o/w and w/o type of emulsions?
4) What are the advantages and disadvantages of emulsions?
5) Comment : For the preparation of emulsions, antioxidants and preservatives are incorporated.
6) Give the primary emulsion ratio for fixed oils, volatile oils and mineral oils.
7) List out the fixed oils, which are used for preparation of emulsion.
8) Give the examples for mineral oil.
9) How much quantity of gum acacia is used for preparation of emulsion containing fixed oil?
10) Explain the mechanism of castor oil emulsion.
11) What is primary emulsion? How it is prepared?
12) What are the methods used for preparation of emulsions?
13) What is the stability of emulsion?
14) What is creaming? How it can be reduced?
15) Enumerate the factors affecting cracking.
16) Comment : Cracking is a reversible process.
17) What is phase inversion ? Why it occurs ?
18) How will you identify the types of emulsions ?
19) What are dispensing aspects for emulsions, meant for internal and external emulsions?
20) Comment : Emulsions should be always stored in a cool place.
21) What is the effect of higher temperature on emulsions?
22) Give the examples for acacia emulsions.
23) Why combination of emulsifying agents is necessary for preparation of emulsions ? Give examples for such emulsions.
24) Give the examples for emulsions, meant for external use.
25) What is the use of Ferric ammonium citrate emulsion and Arachis oil emulsion?
26) How will you prepare Turpentine oil emulsion?
27) Why combination of castor oil and liquid paraffin is used?
28) Comment : "Shake well before use " should be there on the label of emulsions.
29) What is the use of vanillin?
30) How will you prepare mucilage of Methyl cellulose?
31) What is phenolphthalein ? Why it is used in emulsions ?
32) Comment : For the preparation of Liquid paraffin and phenolphthalein emulsion both acacia and agar are used as emulgents.
33) Comment : Syrup is used in preparation of emulsions.
34) What is Calciferol solution ? Why it is formulated as emulsion?

35) Comment : Castor oil or arachis oil is used in the preparation of Calciferol emulsion.
36) What is the mechanism of action of liquid paraffin?
37) Comment : Acacia emulsion can be stabilized by alcohol.
38) Comment : Emulsions are more stable at room temperature.
39) Comment : Creaming is desirable in emulsions.
40) What is the use of Cod-liver oil emulsion? List its ingredients with their uses.
41) What is the meaning of Cochleare minimum and Omni nocte sumendum?
42) What are lime creams? Why they are called so?
43) Give examples for Lime creams.
44) What is use of zinc oxide and calamine?
45) How will you prepare lime water?
46) Comment : For the preparation of Calcium soap emulsion (lime creams), freshly prepared Lime water should be used.
47) Write the meaning of "Applicandus cum gossyp super dolentiparti more dicto ".
48) Briefly enumerate the principle behind the preparation of calcium soap emulsion?
49) What is the synonym for calcium soap emulsion?
50) Comment : Calcium soap emulsion can be used for constipation.
51) What should be the auxilliary label for Lime cream?
52) What is the synonym for oily calamine lotion BP.?
53) What is the difference between Calcium soap emulsion and Calamine soap emulsion?
54) Comment : Wool fat is used in preparation of Oily calamine lotion BP.
55) Why Oleic acid is necessary in Calamine soap emulsion?
56) What is the use of Oily calamine lotion?
57) How will you dispense Oily calamine lotion and calcium soap emulsion?
58) What is an application? What is the latin term for it?
59) What are ingredients used for Benzyl benzoate application?
60) What is Emulsifying wax? How it is prepared?
61) How will you dispense the Benzyl benzoate application?
62) What is the use of Benzyl benzoate application?
63) Define Scabicide, Dermatitis, and Eczema.
64) Define the soothing agents, astringents, protectives with examples.
65) Why wet gum method is used for preparation of emulsion?
66) What are the advantages of dry gum method over wet gum method?
67) How will you prepare the emulsions containing less than 20% of oil phase?
68) Which oils are used in the preparation of emulsions containing less than 20% of oil phase?

32 OINTMENTS

Latin term : Unguentum.

Ointments are semisolid preparations meant for external application to the skin or mucous membrane. They may be medicated or non-medicated. Ointments are generally used for their,

1) Emollient action (Lubricating effect).
2) Protective action.
3) Therapeutic action (Topical effect).
4) Prophylactic action on the skin (to treat skin diseases).

Types of ointments:

1) Non-medicated ointments: These ointments contain only ointment base, does not contain any medicaments, hence they are commonly referred as 'ointment bases' and they are used as such, for emollient or lubricating effect or used as vehicle (base), for the preparation of medicated ointments.

Eg.
- Simple ointment B.P.
- Emulsifying ointment B.P.
- Paraffin ointment,
- Ointment of wool alcohols.

2) Medicated ointments: These ointments contain medicaments, which may be dissolved, suspended or emulsified in the ointment base.

Eg.
- Sulphur ointment
- Boric acid ointment
- Methyl salicylate ointment
- Compound benzoic acid ointment
- Betamethasone ointment.

Characteristics of an ideal ointment:

1) It should be smooth and free from grittiness.
2) It should melt and soften at body temperature.
3) It should be chemically and physically stable.
4) The medicament should be finely divided and uniformly distributed through out the base.
5) The base used for preparation of the ointments should be non-irritating and should not have any pharmacological activity of its own.

Ointment bases: Ointment base is a substance or a part of an ointment, which serves as a carrier or vehicle for the medicament, in the preparation of ointment.

Classification of ointment bases: There are four types of ointment bases such as,

1) Hydrocarbon bases (oleoginous bases).
2) Absorption bases.
3) Emulsion (water miscible) bases.
4) Water soluble bases.

1) Hydrocarbon bases (oleoginous or fatty bases)

These bases consist of water insoluble oils, fats, hydrocarbons and waxes.

Eg.	Hydrocarbons	Vegetable oils	Animal fat
	White soft paraffin	Olive oil	Lard
	Yellow soft paraffin	Cotton seed oil	
	Hard paraffin	Almond oil	
	Liquid paraffin	Coconut oil	

Advantages:

1) These bases have a low capacity to absorb water, hence they are usually used as emollients or as inert vehicles.
2) They are not absorbed by the skin, hence retains on the surface of the skin for prolonged period.
3) These bases are stable to dry heat sterilization, hence suitable for sterile ointments. Eg: Eye ointments
4) These bases do not allow the growth of microorganisms.
5) These bases are used for antibiotics, which are unstable in presence of water.
6) They have high chemical stablity and do not become rancid.

Disadvantages:

1) These are greasy and sticky in nature, hence they are difficult to remove from the skin and cloths.
2) They exert an occlusive effect, by forming a water impermeable layer on the skin, hence retain the body heat, which produce an uncomfortable feeling of warmth, to the patients.
3) They have very low (5-10%) water absorption capacity, hence they have poor capacity to absorb moisture from moist wounds and used for dry skins.

   Eg. Paraffin ointment (Hydrocarbon base).

2) Absorption bases:

Absorption bases are anhydrous in nature and have the capacity to absorb large quantities of water and solutions to give and produce (w/o) emulsions. These bases consist of hydrophobic fatty bases, but due to the presence of a suitable (w/o) emulsifying agent, they get hydrophilic nature.

Eg. For (w/o) emulsifiers: Wool fat (Anhydrous lanolin), Wool alcohols, Bees wax, cholesterol etc.

Advantages:

1) These bases are less occlusive than hydrocarbon bases and spread easily.
2) These bases acts as good emollients.
3) These are relatively heat stable, hence they can be easily sterilized by dry heat.
4) Due to their high water absorption capacity, water-soluble drugs can be easily incorporated.
5) They also assist (helps), in the penetration of oil soluble drugs, through the skin.

Disadvantages: Absorption bases have undesirable property of greasiness, but compared to hydrocarbon bases they are less greasy.

3) Emulsion bases (Water miscible bases):

Emulsion bases are semisolid emulsions, having cream like consistency. They are of two types,

A. w/o type emulsion bases: These bases easier to spread on the skin and they are cosmetically more acceptable than hydrocarbon and absorption bases. But due to their oily external phase, they have little occlusive properties. Since, they have greasy and sticky nature, they are little difficult to remove by water compared to (o/w) type emulsion bases.

Eg.
- Hydrous ointment B.P. (Oily cream)
- Hydrous wool fat B.P. (Lanolin)

B. o/w type emulsion bases:

These bases are cosmetically more elegant and spread easily on the skin. These are easily miscible with exudates from wounds. They have water as external phase, hence easily washed off from the skin, cloth and hair. They are prepared by using (o/w) type of emulsifier.

Eg. Emulsifying ointment: contains an (o/w) type emulsifying agent along with paraffins.

Three compendial water-soluble bases are used for preparation of emulsifying ointments,

Eg. a) Emulsifying ointment B.P. (Containing anionic emulsifying agent)

b) Cetrimide emulsifying ointment B.P. (Containing cationic emulsifying agent)

c) Cetamacrogol emulsifying ointment B.P. (Containing non-ionic emulsifying agent)

These bases are used for preparing o/w creams. These are useful for preparation of scalp ointments.

4) Water soluble bases (Greaseless bases):

These bases are completely water soluble and consist only mixtures of water soluble ingredients like polyethylene glycols (PEG) (carbopol or macrogols, carbowaxes). The molecular weight of PEGs varies from 200 to 6000. Depending on their molecular weights, they are available in different consistencies like liquids, semisolids and waxy solids. Low molecular weight PEGs exit as liquids and high molecular weight PEGs exist as solid. Ointment like consistency is obtained by combining liquid and solid PEGs, in suitable proportions.

Ex. Macrogol ointment B.P.C. consists of combination of following,

Macrogol 300	– 650 g
Macrogol 4000	– 350 g

Advantages:

1) These bases are non-occlusive, non sticky, miscible with exudates and easily removed by washing.
2) They are compatible with wide range of dermatological medicaments and release of medicament, from base is rapid.

3) They can be easily sterilized by heating and do not support microbial growth and rancidity.
4) They show good absorption through skin. Hence they are used for drugs, which should penetrate the skin.

Disadvantages:

1) These bases interact with antimicrobial agents and reduce their activity.

   Eg. Phenols, Hydroxybenzoate and quaternary ammonium compounds.

2) They also react with plastic closures and containers containing polytheneand bakelite.

Other materials used as ointment bases may include:

a) Oils: Vegetable oils like arachis, olive, coconut and castor oil can be used as oleogenous base. eg: Zinc and castor oil ointment, Non-staining Iodine ointment.

b) Fatty alcohols: Higher members of saturated aliphatic monohydric alcohols are also used. eg: Cetyl alcohol, stearyl alcohol, cetostearyl alcohol.

c) Esters of fatty acids: They are used as substitutes for vegetable oils. eg: Isopropyl myristate, Isopropyl palmitate.

d) Silicones: They are used for water repellant properties in the formulation of Barrier ointments. eg: Dimethicone.

Preparation of Ointments: Ointments are prepared by four methods.

1) Trituration method:

This method is used for preparation of soft ointments in small scale. It is used when base is soft in nature, medicament is a solid and insoluble in base and small amount of liquid is to be incorporated in to the base.

The advantage of this method is that, it includes both mixing and size reduction process simultaneously. This results in getting smooth and homogenous ointment.

Trituration is done by using,

a) Ointment slab and spatula (Levigation)

b) Mortar and pestle.

a) Levigation: In this method, ointment is prepared by using ointment slab and ointment spatula, as follows:

Ointment slab (tile)

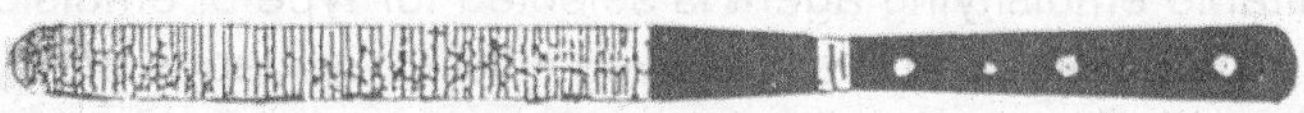

Ointment spatula

1) Finely powder the solid medicaments and place on a cleaned Ointment slab or Tile (30 cm square size).
2) Weigh the required quantity of ointment base and keep it on a different part of the slab. Take a portion of the base of about three times the volume of the drug and levigate with the help of ointment spatula, until there is no sign of any particles of solid. This can be checked by spreading as a thin layer on the slab.

3) Gradually incorporate remaining quantity of ointment base and levigate, to get a homogenous and smooth ointment.

Eg. • Sulphur ointment I.P.,
- Boric acid ointment,
- Whitfield's ointment, are prepared by levigation method.

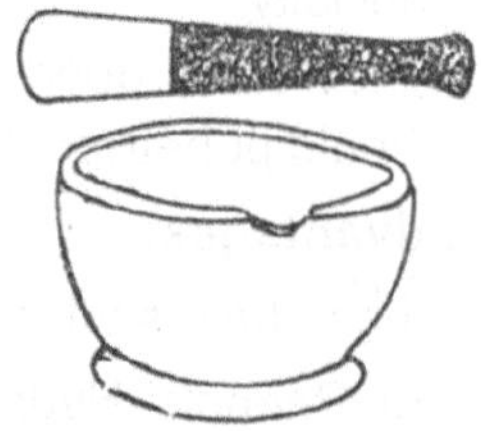

Mortar and pestle

b) Mortar and pestle method: When a large quantity of liquid is to be incorporated in to the base, mortar and pestle are used. But this method is not preferable compared to slab method, because liquid ingredient may slip out of the mortar during trituration, hence leads to improper mixing and recovery (collection) of the product from mortar is difficult.

2) Fusion method: This method is used, when an ointment contains a number of solid (waxy) ingredients, of different melting points like white beeswax, stearic acid, hard paraffin. In small scale, this method is carried out in porcelain dish, which is heated on a water bath.

1) Melt the substance, which has highest melting point first and followed by addition of substances in the decreasing order of their melting point.
2) To this melted mass, incorporate the medicament and stir thoroughly until the mass cools down and a homogenous ointment is formed.
3) If an aqueous liquid ingredient is required to be incorporated, that should also be heated to almost to the same temperature of the melted mass. Otherwise if temperature difference is there, waxy materials separates out, after mixing of two portions.
4) After mixing of two portions, stir the ingredients gently, until it becomes cool.
5) If foreign particles are visible after melting the ingredients, they are removed by decantation or straining.

Eg. • Emulsifying ointment.
- Cetrimide ointment, are prepared by fusion method.

3) Emulsification method:

This method is used for preparation of emulsified ointments and creams.

1) In this method, oil soluble substances are melted together in a china dish on a water bath, at a temperature of 70 °C.
2) Water soluble substances are heated separately, on water bath to a temperature of 70 °C.
3) A suitable emulsifying agent is selected for type of emulsion required (whether o/w type or w/o type) and it is dissolved either in aqueous or oily phase.
4) When both the phases reaches same temperature, aqueous phase is slowly added to the oily phase, with continuous stirring, untill the product becomes cool and semisolid mass is obtained.
5) It is very important to heat both the phases to same temperature before mixing, otherwise high melting point fats and waxes will immediately get solidified when a cold aqueous solution is mixed with the melted mass or vice-versa. Hence a ointment containing lumps will be formed, which gives grittiness to the ointment.

   Eg. Cetrimide cream is prepared by this method.

4) By chemical reaction:

In this method, ointment is prepared by chemical reaction between, the medicament and one or more of ingredients of the base.

Eg. • Non-staining iodine ointment.

• Strong mercuric nitrate ointment are prepared by chemical reaction.

Additives used in Ointments:

In addition to medicament and the base, ointments also consist of other additives like,

Sr.no	Ingredients	Examples
1	Preservatives	Methyl paraben, Propyl paraben. Benzoic acid, Chlorocresol, Phenoxy ethanol, Phenyl mercuric nitrite, Cetrimide, and Alcohol.
2	Anti oxidants	Tocopherol, Ethyl gallate, Propyl gallate, Butylated hydroxy anisole, Butylated hydroxy toluene.
3	Chelating agents	Citric acid, Maleic acid, Tartaric acid.
4	Humectants	Glycerin, Poly ethylene glycol, Sorbitol.

Dispensing: Ointments are dispensed in wide mouthed, glass or plastic bottle or ointment jar (squat pot), having screw cap with impermeable liner. These should be air tight, so that they should prevent contamination of ointment and evaporation of water and volatile constituents.

Now-a-days, flexible plastic collapsible tubes are most widely used, for dispensing of ointments. The internal surface of the metallic tubes should be coated with a suitable lacquer coating, to prevent an interaction of metal, with the contents of the ointment.

Collapsible tubes are generally preferred over wide mouthed jar, to reduce the bacterial contamination during use.

Storage: Since at higher temperature ointment will melt, ointment should be preferably stored in a cool place

Auxilliary label:
- FOR EXTERNAL USE,
- STORE IN A COOL PLACE.

Direction: Label should also bear a suitable direction to the patients, how to apply, how much and how many times to apply.

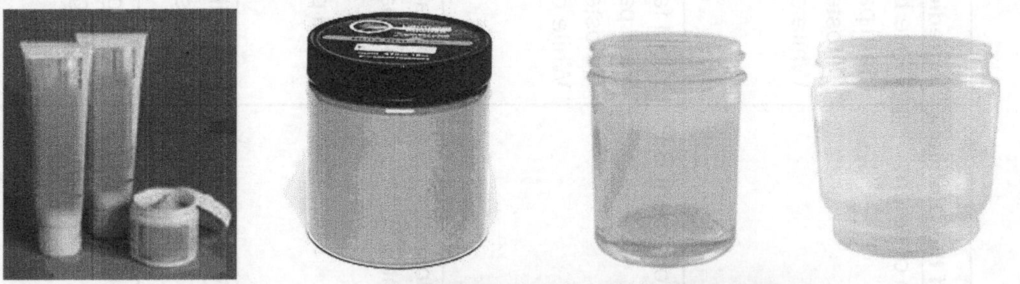

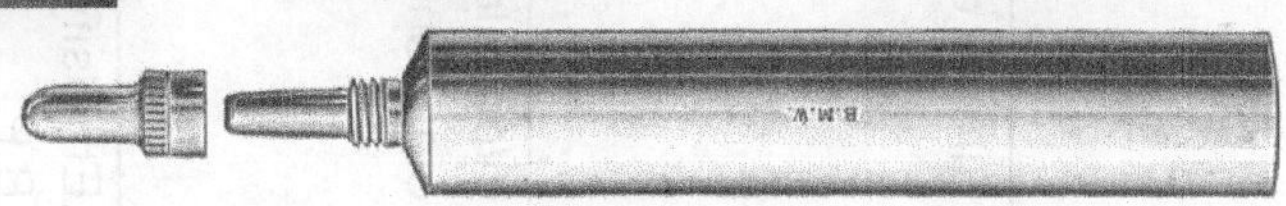

Collapsible tube

Different types of containers used for ointment

(A) EXAMPLES FOR OINTMENT BASES

S.N.	Name of the Ointment	Ingredients (Formulation)	Type and Method of preparation	Uses
1)	Paraffin ointment B.P.C.	White bees wax Hard paraffin Cetosteryl alcohol White or Yellow soft paraffin	Hydrocarbon ointment base, prepared by fusion method.	Used as, ◆ Base for ointments which required prolonged action. ◆ As Ointment base for antibiotics ◆ As Ointment base for Eye ointments. ◆ Emollient.
2)	Simple ointment B.P.	Wool fat Hard paraffin Cetostearyl alcohol White or Yellow soft paraffin	Absorption ointment base, prepared by fusion method.	Used as, ◆ Emollient. ◆ Base for Eye ointments. ◆ Base for ointment, where incorporation of small quantities of aqueous liquids is necessary.
3)	Wool alcohols ointment B.P.	Wool alcohol Hard paraffin Yellow soft paraffin Liquid paraffin	Absorption ointment base, prepared by fusion method	◆ Used as Base for preparation of (w/o) type ointment. ◆ As base, where aqueous liquids and solutions of medicaments to be incorporated.
4)	Emulsifying ointment B.P.	Emulsifying wax White soft paraffin	Emulsion base (Water miscible ointment base) Prepared by fusion method.	Used as, ◆ base for emulsion or (o/w) type of ointments.
5)	Macrogol ointment B.P.C.	Macrogol - 4000 Macrogol - 300	Water soluble ointment base	Used as, ◆ base for medicated ointments, containing water soluble ingredients.

(B) EXAMPLES FOR MEDICATED OINTMENTS

S.N.	Name of the Ointment	Ingredients (Formulation)	Type and Method of Preparation	Uses
1)	Salicylic acid ointment B.P.	Salicylic acid (finely sifted) Wool alcohol ointment	Ointment prepared by fusion and containing a partially soluble solid.	Used as ◆ Keratolytic. ◆ Ointment in the treatment of warts and corns.
2)	Sulphur ointment	Precipitated sulphur Ointment (finely sifted) Simple ointment	Ointment prepared by trituration (levigation) and containing insoluble solid.	Used as, ◆ Antiseptic, Anti parasitic and scabicide. ◆ Also used in the treatment of Acne and dandruff.
3)	Boric acid ointment	Boric acid Paraffin ointment	Ointment prepared by trituration (levigation) and containing insoluble solid.	◆ Used as anti-infective and antiseptic in the treatment of skin infections.
4)	Compound Benzoic acid ointment B.P. (Whitfield ointment)	Benzoic acid (finely sifted) Salicylic acid (finely sifted) Emulsifying ointment	Ointment prepared by levigation and containing insoluble solids	◆ Used as fungicidal and keratolytic.
5)	Ichthammol ointment B.P.C.	Ichthammol Wool fat Yellow soft paraffin	Ointment prepared by fusion and containing a semisolid	◆ Used as antiseptic.
6)	Compound Methyl salicylate ointment B.P.C.	Methyl salicylate Cajuput oil Cincole Water Menthol Wool fat White bees wax	Ointment prepared by fusion containing liquids, miscible with the base	◆ Used as counter irritant. ◆ Also used as analgesic .

S.N.	Name of the Ointment	Ingredients (Formulation)	Type and Method of Preparation	Uses
7)	Calamine and Coal tar ointment B.P.C.	Calamine (finely sifted) Strong coal tar solution Zinc oxide Hydrous wool fat White soft paraffin	Ointment prepared by fusion and containing insoluble solids.	Used as, ◆ Skin protective.
8)	Zinc and Castor oil ointment B.P. Syn.:The Baby cream	Zinc oxide (finely sifted) Castor oil Cetostearyl alcohol White bees wax Arachis oil	Ointment prepared by fusion and containing an insoluble solid.	Used as, ◆ skin protective and emollient for the babies.
9)	Ammoniated mercury and Coal tar ointment B.P.C.	Ammoniated mercury Strong coal tar solution Yellow soft paraffin	Ointment prepared by trituration and containing a solid and liquid.	Used as, ◆ antiseptic and skin protective.
10)	Hamamelis ointment B.P.C.	Hamamelis liquid extract Yellow soft paraffin Wool fat	Ointment prepared by (levigation) trituration and containing a liquid.	Used as, ◆ antiseptic ointment.
11)	Compound Resorcinol ointment B.P.C.	Resorcinol Cod liver oil Zinc oxide (finely sifted) Bismuth subnitrate (finely sifted) Starch (finely sifted) Sodium metabisulphite Hard paraffin Water Wool fat Yellow soft paraffin	Ointment prepared by levigation and containing solids and liquids.	Used as, ◆ antiseptic and skin protective.

S.N.	Name of the Ointment	Ingredients (Formulation)	Type and Method of Preparation	Uses
12)	Strong Iodine ointment	Iodine Wool fat Yellow soft paraffin Potassium iodide Water	Ointment prepared by chemical reaction method and containing free iodine.	Used as, ◆ Treat ring worm infection in cattles.
13)	Non-staining Iodine ointment B.P.C.	Iodine Arachis oil Oleic acid Yellow soft paraffin	Ointment prepared by chemical reaction	Used as, ◆ Analgesic and anti-inflammatory.
14)	Tannic acid ointment	Tannic acid Purified water Wool alcohol ointment	Ointment prepared by emulsification (fusion) method	Used as, ◆ Astringent in the treatment of haemorrhoids.
15)	Cetrimide emulsifying Ointment	Cetrimide White soft paraffin Cetostearyl alcohol Liquid paraffin	Ointment prepared by fusion method	Used as, ◆ Antiseptic and skin protective.
16)	Salicylic and Sulphur ointment B.P.C.	Salicylic acid (finely sifted) Precipitated sulphur Oily cream	Ointment prepared by trituration (levigation) and containing solids	◆ Used as fungicidal, antiseptic and scabicide. Also used in the treatment of acne and dandruff.

HYDROCARBON OINTMENT BASE

Synonyms: Paraffin ointment or Oleogenous base or Fatty base.

Rx	
Cerae bees albae	gr xxx
Paraffinum dura	gr VL
Cetostearyl alcoholis	3 i s
Paraffini mollis albi or flavum	3 xxii ss
Fiat : Unguentum	Mitte : 3 ii ss
Direction: Use this base as emmolient for preparation of eye ointment and other ointments.	

Conversion :

gr xxx → 30 grains

15 grains = 1 g

30 grains = 2 g

gr VL → 45 grains = 3 g

3 i s → 1.25 drachms

1 drachm = 4 g

1.25 drachms = 5 g

3 xxii ss → 22.5 drachms = 90 g

3 ii ss → 2.5 drachms = 10 g

Calculation : 3 ii ss → 2.5 dr = 10 g, but calculate for (10 + 2) = 12 g

White bees wax $= \frac{2}{100} \times 12 = 0.24\text{g}$

Hard paraffin $= \frac{3}{100} \times 12 = 0.36\text{g}$

Cetostearyl alcohol $= \frac{5}{100} \times 12 = 0.6\text{g}$

White soft paraffin $= \frac{90}{100} \times 12 = 10.8\text{g}$

Type	Ingredients	Quantity in imperial	Quantity in metric	Quantity taken
Semi solid hydrocarbon ointment base	White bees wax	30 gr	2 g	0.24 g
	Hard paraffin	45 gr	3 g	0.36 g
	Cetostearyl alcohol	1.25 dr	5 g	0.6 g
	White or yellow soft paraffin	22.5 dr	90 g	10.8 g
	Make: Ointment base Send: 10 g Direction: Use this base as emmolient, for preparation of eye ointment and other ointments.			

Theory:

Paraffin ointment is a hydrocarbon ointment base, because it contains, hard paraffin, white or yellow soft paraffin, and white bees wax, which are hydrophobic in nature. Due to the hydrophobic nature of the base, it is unable to absorb any proportion of water. (White bees wax absorbs small proportion of water, but due to its very small amount, it acts as a hydrocarbon base, instead of absorption base).

Paraffin ointment is sticky and almost inert in nature. It is not absorbed by skin and is immiscible with water. In this preparation, hard paraffin is used, to give stiffness (hardness) to the ointment base. Cetostearyl alcohol is used, to improve the stability and emollient property of the ointment. White soft paraffin is used as protective and as an emollient.

If the hydrocarbon base (paraffin ointment) is used for preparation of ophthalmic ointment, then yellow soft paraffin should be used instead of white soft paraffin, because white soft paraffin is obtained by bleaching of yellow soft paraffin, with oxidizing agents and acids. Hence the traces of oxidizing agents and acids may remain in the white soft paraffin, and can cause irritation to the eyes.

Procedure(By fusion method):

Since there will be little wastage (loss) of ingredients during weighing and preparing, to manipulate these practical losses, calculate the ingredients for at least one or two grams extra, than prescribed.

1) Grate (cut) all the waxy materials and weigh according to the calculation and melt in the descending order of their melting points i.e. Melt bees wax, hard paraffin followed by cetostearyl alcohol and white (yellow) soft paraffin, by placing on a water bath with continuous stirring.
2) After melting, decant the melt into a hot dish, to remove foreign matter, if present.
3) After decantation, stir the mixture, until it becomes cool and a semisolid base is obtained.

Dispensing: Weigh the prescribed quantity of the ointment, on a butter paper and transfer into an ointment jar, close it thoroughly and label.

Storage: Store in a cool place.

Auxilliary label: FOR EXTERNAL USE ONLY.

Uses:

1) Paraffin ointment (hydrocarbon ointment base) is used as base for preparation of ointments, which are required for prolonged action.
2) It is used as ointment base for incorporation of antibiotics, which are unstable in presence of water. It is also used as emollient.
3) It is heat stable, hence used as base for sterile ointments like, eye ointments.

BORIC ACID OINTMENT

Rx	
Acidi borici	gr XV
Paraffinum unguentum... q.s. ...	3 XXV
Fiat : Unguentum	Mitte : 3 ii ss
Signa : Applicanda parti affecatae b.i.d - t.i.d more dicto.	

Conversion :

gr XV → 15 grains   3 XXV → 25 drachms

15 grains = 1 g   1 drachms = 4 g

25 drachms = 100 g

Calculation : 3 ii ss → 2.5 dr = 10 g, but calculate for (10 + 2) = 12 g

Boric acid = $\frac{1}{100} \times 12 = 0.12$ g

Paraffin ointment ...q.s... = 12 g

Type	Ingredients	Quantity in imperial	Quantity in metric	Quantity taken
Ointment containing insoluble solid.	Boric acid	15 gr	1 g	0.12 g
	Paraffin ointment... q.s.	25 dr	100 g	12 g
Prepared using paraffin (hydrocarbon) ointment, as base.	Make: Ointment Send: 10 g Direction: Apply to the affected part two - three times a day, as directed.			

Theory:

Boric acid ointment is used as local antiinfective, which is prepared by levigation method, because boric acid is insoluble in paraffin ointment. Boric acid is white coloured substance. Hence paraffin ointment, prepared with white soft paraffin is used as base.

Boric acid is triturated and passed through sieve number 180 to get a very fine powder, to prevent the grittiness, after the application of ointment.

Procedure:

Since there will be little wastage (loss) of ingredients during weighing and preparing, to manipulate these practical losses, calculate the ingredients for at least one or two grams extra, than prescribed.

1) Triturate the boric acid into a fine powder and pass through the sieve no. 180.
2) Weigh the required amount of finely sifted boric acid and place on a cleaned ointment slab.
3) Weigh the paraffin ointment on a butter paper, to prevent it sticking to the balance and place it on other part of ointment slab.
4) Take a portion of the base, of about three times the volume of the boric acid and levigate with the help of ointment spatula, until there is no sign of any particles of boric acid. (Because with a little base, a smooth dispersion is obtained, with minimum efforts)
5) Gradually incorporate the remaining portion of paraffin ointment and levigate to get a homogenous and smooth ointment.

Dispensing: Weigh the prescribed quantity of the ointment on a butter paper and transfer into an ointment jar or collapsible tube, seal and label.

Direction: Apply to the affected part, two - three times a day, as directed.

Storage: Store in a cool place.

Auxilliary label: FOR EXTERNAL USE ONLY.

Uses: Boric acid acts as anti-infective and antiseptic, hence this ointment is used as local anti-infective, in the treatment of skin infections.

Caution: Not to be applied on open wounds.

SIMPLE OINTMENT B.P. / I.P.

Rx	
Adipis lanae	3 i s
Paraffinum dura	3 i s
Alcoholis cetostearyl	3 i s
Paraffinum mollis albi or flavum	3 xxi s
Fiat : Unguentum	Mitte : 3 vii ss
Signa : Apply to the affected part as directed and use as base in the preparation of eye ointment and other ointments.	

Conversion :

3 i s → 1.25 drachms 3 xxi s → 21.25 drachms = 85 g

1 drachm = 4 g

1.25 drachms = 5 g

Calculation : 3 vii ss → 7.5 dr = 30 g, but calculate for (30 + 2) = 32 g

Wool fat = $\frac{5}{100} \times 32 = 1.6\,g$

Hard paraffin = $\frac{5}{100} \times 32 = 1.6\,g$

Cetostearyl alcohol = $\frac{5}{100} \times 32 = 1.6\,g$

White soft paraffin = $\frac{85}{100} \times 32 = 27.2\,g$

Type	Ingredients	Quantity in imperial	Quantity in metric	Quantity taken
Semi solid absorption type ointment base	Wool fat	1.25 dr	5 g	1.6 g
	Hard paraffin	1.25 dr	5 g	1.6 g
	Cetostearyl alcohol	1.25 dr	5 g	1.6 g
	White or Yellow soft paraffin	21.25 dr	85 g	27.2 g
	Make: Ointment	Send: 30 g		
	Direction: Apply to the affected part as directed and use as base in the preparation of eye ointment and other ointments.			

Theory:

Simple ointment is an absorption type ointment base, which is prepared by fusion method. It consists of hydrophobic fatty bases like hard paraffin, cetostearyl alcohol and white or yellow soft paraffin.

Wool fat acts as an w/o type of emulsifying agent, hence it ensures satisfactory emulsification of aqueous solution of the medicament. Therefore base gets hydrophilic nature and capacity, to absorb large quantity of water.

In this preparation, hard paraffin is used to stiffen the ointment base. Cetostearyl alcohol improves the stability and emollient property of the ointment. Soft paraffin gives spreadability and emollient nature to the preparation. If the medicament is white or colourless then white soft paraffin can be used.

If the simple ointment is used for preparation of ophthalmic ointment, then yellow soft paraffin should be used instead of white soft paraffin, because white soft paraffin is obtained by bleaching of yellow soft paraffin with oxidizing agents and acids. Hence the traces of oxidizing agents and acids may remain in the white soft paraffin, and cause irritation to the eyes.

Simple ointment absorbs about 15% of its weight of water and forms an w/o type emulsion.

Procedure: (By fusion method)

Since there will be little wastage (loss) of ingredients during weighing and preparing, to manipulate these practical losses, calculate the ingredients for at least one or two grams extra, than prescribed.

1) Weigh all the ingredients according to calculation.
2) Melt hard paraffin and cetostearyl alcohol in a porcelain dish, by keeping on a water bath.
3) To this melt, incorporate wool fat and white soft paraffin, stir well during melting.
4) After melting of all the ingredients, remove the foreign matter if present by decanting or straining into another hot dish. Stir the mixture thoroughly, until it becomes cooled and a semisolid base is obtained.

Dispensing: Weigh the prescribed quantity of the ointment, on a butter paper and transfer into an ointment jar, close it thoroughly and label.

Storage: Store in a cool place.

Auxilliary label: FOR EXTERNAL USE ONLY.

Uses: Simple ointment is used as an emollient. It is also used as ointment base for preparation of eye ointments and other ointments. It is used as base, when incorporation of small quantities of aqueous liquids is necessary.

SULPHUR OINTMENT B.P.

Rx
Sulphuris praecipitati 3 ii ss
Simple unguentum 3 xxii ss
Fiat : Unguentum Mitte : 3 ii ss
Signa :Applicandus unguentum party affectae,
S.O.S. more dicto.

Conversion :

3 ii ss → 2.5 drachms 3 xxii ss → 22.5 dr = 90 g
1 drachm = 4 g
2.5 drachms = 10 g

Calculation : 3 ii ss → 2.5 dr = 10 g, but calculate for (10 + 2) = 12 g

$$\text{Precipitated sulphur} = \frac{10}{100} \times 12 = 1.2\,g$$

$$\text{Simple ointment} = \frac{90}{100} \times 12 = 10.8\,g$$

Type	Ingredients	Quantity in imperial	Quantity in metric	Quantity taken
Ointment containing insoluble solids, prepared using simple ointment, as base.	Precipitated sulphur (Finely sifted)	2.5 dr	10 g	1.2 g
	Simple ointment	22.5 dr	90 g	10.8 g
	Make: Ointment Send: 10 g Direction: Apply the ointment to the affected area, when ever neccessary, as directed.			

Theory:

This is an ointment containing solid medicament like- Precipitated sulphur, which is insoluble in the base. Because precipitated sulphur is hydrophobic in nature but simple ointment is an absorption base, which is hydrophilic in nature. Therefore precipitated sulphur is incorporated (dispersed) in to the base, by levigation method.

In this prescription, precipitated sulphur is preferred than sublimed sulphur for the preparation of ointment, because it is amorphous in nature and hence it gives a smooth ointment, than sublimed sulphur.

Sulphur is pale yellow in colour, therefore to mask this colour, simple ointment prepared by white soft paraffin is used as base.

Procedure:

Since there will be little wastage (loss) of ingredients during weighing and preparing, to manipulate these practical losses, calculate the ingredients for at least one or two grams, extra than prescribed.

1) Calculate the ingredients according to the calculation.
2) Pass precipitated sulphur through the sieve no. 180 to get very fine powder.
3) Weigh required amount of precipitated sulphur and place on a cleaned ointment slab.
4) Weigh required amount of simple ointment on a piece of butter paper, to prevent it sticking to the balance and place it on a different part of the slab.
5) Take a portion of the base of about three times the volume of the sulphur and levigate with sulphur with the help of ointment spatula, until there is no sign of any particles of sulphur. This can be checked by spreading as a thin layer on the slab.
6) Gradually incorporate remaining quantity of simple ointment and levigate, to get a homogenous and smooth ointment.

Dispensing: Precipitated sulphur is sensitive to the light. Hence transfer the prescribed quantity of ointment, to a light resistant ointment jar or collapsible tube, close it thoroughly and label.

Direction: Apply the ointment to the affected area, when ever neccessary, as directed.

Storage: Store in a cool and dark place.

Auxilliary label:
- FOR EXTERNAL USE ONLY.
- STORE IN COOL AND DARK PLACE.

Uses: Precipitated sulphur acts as an antiseptic and parasiticidal and scabicidal, hence sulphur ointment is used, in the treatment of scabies, acne and other skin disorders.

WOOL ALCOHOL OINTMENT (BASE)

Rx	
Lanae alcoholis	3 i ss
Paraffinum dura	3 Vi
Paraffinum molle flavum	3 ii ss
Liquidi paraffinum	3 XV
Fiat : Unguentum	Mitte : 3 V
Signa: Use as base, for preparation of ointment and cream.	

Conversion :

3 i = 4 g therefore,

3 i ss → 1.5 drachms = 6 g   3 ii ss → 2.5 drachms = 10 g

3 Vi → 6 drachms = 24 g   3 XV → 15 drachms = 60 g

Calculation : For 3 V → 5 dr = 20 g, but calculate for (20 + 2) = 22 g

Wool alcohol = $\frac{6}{100} \times 22 = 1.32\text{g}$

Hard paraffin = $\frac{24}{100} \times 22 = 5.28\text{ g}$

Yellow soft paraffin = $\frac{10}{100} \times 22 = 2.2\text{ g}$

Liquid paraffin = $\frac{60}{100} \times 22 = 13.2\text{g}$

Type	Ingredients	Quantity in imperial	Quantity in metric	Quantity taken
Absorption type ointment base	Wool alcohol	1.5 dr	6 g	1.32 g
	Hard paraffin	6 dr	24 g	5.28 g
	Yellow soft paraffin	2.5 dr	10 g	2.2 g
	Liquid paraffin	15 dr	60 g	13.2 g
	Make: Ointment	Send: 20 g		
	Direction: Use as base, for preparation of ointment and cream.			

Theory:

It is an absorption type ointment base and has the capacity, to absorb large quantities of aqueous liquid, to form (w/o) type emulsion. Wool alcohol consists not less than 30% of cholesterol, which can emulsify several times its own weight of an aqueous liquid and it can emulsify about half of its own weight of water, when mixed with fats like soft paraffin.

Therefore, wool alcohol ointment is used as emulsifying agent, in the preparation of (w/o) type emulsions. It also used to improve texture, stability and emollient properties of (o/w) type emulsions.

Wool alcohol is very sticky in nature, when used alone. Hence it is usually mixed with hydrocarbons like hard paraffin, yellow soft paraffin and liquid paraffin, in suitable proportions for the preparation of ointment base.

Procedure (By fusion method):

Since there will be little wastage (loss) of ingredients during weighing and preparing, to manipulate these practical losses, calculate the ingredients for at least one or two grams extra than prescribed.

1) Weigh wool alcohol, hard paraffin and soft paraffin, separately.
2) Grate (cut) the wool alcohol and hard paraffin into small pieces and melt in china dish. To this melt, add yellow soft paraffin and liquid paraffin.
3) Heat the above contents in china dish over a water bath with continuous stirring, until they melts.
4) After melting, stop heating and stir continuously until it becomes cool and a semisolid mass is formed.

Dispensing: Weigh the prescribed quantity of the ointment on a butter paper and transfer into an ointment jar, close it throughly and label.

Storage: Store in a cool place.

Auxilliary label: FOR EXTERNAL USE ONLY.

Uses: Wool alcohol ointment is used as vehicle (base) for preparation of (w/o) type ointments, where aqueous liquids and solutions of medicaments are to be incorporated.

Eg. Tannic acid ointment.

It spreads easily on the skin and comparatively less occlusive than hydrocarbon base.

TANNIC ACID OINTMENT

Rx	
Acidi tannici	3 V
Aquam	3 X
Lanae alcoholis unguentum	3 X
Fiat : Unguentum	Mitte : 3 ii ss
Signa : Applicandus super dolenticus cutis more dicto.	

Conversion :

3 i → 1 dr = 4 g

3 V → 5 drachms = 20 g

3 X → 10 drachms = 40 g

3 ii ss → 2.5 drachms = 10 g

Calculation : 3 ii ss → 2.5 dr = 10 g, but calculate for (10 + 2) = 12 g

Tannic acid $= \frac{20}{100} \times 12 = 2.4$ g

Water $= \frac{40}{100} \times 12 = 4.8$ g

Wool alcohol ointment $= \frac{40}{100} \times 12 = 4.8$ g

Type	Ingredients	Quantity in imperial	Quantity in metric	Quantity taken
Ointment containing soluble substance, Prepared using wool alcohol ointment, as base.	Tannic acid	5 dr	20 g	2.4 g
	Distilled water	10 dr	40 g	4.8 g
	Wool alcohol ointment	10 dr	40 g	4.8 g
	Make: Ointment	Send: 10 g		
	Direction: Apply on the affected area of the skin, as directed.			

Theory:

Tannic acid is soluble in water and acts as astringent. This ointment is prepared by using absorption base like, Wool alcohol ointment, which has the capacity to absorb large quantities of aqueous liquid to form (w/o) type emulsion.

Wool alcohol ointment consists of wool alcohol and hydrocarbons like hard paraffin, liquid paraffin and yellow soft paraffin. In which wool alcohol acts as (w/o) type emulsifying agent. Hence tannic acid ointment is prepared by emulsification method.

Procedure: (By emulsification method)

Since there will be little wastage (loss) of ingredients during weighing and preparing, to manipulate these practical losses, calculate the ingredients for at least one or two grams extra, than prescribed.

1) Weigh wool alcohol ointment base and melt in china dish, on a water bath at temperature 60-70 °C.
2) Weigh the tannic acid and dissolve it in distilled water in a beaker. Warm it to a temperature, up to 60-70 °C on a water bath.
3) When both aqueous and oily phases reaches same temperature (60-70 °C), add tannic acid solution gradually to the melted base with continuous stirring, until it become cool and a semisolid mass is formed.

Dispensing: Tannic acid reacts with iron and causes the formation of black coloured iron tannate, which would discolour (darken) the preparation. Therefore iron containers or spatula should not be used for storage or for preparation of tannic acid ointment.

Hence transfer the prescribed quantity of tannic acid ointment to a plastic collapsible tube, seal and label.

Direction: Apply on the affected area of the skin, as directed.

Storage: Store in a cool place.

Auxilliary label:
- FOR EXTERNAL USE ONLY.
- STORE IN A COOL AND DARK PLACE.

Uses: Tannic acid ointment is used as an astringent in the treatment of haemorrhoids.

Similar example:

Salicylic acid ointment B.P.

Salicylic acid (finely sifted)	---	20 g
Wool alcohols ointment	---	980 g

Uses: Salicylic acid has keratolytic, bacteriostatic and germicidal properties. Hence it is used in the treatment of warts and corns. It can also be used as anti dandruff agent.

EMULSION BASE

Synonym : Emulsifying ointment B.P.C

Rx	
Cerae emulsif	3 Vii ss
Paraffini mollis albi	3 Xii ss
Liquidi paraffinum	3 V
Fiat : Unguentum	Mitte : 3 ii ss
Signa: Use as base, for preparation of whitfield ointment and aqueous cream.	

Conversion : 3 i → 1 dr = 4 g

3 Vii ss → 7.5 drachms = 30 g

3 Xii ss → 12.5 drachms = 50 g

3 V → 5 drachms = 20 g

Calculation : 3 ii ss → 2.5 dr = 10 g, but calculate for (10 + 2) = 12 g.

$$\text{Emulsifying wax} = \frac{30}{100} \times 12 = 3.6\,\text{g}$$

$$\text{White soft paraffin} = \frac{50}{100} \times 12 = 6\,\text{g}$$

$$\text{Liquid paraffin} = \frac{20}{100} \times 12 = 2.4\,\text{g}$$

Type	Ingredients	Quantity in imperial	Quantity in metric	Quantity taken
Ointment base (Emulsion base)	Emulsifying wax	7.5 dr	30 g	3.6 g
	White soft paraffin	12.5 dr	50 g	6 g
	Liquid paraffin	5 dr	20 g	2.4 g
	Make: Ointment	Send: 10 g		
	Direction: Use as base, for preparation of whitfield ointment and aqueous cream.			

Theory:

Emulsifying ointment is a water miscible base prepared by fusion method, which is used as a base for preparation of emulsion type ointments usually o/w type.

Emulsifying wax is a synthetic wax consists of a combination of water soluble surfactant - sodium lauryl sulphate and oil soluble surfactant - cetostearyl alcohol (1:9), hence it is responsible for the formation of oil in water type emulsion.

Procedure:

A) Procedure for preparation of Emulsifying wax

Formula for emulsifying wax:

Sodium lauryl sulphate	---	10 g
Cetostearyl alcohol	---	90 g

1) Weigh the required amount of sodium lauryl sulphate and cetostearyl alcohol.
2) Melt cetostearyl alcohol in a dish on water bath, to this melt incorporate sodium lauryl sulphate by continuous stirring, until it becomes cool.
3) Use this emulsifying wax, for the preparation of emulsifying ointment.

B) Procedure for preparation of Emulsifying ointment B.P. (By fusion method)

Since there will be little wastage (loss) of ingredients during weighing and preparing, to manipulate these practical losses, calculate the ingredients for at least one or two grams extra, than prescribed.

1) Melt emulsifying wax in a porcelain dish, on a water bath. To this melt, incorporate liquid paraffin and white soft paraffin with continuous stirring.
2) Remove the foreign particles if present, by decanting or straining to a hot vessel and stir until, product becomes cool and a semisolid mass is obtained.

Dispensing: Weigh the prescribed quantity of the ointment on a butter paper and transfer into an ointment jar, close it thoroughly and label.

Direction: Use as base, for preparation of Whitfield's ointment and aqueous cream.

Storage: Store in a cool place.

Auxilliary label: FOR EXTERNAL USE ONLY.

Uses: Emulsifying ointment is used as a base, for the preparation of emulsion type (o/w type) of ointments.

Eg. Compound benzoic acid ointment B.P. (Whitfield's ointment, see page no. 344)
Aqueous cream B.P., see page no. 353)

COMPOUND BENZOIC ACID OINTMENT B.P.

Synonym: Whitfield's ointment

Rx	
Acidi benzoici	3 i ss
Acid salicylic	3 i
Emulsif unguentum	3 xxii ss
Fiat : Unguentum	Mitte : 3 ii ss
Signa : Apply sparingly to the affected area but do not apply to the broken or inflamed skin.	

Conversion : 3 i → 1 dr = 4 g

3 i ss → 1.5 drachms = 6 g

3 xx ii ss → 22.5 drachms = 90 g

Calculation : 3 ii ss → 2.5 dr = 10 g, but calculate for (10 + 2) = 12 g

Benzoic acid = $\frac{6}{100} \times 12 = 0.72$ g

Salicylic acid = $\frac{4}{100} \times 12 = 0.48$ g

Emulsifying ointment = $\frac{90}{100} \times 12 = 10.8$ g

Type	Ingredients	Quantity in imperial	Quantity in metric	Quantity taken
O/W emulsion type ointment.	Benzoic acid (fine)	1.5 dr	6 g	0.72 g
	Salicylic acid (fine)	1 dr	4 g	0.48 g
	Emulsifying ointment	22.5 dr	90 g	10.8 g
Prepared using, emulsifying ointment as base	Make: Ointment Send: 10 g Direction: Apply sparingly to the affected area but do not apply to the broken or inflamed skin.			

Theory:

Whitfield's ointment contains, benzoic acid and salicylic acid in emulsifying ointment, which is used as base. Both benzoic acid and salicylic acids are insoluble in emulsifying ointment, because it is water miscible base. Hence this ointment is prepared by levigation method.

Benzoic acid acts as antifungal and salicylic acid acts as keratolytic.

Procedure (By levigation method):

Since there will be little wastage (loss) of ingredients during weighing and preparing, to manipulate these practical losses, calculate the ingredients for at least one or two grams extra, than prescribed.

1) Separately pass the benzoic acid and salicylic acid through the sieve number 180, to get very fine powder.
2) Weigh the required quantity of sifted salicylic acid and benzoic acid and mix them uniformly.
3) Place this powder mixture on a cleaned ointment slab.
4) Weigh the emulsifying ointment on a butter paper and transfer to an other part of the ointment slab.
5) Levigate the base with about three times the volume of powder mixture, until there is no sign of solid particles of benzoic acid and salicylic acid. The base when used in little amounts give a smooth and uniform dispersion with minimum efforts.
6) Gradually incorporate the remaining portion of base and levigate until a smooth and uniform homogenous ointment is obtained.

Dispensing: Since salicylic acid will react with metallic containers and is sensitive to the light, transfer the prescribed quantity of ointment to a wide mouthed, amber coloured jar with a grease proof paper disc or dispense in a plastic collapsible tube, seal and label.

Direction: Apply sparingly to the affected area as directed. Not to be applied to the broken or inflamed skin.

Storage: Store in a cool and dark place.

Auxilliary label:
- FOR EXTERNAL USE ONLY.
- STORE IN A COOL AND DARK PLACE.

Uses: Whitfield ointment is used, as a fungicidal ointment.

Note: Salicylic acid is very irritant to the respiratory tract, hence precautions should be taken, to avoid inhalation.

Marketed preparations by:

1. Sallderm skin ointment, Dermocare Labs, Ahmedabad.
2. Whitfield's ointment, Jilichem Labs (India) Ltd., Ahmedabad.

PREPARATION OF OINTMENTS BY CHEMICAL REACTION

Certain ointments are prepared by chemical reaction between medicament and other ingredients of the ointment.

Eg.
- Strong iodine ointment BPC
- Non-staining iodine ointment.
- Strong mercuric nitrate ointment.
- Oleate mercury ointment.

(1) STRONG IODINE OINTMENT B.P.C. (OINTMENT CONTAINING FREE IODINE)

Strong iodine ointment B.P.C. can be prepared using two formulas,

(A)		(B)	
Iodine	- 2 g	Iodine	- 4 g
Potassium iodide	- 2 g	Potassium iodide	- 4 g
Wool fat	- 2 g	Wool fat	- 4 g
Water	- 6 ml	Yellow bees wax	- 4 g
Yellow soft paraffin	- 38 g	Glycerin	- 12 ml
		Yellow soft paraffin	- 72 g

Theory:

Iodine is only slightly soluble in most of the fats and oils. But it is freely soluble in concentrated aqueous solution of potassium iodide, because iodine reacts with potassium iodide in presence of water and forms molecular complexes (polyiodides). These polyiodides are readily soluble in water, glycerin and alcohol.

$$I_2 + KI \xrightarrow{H_2O} KI.I_2 \quad \text{Potassium monoiodide}$$

$$2I_2 + KI \xrightarrow{H_2O} KI.2I_2 \quad \text{Potassium diiodide}$$

$$3I_2 + KI \xrightarrow{H_2O} KI.3I_2 \quad \text{Potassium triiodide}$$

Iodine Potassium iodide Polyiodides

Therefore for preparation of strong iodine ointment, water, glycerin or alcohol may be used as vehicle. But the selection of solvent (vehicle) is very important, because after application of the ointment, solvent evaporates and iodine will crystallizes into fine particles. These fine crystals cause irritation to the skin. Therefore vehicle should be non-volatile in nature.

Hence for most of the time, Strong iodine ointment is prepared by using glycerin as vehicle instead of water. Glycerin is non-volatile in nature and also gives demulscent (soothing) effect and also acts as humectant. Yellow soft paraffin and wool fat are used as base for the preparation of ointment.

Uses: Iodine acts as antiseptic, hence this ointment is used to treat ring worm infection in cattles. Previously this ointment was also used in human beings. But due to the availability of free iodine in the ointment, it badly stains the skin and cloths, with deep red colour. Therefore this ointment has not became more popular.

Remedy: To avoid the problem of staining by free iodine, Combined iodine ointment (Non-staining iodine ointment) is prepared.

NON-STAINING IODINE OINTMENT I.P./B.P.C.

Synonym : Combined Iodine ointment

Rx	
Iodine	gr xx
Acidi oleici	gr XL
Olei recini (or Olei arachisi)	gr LX
Paraffinum mole flavum…. q.s…	3 vii ss
Fiat: Unguentum	Mitte: 3 ii ss
Signa : Applicandus delontiparti, S.O.S.	

Conversion : 15 grains = 1 g therefore,

gr xx → 20 grains = 1.2 g 3 vii ss→ 7.5 drachms

gr XL → 40 grains = 2.4 g 1 drachm = 4 g

gr LX → 60 grains = 3.6 g 7.5 drachms = 30 g

Calculation: 3 ii ss → 2.5 dr = 10 g, but calculate for (10 + 2) = 12 g

Iodine $= \frac{1.2}{30} \times 12 = 0.48$ g

Oleic acid $= \frac{2.4}{30} \times 12 = 0.96$ g

Castor oil (or Arachis oil) $= \frac{3.6}{30} \times 12 = 1.44$ g

Yellow soft paraffin….q.s…. = 12 g

Type	Ingredients	Quantity in imperial	Quantity in metric	Quantity taken
Ointment prepared, by chemical reaction.	Iodine	20 gr	1.2 g	0.48 g
	Oleic acid	40 gr	2.4 g	0.96 g
	Castor oil (Arachis oil)	60 gr	3.6 g	1.44 g
	Yellow soft paraffin …q.s…	7.5 dr	30.0 g	12.0 g
	Prepare: Ointment	Send: 10 g		
	Direction: Apply to the affected part, when ever necessary.			

Theory:

Non-staining iodine ointment is an ointment prepared by chemical reaction, which is used as an local analgesic and anti-inflammatory. Fixed oils and fats obtained from vegetable source like arachis oil, castor oil, oleic acid contains unsaturated fatty acids (i.e fatty acids contain double or triple bond linkages). Iodine combines with these linkages of fatty acids and form complex.

Though the prepared (obtained) ointment is greenish – black in colour, even then it does not leaves stain when rubbed on the skin, due to non-availability of free iodine. Therefore combined iodine ointment is called as "Non-staining iodine ointment".

Eg.

$$CH_3(CH_2)_7 - CH = CH - (CH_2)_7 - COOH + I_2 \rightarrow CH_3(CH_2)_7 - CHI - CHI - (CH_2)_7 - COOH$$

Oleic acid — Iodine — Di-iodo stearic acid

- For preparation of ointment, arachis oil alone cannot be used, because it does not contain sufficient unsaturated linkages, to make complex with iodine. Therefore oleic acid is used, along with arachis oil, which provides sufficient unsaturated fatty acids and has oleoginic linkages. These linkages make complex with iodine and forms di-iodo stearic acid (olien or glyceryl ester of oleic acid).
- Instead of arachis oil, any of paraffin like, hard paraffin, soft paraffin or liquid paraffin alone cannot be used. Because they consists almost saturated fatty acids, hence they are unable to absorb more than 2% of Iodine. Therefore paraffins are used as base, for preparation ointment along with fixed oils.
- Under normal conditions employed for preparation of ointment, the maximum absorption (complexation) of iodine is not possible. Hence the amount of oil (oils) used, is usually much excess than theoretical quantity.
- The addition of yellow soft paraffin in the initial stage i.e. along with arachis oil and oleic acid, slows down the reaction between fatty acids and iodine. Therefore yellow soft paraffin should be melted separately and added at the end of the preparation.
- Iodine is volatile in nature. Therefore ointment should be prepared in closed vessel and heating should not be done above 50 °C.
- At room temperature, reaction between oil and iodine is very slow. Therefore reaction is hastened by heating the reaction mixture. At the initial stage mixture shows brown colour, but at the final stage it turns to greenish black colour due to complete complexation between fatty acids and iodine. It may requires several hours (2 to 4 hours) for completion of reaction.

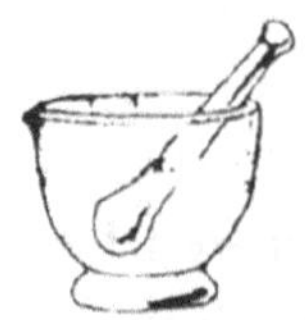

Glass mortar and pestle

Procedure: Since there will be little wastage (loss) of ingredients during weighing and preparing, to manipulate these practical losses, calculate the ingredients for at least one or two grams extra, than prescribed.

1) Finely powder the iodine in a glass mortar and add the required amount of iodine to the glass stoppered bottle containing arachis oil and oleic acid and stir well.
2) Close the bottle with stopper and heat at 50 °C in a thermo statistically controlled water bath, with occasional stirring, until brown colour changes to, greenish black colour (This may make take 2-4 hours).
3) Warm the yellow soft paraffin to 50 °C, on a water bath. To this melt, add iodised oil with continuous stirring. (More heating should not be applied, because it cause deposition of a resinous substance.)

Dispensing: Iodine is sensitive to the light, therefore, pour the mixed mass into a warm, light resistant (greenish or amber coloured) wide mouthed small glass jar and allow to cool without stirring, to avoid entrapment of air and makes the product opaque. After cooling close throughly with plastic screw cap, polish and label.

Direction: Apply to the affected part, when ever necessary.

Storage: Store in a cool and dark place.

Auxillary label: FOR EXTERNAL USE ONLY.

Uses: This ointment is used as, local analgesic and anti inflammatory.

Note:

1. Iodine stains as brown color to the skin, cloth, and containers made up of porcelain and metals. Therefore for the trituration of iodine glass mortar should be used instead of porcelain.
2. Metal spatula should not be used for handling of iodine and metallic containers should not be used for storing of iodine preparations, because iodine being an oxidizing agent, it oxidizes iron and converts in to ferrous iodide.

   $$Fe + I_2 \longrightarrow FeI_2$$

   Hence plastic spoons are used for handling and containers made up of plastic or glass are used to store iodine preparations.
3. If necessary, iodine stain can be removed by using sodium thiosulphate solution.

Student's exercise:

1) Define Ointments. For what purpose they are used?
2) Classify the ointments with examples.
3) What should be the ideal properties of ointments?
4) What is ointment base? Classify with examples.
5) What are the ideal properties of ointment bases?
6) Differentiate between hydrocarbon bases and absorption bases.
7) What are macrogols? How they are useful in the preparation of ointments.
8) What are the advantages and disadvantages of water soluble bases (macrogols)?
9) Which are the methods used for preparation of ointments?
10) What is levigation? When this method is used?
11) In which situation, mortar and pestle method is used for preparation of ointments?
12) Comment : For preparation of ointments, levigation method is preferred than mortar and pestle method.
13) Define fusion method. Briefly explain this process.
14) Comment : In emulsification method, both oily phase and aqueous phase should be heated to the same temperature, before mixing.

15) Give the examples for ointments, which are prepared by chemical reaction.
16) Which are the additives used in ointments? Give examples.
17) How will you dispense ointments?
18) Comment : Now-a-days. Collapsible tubes are preferred, than the wide mouthed containers, for packing of the ointments.
19) Comment : For preparation of eye ointment, yellow soft paraffin is used instead of white soft paraffin.
20) Why hydrocarbon bases are greasy in nature ?
21) What are uses of hydrocarbon bases?
22) What are uses of boric acid and sulphur ointments?
23) Mention the ingredients for eye ointment.
24) Comment : Wool fat and Cetostearyl alcohol are used in preparation of ointments.
25) Define: Acne, scabies, psoriasis.
26) What is Wool alcohol? what is its use?
27) What for Wool alcohol ointment is used?
28) Define Keratolytic, warts and corns.
29) What is whitfield's ointment ? What for it is used ?
30) What is the use of Strong iodine ointment? Why it is not used for human beings?
31) Comment : Glycerin is preferred as a vehicle, in the preparation of iodine ointments, than water and alcohol.
32) Why Iodine ointment is called as Non-staining iodine ointment?
33) Comment : Oleic acid is used in the preparation of non-staining iodine ointment.
34) Comment : Iodine ointments are dispensed in aluminium collapsible tube.
35) Comment : Yellow soft paraffin is added at the end of the preparation of non staining iodine ointment.
(36) What is the use of Non-staining iodine ointment ? Name it's marketed products.
(37) Comments : For handling of iodine, always plastic spoon should be used.
(38) Comment : For preparation of Eye ointments, hydrocarbon bases are preferred than other bases.

33 CREAMS

Latin term: Cremor

Creams are viscous emulsions of semisolid consistency, intended for external application to the skin or mucous membrane. They are of two types,

(1) (W/O) type creams (oily creams)

(2) (O/W) type creams (aqueous creams)

If creams consist medicinally (therapeutic) active agents, they are called as "medicated creams". Creams are used for protective, therapeutic, prophylactic purposes.

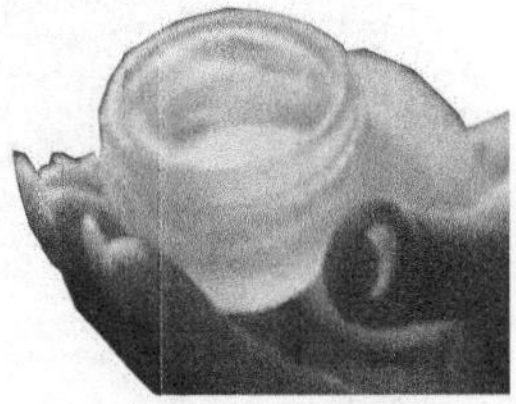

For any cream, basically three things are required such as aqueous phase, oily phase, and emulsifying agent. Volume of phase decides, the type of emulsion or cream. The phase, which is in large amount, will always form the continuous (dispersion) phase. The nature of emulsifying agent also depends up on, the type of emulsion. An emulsifying agent can be added as, one of the ingredients or can be prepared in-situ.

Due to the presence of water soluble components, aqueous creams are comparatively easier to remove from the skin and cloths, by washing with water. Due to the presence of aqueous phase, creams have a tendency of bacterial and mold growth. Therefore preservatives must be incorporated to the creams. Otherwise, the cream, which is contaminated with microorganisms produce infections, when applied to the broken skin.

Examples for the medicated creams:

- Cetrimide cream,
- Salicylic acid - sulphur cream,
- Zinc and ichthammol cream,
- Zinc oxide calamine cream.

Examples for the cosmetic creams:

(O/W) type cream

- Vanishing cream.
- Shaving cream.
- Hand cream.

(W/O) type cream

- Cold cream.
- Cleansing cream.
- Emollient cream.

Oily creams consist a w/o type emulsifying agent Eg. wool fat, wool alcohol, fatty acid, esters of sorbitans or divalent soap,.etc.

Aqueous creams consist of (o/w) type emulsifying agents. Eg. Emulsifying wax, Triethanol amine soap, Tweens, Monovalent soap (alkali soap), Polyethylene glycol derivatives , Fatty acid ester,.etc.

Dispensing: Creams are dispensed in small, wide mouthed, plastic or glass containers, closed with coloured, plastic screw cap with impermeable liner, which facilitate the easy removal of cream.

Now-a-days creams are dispensed in plastic or metallic collapsible tubes, which are suitable to reduce the evaporation of aqueous phase and contamination by micro-organisms, compared to the wide mouthed bottles.

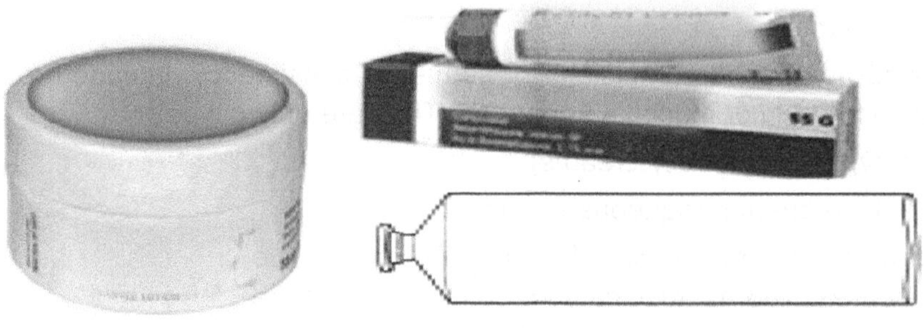

Container for cream

Storage: Creams should be stored in a cool place, but they should not be allowed to freeze, because it may leads to cracking of creams.

Label: Label should bear all necessary requirements. In addition, it should contain auxilliary label like:

- FOR EXTERNAL USE ONLY,
- STORE IN A COOL PLACE, BUT DO NOT ALLOW TO FREEZE.

AQUEOUS CREAM B.P.

Rx	
Emulsif unguentum	℥ vii ss
Phenoxy ethanol	M xv
Aquam	fl. ℥ xvii ss
Fiat : Cremor	Mitte : ℥ v
Signa : Applicandus cutis si opos sit (S.O.S).	

Conversion :

℥ vii ss → 7.5 drachms　　fl. ℥ xvii ss → 17.25 fl. drachms

1 drachm = 4 g　　1 fl. drachm = 4 ml

7.5 drachms = 30 g　　17.25 fl. drachms = 69 ml

M xv → 15 minims = 1 ml

Calculation : ℥ v → 5 drachms = 20 g, but calculate for (20 + 2) = 22 g.

$$\text{Emulsifying ointment} = \frac{30}{100} \times 22 = 6.6 \text{ g}$$

$$\text{Phenoxy ethanol} = \frac{1}{100} \times 22 = 0.22 \text{ml}$$

$$\text{Purified water} = \frac{69}{100} \times 22 = 15.2 \text{ ml}$$

Type	Ingredients	Quantity in imperial	Quantity in metric	Quantity taken
O/W type of cream	Emulsifying ointment	7.5 gr	30 g	6.6 g
	Phenoxy ethanol	15 minims	1 ml	0.22 ml
	Purified water	17.5 fl. dr	69 ml	15.2 ml
	Make: Cream	Send: 20 g		
	Direction: Apply to skin, when ever necessary.			

Theory:

Aqueous cream is an (O/W) type emulsion. For preparation of aqueous cream, emulsifying ointment is used as base. Emulsifying ointment is prepared by using emulsifying wax, white soft paraffin and liquid paraffin.

Emulsifying wax is a synthetic wax, consists a blend of 10% of water soluble surfactant- sodium lauryl sulphate and 90% of oil soluble surfactant --cetostearyl alcohol, hence it is responsible for the formation of oil in water type emulsion.

Phenoxy ethanol is a viscous, water soluble liquid, act as antimicrobial preservative. To reduce the risk of microbial contamination, freshly boiled and cooled water should be used, for preparation of the cream.

Procedure:

Since there will be little wastage (loss) during weighing and preparing, to manipulate these practical losses, calculate the ingredients for at least one or two grams extra, than prescribed.

1) Weigh the emulsifying ointment on a piece of butter paper and melt it in a china dish, on water bath to 60 °C.
2) Dissolve phenoxyethanol in freshly boiled and cooled water and warm up to 60 °C, on water bath.
3) When both aqueous phase and oily phases reaches the 60 °C, add aqueous phase to the melted emulsifying ointment base, with continuous stirring.
4) Remove china dish from the water bath and stir continuously, until it becomes cool and a semi-solid mass is obtained.

Dispensing: Weigh the prescribed quantity of the cream on a butter paper and transfer to a small, wide mouthed glass container (ointment jar or collapsible tube), close it thoroughly with plastic screw cap, polish and label.

Direction: Apply to skin, when ever necessary.

Storage: Store in a cool place but do not allow to freeze.

Auxilliary label: FOR EXTERNAL USE ONLY.

Uses: Aqueous cream is used as an emollient. It is also used as base (diluent), for other creams.

Note: To reduce the risk of microbial contamination, all equipments used for preparations, should be well washed and dried before use.

OILY CREAM

Synonym : Hydrous Ointment B.P.

Rx	
Lanae alcoholis unguentum	3 xii ss
Phenoxy ethanol	M xv
Sicci magnesii sulphatis	3 i s
Aquam	fl. 3 xi
Fiat : Cremor	Mitte : 3 v
Signa : Applicandus cutis si opos sit (S.O.S).	

Conversion :

3 xii ss → 12.5 drachms　　fl. 3 xi → 11 fluid drachms

1 drachm = 4 g　　1 fluid drachm = 4 ml

12.5 drachms = 50 g　　11 fluid drachms = 44 ml

3 i s → 1.25 drachms = 5 g

Calculation : 3 v → 5 drachms = 20 g, but calculate for (20 + 2) = 22 g.

Wool alcohol ointment $= \frac{50}{100} \times 22 = 11\text{ g}$

Phenoxy ethanol $= \frac{1}{100} \times 22 = 0.22\text{ml}$

Dried magnesium sulphate $= \frac{5}{100} \times 22 = 1.1\text{ g}$

Purified water $= \frac{44}{100} \times 22 = 9.68\text{ml}$

Type	Ingredients	Quantity in imperial	Quantity in metric	Quantity taken
W/O type of cream	Wool alcohol ointment	12.5 dr	50 g	11 g
	Phenoxy ethanol	15 minims	1 ml	0.22 ml
	Dried magnesium sulphate	1.25 dr	5 g	1.1 g
	Purified water	11 fl.dr	44 ml	9.68 ml
	Make: Cream Send: 20 g Direction: Apply to skin, when ever necessary.			

Theory:

Oily cream is (w/o) type cream, prepared by using Wool alcohol ointment, as base. Wool alcohol ointment is made up of wool alcohol, liquid paraffin, hard paraffin and yellow or white soft paraffin. The wool alcohol acts as a w/o type emulsifying agent.

The addition of dried magnesium sulphate, enhances the stability and appearance of the cream. Phenoxyethanol is a viscous liquid, which is used as a preservative. To prevent any contamination with microorganisms, freshly boiled and cooled water should be used, for preparation of the cream.

Procedure: (By emulsification method)

Since there will be little wastage (loss) during weighing and preparing, to manipulate these practical losses, calculate the ingredients for at least one or two grams extra, than prescribed.

1) Weigh all the ingredients, according to calculation.
2) Weigh Wool alcohol ointment on a sheet of butter paper, transfer to a chinadish and melt on a water bath, to 60 °C to 70 °C.
3) Boil the purified water, dissolve the phenoxyethanol and dried magnesium sulphate and allow this mixture to attain 60 °C.
4) When both the phases reaches same temperature (60 °C to 70 °C), gradually add the aqueous solution, to the melt of Wool alcohol ointment with continuous stirring, until it becomes cool and a smooth cream is formed.

Dispensing: Weigh the prescribed quantity of cream on a butter paper and transfer to an ointment jar or metallic / plastic collapsible tube, close it thoroughly and label.

Direction: Apply to skin, when ever necessary.

Storage: Store in a cool place, but do not allow to freeze.

Auxilliary label: FOR EXTERNAL USE ONLY.

Uses: Oily cream is used as emollient in treating dry skin conditions. It is also used as base for the preparation of ointments and creams.

CETRIMIDE CREAM B.P.C.

Rx	
Cetrimide	gr vii ss
Cetostearyl alcoholis	ʒ s
Liquidi paraffinum	fl. ʒ xii ss
Aquam	fl. ʒ xi
Fiat : Cremor	Mitte : ʒ v
Signa : Applicandus dolentiparti, more dicto.	

Conversion :

gr vii ss → 7.5 grains	ʒ i s → 1.25 drachms
15 grains = 1 g	1 drachm = 4 g
7.5 grains = 0.5 g	ʒ i s → 1.25 drachms = 5 g
	fl. ʒ xii ss → 12.5 fl. drachms = 50 ml
	fl. ʒ xi → 11 fl. drachms = 44 ml

Calculation : ʒ v → 5 drachms = 20 g, but calculate for (20 + 2) = 22 g.

Cetrimide $= \frac{0.5}{100} \times 22 = 0.11 g$

Cetostearyl alcohol $= \frac{5}{100} \times 22 = 1.1 g$

Liquid paraffin $= \frac{50}{100} \times 22 = 11 ml$

Purified water $= \frac{44}{100} \times 22 = 9.7 ml$

Type	Ingredients	Quantity in imperial	Quantity in metric	Quantity taken
W/O type of emulsion.	Cetrimide	7.5 gr	0.5 g	0.11 g
	Cetostearyl alcohol	1.25 dr	5 g	1.1 g
	Liquid paraffin	12.5 fl. dr	50 ml	11 ml
Medicated cream.	Purified water	11 fl. dr	44 ml	9.7 ml
	Make: Cream	Send: 20 g		
	Direction: Apply to the affected part, as directed.			

Theory:

It is a medicated cream. Cetrimide has antiseptic action and it also acts as cationic emulsifier. It is freely soluble in water, but highly soluble in warm water. Since cetrimide is quaternary ammonium compound, it cannot acts as good emulsifier, if it is used alone.

Hence it is combined with another emulsifier, cetostearyl alcohol. This combination improves the stability and emollient property of the cream.

Liquid paraffin is used to give a smooth consistency to the cream. Cream is prepared by emulsification method.

Procedure (By emulsification method):

Since there will be little wastage (loss) during weighing and preparing, to manipulate these practical losses, calculate the ingredients for at least one or two grams extra, than prescribed.

1) Weigh cetostearyl alcohol and liquid paraffin, transfer to a china dish and melt on a water bath, to 60 °C to 70 °C.
2) Dissolve cetrimide in a freshly boiled and cooled water and warm to the 60 °C to 70 °C, on a water bath.
3) When both aqueous and oily phases reaches the same temperature (60°C to 70°C), gradually add, cetrimide solution into the oily phase, with continuous stirring.
4) Remove the china dish from the water bath and stir, until it becomes cool and a smooth cream is formed.

Dispensing: Weigh the prescribed quantity of cream on a butter paper and transfer to an ointment jar or metallic / plastic collapsible tube, close it thoroughly and label.

Direction: Apply to the affected part, as directed.

Storage: Store in a cool place, but do not allow to freeze.

Auxilliary label: FOR EXTERNAL USE ONLY.

Uses: This cream is used as an antiseptic cream.

Advice for patients, while dispensing: The cream should not be applied repeatedly and, wet dressings should not be used for its application.

Precaution: Excessive stirring of cetrimide solution should be avoided as this may leads to froth fromation, which is difficult to remove.

COLD CREAM

Rx	
Cerae albae	3 ii ss
Liquidi paraffinum	3 vii ss
Boracis	gr vii ss
Olei rosae	M i ss
Aquam	fl. 3 ii ss
Fiat : Gelidae cremor	Mitte : 3 v
Signa : Applicandus cutis, frequenter.	

Conversion :

3 ii ss → 2.5 drachms	gr vii ss → 7.5 grains
1 drachm = 4 g	15 grains = 1 g
2.5 drachms = 10 g	7.5 grains = 0.5 g
3 vii ss → 7.5 drachms = 30 g	M i ss → 1.5 Minims
	15 Minims = 1 ml.
	1.5 Minims = 0.1 ml.

Calculation : 3 v → 5 drachms = 20 g, but calculate for (20 + 2) = 22 g.

White bees wax = $\frac{10}{50} \times 22 = 4.4$ g

Liquid paraffin = $\frac{30}{50} \times 22 = 13.2$ g

Borax = $\frac{0.5}{50} \times 22 = 0.22$ g

Rose oil = $\frac{0.1}{50} \times 22 = 0.044$ ml

Water = $\frac{10}{50} \times 22 = 4.4$ ml

Type	Ingredients	Quantity in imperial	Quantity in metric	Quantity taken
W/O type, Borax soap emulsion.	White bees wax	2.5 dr	10 g	4.4 g
	Liquid paraffin	7.5 dr	30 g	13.2 g
	Borax	7.5 gr	0.5 g	0.22 g
	Rose oil	1.5 minims	0.1 ml	0.044 ml
	Water	2.5 fl. dr	10 ml	4.4 ml
	Make: Cold cream	Send: 20 g		
	Direction: Apply to the skin, frequently.			

Theory:

Cold cream is W/O type of emulsion, which when applied to the skin, a cooling effect is produced, due to the slow evaporation of water, present in emulsion. Cold cream is prepared by saponification reaction between beeswax and alkali-borax. i.e borax reacts with free fatty acids of bees wax and produce borax soap in-situ (ester of fatty acid). This soap acts as, emulsifying agent.

In cold cream, the internal phase is oil and external phase is water, hence it forms o/w type of emulsion. But after application on the skin, water evaporates and leads to phase inversion from o/w type to w/o type emulsion. Therefore oily phase, which is remaining (left) on the skin gives emolient nature.

Liquid paraffin is used as emollient and rose oil is used as perfume, to give a pleasant flavour to the cream.

> **Note:** Triethanolamine can be used as alkali, instead of borax if required. But cold creams prepared with borax is white, smooth and more stable than, if it is prepared with other alkalies.

Procedure:

Since there will be little wastage (loss) during weighing and preparing, to manipulate these practical losses, calculate the ingredients for at least one or two grams extra, than prescribed.

1) Grate the white beeswax in to small pieces. Weigh the required quantity of white beeswax and liquid paraffin and melt in china dish, by heating on a water bath up to 70°C.
2) In a glass beaker, dissolve borax in water and heat up to 70°C.
3) When both oily and aqueous phases reaches the same temperature (70°C), gradually add borax solution to the melt of beeswax drop by drop, with constant stirring.
4) Stir continuously until it becomes cool. When the temperature loweres to 40- 45 °C, incorporate rose oil and mix uniformly, until a homogenous semi solid mass is obtained.

Dispensing: Weigh the prescribed quantity of cream on a butter paper and transfer to an ointment jar or metallic / plastic collapsible tube, close it thoroughly and label.

Direction: Apply to the skin, frequently.

Storage: Store in a cool place, but do not allow to freeze.

Auxilliary label: FOR EXTERNAL USE ONLY.

Uses: Cold cream is used as an emollient, for the treatment of dry skin. Hence this cream become quite popular, in winter season.

Other similar formulas for Cold cream

1) **Rx**

Bees wax	5 g
Liquid paraffin	45 g
White soft paraffin	10 g
Hard paraffin	7 g
Borax	0.2 g
Water	32.8 ml
Perfume and preservative	..q.s..

2) **Rx**

Bees wax	5 g
Glyceryl mono stearate	2.5 g
Lanolin	10 g
White soft paraffin	10 g
Liquid paraffin	30 g
Borax	0.5 g
Water	19 g
Perfume and preservative	..q.s..

3) **Rx**

Spermaceti	4 g
White bees wax	15 g
Mineral oil	56 g
Borax	0.8 g
Water	23.7 g
Perfume and preservative	0.5 g

VANISHING CREAM

Synonym: Foundation cream.

Rx	
Stearic acid	3 vi s
Potassii hydroxidi	gr xii
Glyerini	fl. 3 ii ss
Methyl paraben	gr iii
Perfume	...q.s..
Aquam	fl. 3 xvi
Fiat : Cremor	Mitte : 3 v
Signa : Applicandus cutis, S.O.S.	

Conversion :

3 vi s → 6.25 drachms	gr xii → 12 grains	fl. 3 ii ss → 2.5 fl.dr
1 drachm = 4 g	15 grains = 1 g	1 fl. dr = 4 ml
6.25 drachms = 25 g	12 grains = 0.8 g	2.5 fl.dr = 10 ml
3 v → 5 drachms = 20 g	gr iii → 3 grains = 0.2 g	16 fl.dr = 64 ml

Calculation : For 3 v → 5 drachms = 20 g, But calculate for (20 + 2) = 22 g.

Stearic acid $= \frac{25}{100} \times 22 = 5.5$ g

Potassium hydroxide $= \frac{0.8}{100} \times 22 = 0.176$g

Glycerin $= \frac{10}{100} \times 22 = 2.2$ ml

Methyl paraben $= \frac{0.2}{100} \times 22 = 0.044$g

Perfume = ...q.s.....

Water $= \frac{64}{100} \times 22 = 14.08$ ml

Type	Ingredients	Quantity in imperial	Quantity in metric	Quantity taken
o/w type emulsion.	Stearic acid	6.25 dr	25 g	5.5 g
	Potassium hydroxide	12 gr	0.8 g	0.176 g
	Glycerin	2.5 fl. dr	10 ml	2.2 ml
Vanishing / foundation cream.	Methyl paraben	3 gr	0.2 g	0.044 g
	Perfume	..q.s..	..q.s..	..q.s..
	Water	16 fl.dr	64 ml	14.08 ml
	Make: Cream	Send: 20 g		
	Direction : Apply to skin, when ever necessary.			

Theory:

Vanishing cream is o/w type emulsion, which when applied to the skin, it vanishes and leaves an almost invisible layer on it. Hence it is called as "vanishing cream". The layer left behind after application, acts as a base or foundation, for facial make up. Hence vanishing creams are also called as "foundation creams". Since water is an external phase, it will be quickly washed off with water.

The main ingredients of vanishing creams are stearic acid, alkali and water. Stearic acid gives a pearly white shining appearance to the cream, which on application gives a thin white film of free stearic acid. Soap is prepared in-situ by the chemical reaction between alkali and stearic acid, which is used as emulsifying agent.

For preparation of vanishing cream, various types of alkalies are used such as Potassium hydroxide, Sodium hydroxide, Aqueous ammonia, Potassium carbonate, Sodium carbonate, Borax and Triethanolomine.

- Out of these alkalies potassium hydroxide is most widely used, because it makes a cream of fine texture and excellent consistency. Otherwise, borax can be used in combination with potassium hydroxide or triethanolamine, to get smooth and white cream.
- If sodium hydroxide is used alone, it makes the cream hard. Hence it should be used in combination with potassium hydroxide.
- Carbonates are generally not used, because they liberate carbon dioxide and makes the cream spongy.
- Aqueous ammonia is also used as effective alkali, but due to it's objectionable odour and volatility, it is difficult to handle. Ammonia creams also tend to turn yellow in colour, with age (during storage).

  Therefore selection of an alkali becomes an important criteria in preparing vanishing creams.

Vanishing creams are o/w type emulsions, there is a possibility of evaporation of water from the external phase of emulsion. Therefore, Glycerin, polyethyleneglycol or alcohol are incorporated as humectants, to prevent the drying out of cream, Since external phase of vanishing cream is aqueous, it should be protected from the contamination, from microorganisms by adding suitable preservatives, like methyl paraben or propyl paraben. These creams are also be scented pleasantly, using suitable perfumes in small quantities.

Procedure : (By emulsification method)

Since there will be little wastage (loss) during weighing and preparing, to manipulate these practical losses, calculate the ingredients for at least one or two grams extra, than prescribed.

1) Melt stearic acid in china dish on a water bath upto 70 °C.

2) In a beaker, dissolve potassium hydroxide and methyl paraben (methyl para hydroxybenzoate) in water, add glycerin to it. Heat this aqueous solution upto 70 °C, on water bath.
3) When both aqueous and oily phases reaches the same temperature (70 °C), add aqueous phase to the melted stearic acid, with continuous stirring.
4) Remove the dish from heat and continue the stirring. When the temperature reaches 40°C, add perfume and mix uniformly until it becomes cool and a homogenous (smooth) cream is obtained.

Dispensing: Weigh the prescribed quantity of cream on the butter paper and transfer to a wide mouthed, small, screw capped plastic or glass bottle or to collapsible tube. seal and label.

Direction: Apply to skin, when ever necessary.

Storage : Store in a cool place.

Auxilliary label : FOR EXTERNAL USE ONLY.

Uses : Vanishing cream is used as foundation, for holding the make-up preparation, for longer period of time.

Other similar formulas for Vanishing cream

1) Rx

Stearic acid	:	15.8 %
Potassium hydroxide	:	1 %
Cetyl alcohol	:	0.5 %
Methyl paraben	:	0.2 %
Glycerin	:	5 %
Purified water	:	77.5 %
Perfume	:	...q.s..

2) Rx

Stearic acid	:	18 g
Lanolin	:	2 g
Triethanolamine	:	1 g
Glycerin	:	3 g
Preservative	:	1 g
Water	:	80 ml

3) Rx

Stearic acid	:	18 g
Sodium hydroxide	:	0.18 g
Potassium hydroxide	:	0.52 g
Cetyl alcohol	:	0.50 ml
Glycerin	:	18 g
Preservative and perfume	:	...q.s..
Water	:	62.2 ml

Student's exercise:

1) Define creams. What is the Latin term for creams?
2) What are the basic ingredients of creams?
3) For what purposes creams are used ?
4) Classify the creams, with examples.
5) Give the examples for medicated creams.
6) Why creams are dispensed in wide mouthed containers ?
7) Comment : Creams are also dispensed in collapsible tubes.
8) Comment : Creams should be stored in a cool place.
9) Which auxilliary label will you write on the label of creams?
10) What is aqueous cream?
11) Write the ingredients of emulsifying ointment.
12) What is emulsifying wax and phenoxy ethanol? Why they are used in ointments?
13) What is the name for Oily cream? Why it is called so?
14) Write the ingredients of Wool alcohol ointment.
15) Comment : Freshly boiled and cooled water should be used for preparation of creams.
16) What are the uses of Oily cream?
17) What is cetrimide? Explain its uses.
18) Why Cetostearyl alcohol is used in preparation of cetrimide cream ?
19) What are the ingredients used in cold creams ? Why it is called so ?
20) Which reaction is used for preparation of Cold cream? Explain.
21) Which alkali can be used instead of borax for preparation of cold cream and why?
22) Comment : Vanishing cream is also called as Foundation cream ?

23) Why Stearic acid is used in the preparation of Vanishing cream?
24) Comment : In the preparation of Vanishing cream soap is prepared in-situ.
25) List out the different types of alkaloids used for the preparation of vanishing cream. Give reason for each.
26) Why carbonates are not used generally, for the preparation of vanishing creams ?
27) Define humectants. Which humectants are used in vanishing cream?
28) Why preservatives are necessary for preparation of vanishing cream, Give examples.
29) Briefly explain the procedure used for preparation of vanishing cream.
30) Why temperature of both aqueous and oily phases should be maintained to equal before mixing ?
31) Give the other two similar formulas for vanishing cream. Explain the use of each ingredient, with reason.

34 PASTES

Latin term: Pasta

Pastes are semisolid preparations, intended for topical application containing high proportion (20-60 %) of finely powdered, insoluble, solid medicaments like starch, zinc oxide and calcium carbonate in a suitable base.

Due to higher concentration of powdered ingredients, pastes are thick and stiff in nature than ointments, but less greasy than ointments, hence they form a protective layer at the site of application. For the same reason they are more absorptive, and hence they are used in the treatment of oozing lesions, where they act by absorbing serous secretions (exudate).

Pastes are mainly used as absorbents, antiseptics, protectives, for soothing the broken skin surfaces. They are usually intended to be applied to the small localized areas of the skin. They soothen the inflamed and raw surfaces of the skin and minimizes the damage, done by scratching, in itchy conditions like chronic eczema. But they are not suitable for application to the scalp (hairy portion), because they form a densely matted mass, which is very difficult to remove from the hair.

Pastes can be applied to the affected part, with the help of a spatula or they may be spread on any dressing material (lint) and then applied, which is not removed from the site of application for a longer time.

Bases used for pastes: Pastes are prepared by levigation method, i.e.dispersing the finely divided powder (medicament) in a suitable base. The following bases are used for preparation of pastes.

1) Hydrocarbon bases:

   Eg.
   - Soft paraffin
   - Liquid paraffin

   These are most widely used as hydrocarbon bases, for the preparation of pastes either alone or in combination.

2) Water miscible bases:

   Eg.
   - Emulsifying wax
   - Emulsifying ointment
   - Glycerin

3) Water soluble bases:

   Eg.
   - Polyethylene glycols

   Suitable combinations of high and low molecular weight polyethylene glycols (macrogols) are used as water soluble bases. In some cases, to get stiffness in the paste, thickening agents such as sodium carboxy methylcellulose, pectin, and gelatin are incorporated.

Preparation of pastes: Pastes are generally prepared by fusion and trituration methods.

Ointment slab (tile)

Ointment spatula

Dispensing: Pastes are dispensed in wide mouthed, glass or plastic bottles with tight screw cap with a liner, to prevent evaporation of water, because evaporation of water hardens the paste, which is found very difficult to spread over a lint.

Now-a-days, paste is dispensed in metallic or plastic collapsible tube, to prevent the microbial contamination and loss of water, by evaporation.

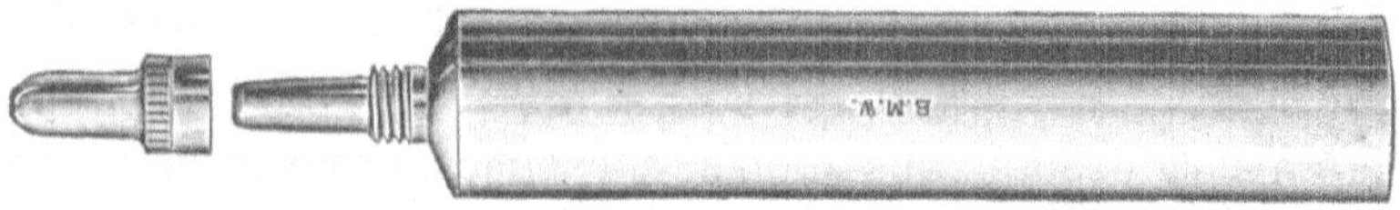

Collapscible tube

Storage: Pastes should be stored in a cool temperature, to prevent the evaporation of aqueous phase (water), at higher temperature.

Label: Label should bear all necessary requirements. In addition, it should contain auxilliary label:

- FOR EXTERNAL USE ONLY,
- STORE IN A COOL PLACE.

EXAMPLES FOR PASTES

S.N.	Name of the Paste	Ingredients (Formulation)	Type and Method of preparation	Uses
1)	Compound Zinc paste B.P.C.	Zinc oxide (finely sifted) Starch White soft paraffin	Paste with semisolid base, prepared by fusion and trituration method	Used as astringent, protective, also used in dermatological conditions like eczema and psorasis.
2)	Zinc-Gelatin paste Syn. : Unnas paste	Zinc oxide Gelatin Glycerin Water	Paste with semisolid base, prepared by fusion method.	Used as astringent and protective.
3)	Zinc and salicylic acid paste Syn. : Lassar's paste	Zinc oxide (Finely sifted) Salicylic acid " Starch " White soft paraffin	Paste with semisolid base, prepared by combined fusion and trituration method.	Used as antifungal and topical protective.
4)	Zinc and Coaltar paste B.P.C.	Zinc oxide (finely sifted) Coal tar Starch Emulsifying wax Yellow soft paraffin	Paste with semisolid base, prepared by fusion method.	Used as astringent and protective.
5)	Compound Aluminium paste B.P.C.	Aluminium Powder Zinc oxide finely sifted Liquid Paraffin	Paste with liquid vehicle, prepared by trituration method.	Used as antiseptic, astringent and protective.
6)	Resorcinol and Sulphur paste	Resorcinol (finely sifted) Precipitated sulphur Zinc oxide (finely sifted) Emulsifying ointment	Paste with semisolid base, prepared by trituration.	Used as antiseptic and scabicide.
7)	Magnesium sulphate paste B.P.C.	Magnesium sulphate (dried) Phenol Glycerin	Paste with liquid vehicle prepared by trituration.	Used as bacteriostatic and skin protective.

COMPOUND ZINC OXIDE PASTE B.P.C.

Rx	
Zinci oxidi (sifted)	ʒ vi s
Amyli pulverati (sifted)	ʒ vi s
Paraffini mollis albae	ʒ xii ss
Fiat : Pasta	Mitte : ʒ v
Signa : Spred pasta super lintum et applicantus, dolentiparti.	

Conversion :

ʒ vi s → 6.25 drachms　　ʒ xii ss → 12.5 drachms = 50 g

1 drachm = 4 g　　ʒ v → 5 drachms = 20 g

6.25 drachms = 25 g

Calculation : ʒ v → 5 drachms = 20 g, but calculate for (20 + 2) = 22 g.

Zinc oxide $= \frac{25}{100} \times 22 = 5.5$ g

Starch $= \frac{25}{100} \times 22 = 5.5$ g

White soft paraffin $= \frac{50}{100} \times 22 = 11$ g

Type	Ingredients	Quantity in imperial	Quantity in metric	Quantity taken
Paste with semisolid base.	Zinc oxide (finely sifted)	6.25 dr	25 g	5.5 g
	Starch (finely sifted)	6.25 dr	25 g	5.5 g
	White soft paraffin	12.5 dr	50 g	11 g
Prepared by fusion and trituration method	Make: Paste　　Send: 20 g Direction: Spread the paste upon lint and apply, to the affected part as directed.			

Theory:

It is a paste prepared with white soft paraffin, which acts as hydrocarbon base. Zinc oxide acts as astringent and skin protective. Starch powder is used, to give absorptive and stiff nature to the paste.

Both zinc oxide and starch are insoluble in white soft paraffin. Hence paste is prepared by combined fusion and trituration method.

To prevent the grittiness, zinc oxide and starch should be passed through sieve number 120, to get a fine powder.

Procedure:

Since there will be little wastage (loss) during weighing and preparing, to manipulate these practical losses, calculate the ingredients for at least one or two grams extra, than prescribed.

1) Weigh zinc oxide and starch, pass separately through sieve number 120 and mix them uniformly, in a warmed mortar.
2) Melt white soft paraffin on a water bath. Add this melted base, to the powder in small portions and triturate until a smooth paste is obtained. Add remaining amount of melted base gradually with continous trituration, until it becomes cold and semisolid mass is obtained.

Dispensing: Weigh the prescribed quantity of paste and transfer to a plastic or metallic collapsible tube, seal and label.

Direction: Spread the paste upon lint and apply, to the affected part, as directed.

Storage: Store in a cool place.

Auxilliary label: FOR EXTERNAL USE ONLY.

Uses: This paste is used as astringent, for the treatment of variety of dermatological conditions, including eczema and psoriasis.

ZINC GELATIN PASTE B.P.

Synonym: Unna's paste

Rx	
Zinci oxidi (sifted)	3 iii sss
Gelatini	3 iii sss
Glyerini	fl. 3 viii sss
Aquam	fl. 3 viii sss
Fiat : Pasta	Mitte : 3 vii ss
Signa : Melt the pieces of paste, cool and apply with brush to the affected part, before covering with a gauze bandage	

Conversion :

3 iii sss → 3.75 drachms = 15 g   fl. 3 viii sss → 8.75 fl.dr = 35 ml

3 viii sss → 8.75 drachms = 35 g

Calculation : 3 vii ss → 7.5 dr = 30 g, but calculate for (30 +2) = 32 g.

Zinc oxide $= \frac{15}{100} \times 32 = 4.8$ g

Gelatin $= \frac{15}{100} \times 32 = 4.8$ g

Glycerin $= \frac{35}{100} \times 32 = 11.2$ ml

Water $= \frac{35}{100} \times 32 = 11.2$ ml

Type	Ingredients	Quantity in imperial	Quantity in metric	Quantity taken
Paste with gelatin base.	Zinc oxide (finely sifted)	3.75 dr	15 g	4.8 g
	Gelatin	3.75 dr	15 g	4.8 g
	Glycerin	8.75 fl.dr	35 ml	11.2 ml
Prepared by fusion method	Water	8.75 fl. dr	35 ml	11.2 ml
	Make: Paste Send: 30 g Direction: Melt the pieces of paste, cool and apply with brush to the affected part, before covering with a gauze bandage.			

Theory:

It is a paste prepared with gelatin as a base, because a hot solution containing gelatin reforms as gel (jelly) upon cooling, hence it gives stiffness to the paste, which is applied in a melted condition with a stiff brush. Glycerin is used as preservative to prevent putrefaction of gelatin, it also acts as non-volatile hygroscopic emollient.

Gelatin paste is medicated with zinc oxide, which acts as astringent and skin protective. This paste preparation is harder and firmer in consistency. Hence it cannot be used, as such. Therefore, the molten mass is poured into a tray, just before setting and when it is going to be set, cut into small pieces about ¼th in square with a sharp knife. These pieces are placed in wide mouthed jar or an ointment pot. Whenever required for use, appropriate number of pieces are melted and applied with brush, each time.

Gelatin may be used, in the form of gelatin sheet or gelatin powder. If gelatin sheet is used, it should be cut into small pieces with scissor, before placing in water. If powdered gelatin is used, it should be carefully sprinkled, on the surface of the water and stirred to avoid the formation of lumps, which may be difficult to disperse.

Procedure:

Since there will be little wastage (loss) during weighing and preparing, to manipulate these practical losses, calculate the ingredients for at least one or two grams extra, than prescribed.

1) Heat the glycerin to 100°C in a china dish, on a water bath.
2) Heat the purified water to boiling. After boiling, remove it from the heat and add weighed quantity of gelatin and stir gently to dissolve.
3) Add hot glycerin solution to the aqueous solution of gelatin and take the weight of the content of the dish and stir gently, until gelatin dissolves completely and jelly is formed. (avoid entrapment of air bubbles in the solution.)
4) Maintain this glycero-gelatin base at 100 °C for 1 hour, to remove (kill) possible contaminating viable microorganisms.
5) When solution completes, weigh the content of the dish. If necessary, add the hot purified water to adjust the original weight, which lost during heating due to evaparation.
6) Sift the zinc oxide through sieve no.120 and incorporate to the molten base in small portions. Continue the stirring without aeration, until the preparation is viscous enough, to hold the powder in suspension and pourable.
7) Then pour into a shallow tray and allow it to set.
8) After setting, with the help of sharp knife, cut into small pieces of about ¼th in square.

Dispensing: Transfer these pieces to a wide mouthed glass jar, close it tightly with plastic screw cap, label and supply with a brush.

Direction: Melt appropriate number of pieces of the paste, cool and apply with a brush to the affected part, in several layers before covering with a gauze bandage.

Storage: Store in a cool place.

Auxilliary label:
- FOR EXTERNAL USE ONLY.
- STORE IN A COOL PLACE.

Uses: It is used as, mild astringent and protective.

ZINC AND SALICYLIC ACID PASTE

Synonym: Lassar's paste.

Rx	
Acidi salicylici	gr xxx
Zinci oxidi	3 vi
Amyli	3 vi
Paraffini mollis albi	3 xii ss
Fiat : Pasta	Mitte : 3 v
Signa : Applicandus pasta dolentiparti t.i.d - q.i.d.	

Conversion :

gr xxx → 30 grains
15 grains = 1 g
30 grains = 2 g

3 vi → 6 drachms
1 drachm = 4 g
6 drachms = 24 g
3 xii ss → 12.5 drachms = 50 g

Calculation : 3 v → 5 drachms = 20 g, but calculate for (20 + 2) = 22 g.

Salicylic acid = $\frac{2}{100} \times 22 = 0.44\,g$

Zinc oxide = $\frac{24}{100} \times 22 = 5.30\,g$

Starch = $\frac{24}{100} \times 22 = 5.30\,g$

White soft paraffin = $\frac{50}{100} \times 22 = 11\,g$

Type	Ingredients	Quantity in imperial	Quantity in metric	Quantity taken
Paste with semisolid base.	Salicylic acid, finely sifted	30 gr	2 g	0.44 g
	Zinc oxide, finely sifted	6 dr	24 g	5.3 g
	Starch, finely sifted	6 dr	24 g	5.3 g
Prepared by fusion and trituration.	White soft paraffin	12.5 dr	50 g	11 g
	Make: Paste	Send: 20 g		
	Direction: Apply paste to the affected part, three - four times a day.			

Theory:

Zinc and salicylic acid paste is also called as Lassar's paste. It is a medicated paste, consists two medicaments like Salicylic acid and Zinc oxide, where salicylic acid acts as antifungal and zinc oxide acts as astringent, soothing agent and topical protectant.

Starch acts as adsorbent and gives stiffness to the paste. White soft paraffin is used as, semisolid hydrocarbon base.

Zinc oxide, salicylic acid and starch are insoluble in white soft paraffin. Therefore Lassar's paste is prepared by, combined fusion and trituration method.

Procedure:

Since there will be little wastage (loss) during weighing and preparing, to manipulate these practical losses, calculate the ingredients for at least one or two grams extra, than prescribed.

1) Pass zinc oxide, salicylic acid and starch through the sieve number 120, to get fine powder and mix them uniformly.
2) Melt white soft paraffin, in a china dish on water bath.
3) To the melt, incorporate the powder mixture of zinc oxide, salicylic acid and starch gradually with stirring, until it becomes cool and a homogeneous paste is formed.

Dispensing: Weigh the prescribed quantity of paste and transfer to a plastic/metallic collapsible tube, seal and label.

Direction: Apply paste to the affected part, three - four times a day.

Storage: Store in a cool place.

Auxilliary label: FOR EXTERNAL USE ONLY.

Uses: Lassar's paste is used, as antifungal and topical protective.

COMPOUND ALUMINUM PASTE B.P.C.

Synonym: Baltimore paste.

Rx	
Aluminium powder	3 v
Zinci oxidi	3 x
Liquidi Paraffinum	fl. 3 x
Fiat : Pasta	Mitte : 3 v
Signa : Spread pasta super lintum at applicantus dolentiparti.	

Conversion : 3 v → 5 drachms = 20 g, but calculate for (20 + 2) = 22 g.

3 V → 5 drachms

1 drachm = 4 g

5 drachms = 20 g

fl. 3 x → 10 fl. drachms = 40 ml

Calculation : For (20 + 2) = 22 g.

Aluminium powder = $\frac{20}{100} \times 22 = 4.4$ g

Zinc oxide = $\frac{40}{100} \times 22 = 8.8$ g

Liquid paraffin = $\frac{40}{100} \times 22 = 8.8$ g

Type	Ingredients	Quantity in imperial	Quantity in metric	Quantity taken
Paste with liquid base, prepared by trituration.	Aluminium powder	5 dr	20 g	4.4 g
	Zinc oxide	10 dr	40 g	8.8 g
	Liquid paraffin	10 fl. dr	40 ml	8.8 ml
	Make: Paste Send: 20 g Direction: Spread the paste upon lint and apply to the affected part.			

Theory:

Compound aluminium paste is also called as 'Baltimore paste', which is prepared by using liquid paraffin as base. Aluminium powder acts as antiseptic and zinc oxide acts as astringent, protective and soothing agent.

Paste is prepared by triturating both aluminium and zinc oxide with liquid paraffin.

Procedure:

Since there will be little wastage (loss) during weighing and preparing, to manipulate these practical losses, calculate the ingredients for at least one or two grams extra, than prescribed.

1) Weigh aluminium powder and zinc oxide, pass through the sieve number 120, mix them uniformly in a mortar.
2) Incorporate liquid paraffin in small portions by trituration, until a smooth paste is obtained.

Dispensing: Weigh the prescribed quantity of paste and transfer to a wide mouthed, glass bottle or aluminium collapsible tube, seal and label.

Direction: Spread the paste upon lint and apply to the affected part.

Storage: Store in a cool place.

Auxilliary label: FOR EXTERNAL USE ONLY.

Uses: Baltimore paste is used as antiseptic, astringent and protective.

Student's exercise:

1) Define pastes, what is its Latin term? What are the uses of pastes?
2) Comment : Pastes are thick and stiff in nature, than ointment.
3) How pastes are applied? How the pastes acts in preventing of skin infections.
4) Classify the bases used for pastes, with examples.
5) What is levigation ? Give an example for paste prepared by levigation method.
6) Explain why levigation method is used for preparation of pastes?
7) How will you dispense the paste?
8) Which auxilliary label is necessary for paste?
9) How Compound zinc oxide paste is prepared and why?
10) Define Eczema and psoriasis.
11) What is Unna's paste? What are its ingredients?
12) How the Unna's paste is applied ?
13) Comment : For preparation of Unna's paste, Heating of glycero-gelatin base, at 100°C for 1 hour is necessary.
14) Briefly enumerate the procedure, followed for preparation of zinc gelatin paste.
15) What is the synonym, for zinc oxide and salicylic acid paste?
16) What are ingredients of Lasser's paste? Explain their uses.
17) What is the use of Lasser's paste?
18) What is Baltimore paste? What for it is used?

35 JELLIES (GELS)

Synonym: Gelatina

Jellies are thin transparent or translucent, non-greasy, semi-solid preparations, meant for external application to the skin or mucous membrane. They are mainly used for medication and lubrication purposes. They are prepared from natural gums or from synthetic derivatives of natural substances.

Jellies are similar to the muscilages, but they differ from mucilages in having jelly like consistency.

Classification of jellies: Jellies are classified according to their uses as,

1) **Medicated jellies:** These are mainly used for skin and mucous membrance, for their local anaesthetic, antiseptic, antiinfective and spermicidal properties. These medicaments are soluble in water, hence these jellies contain sufficient water, which will evaporate after application and provides, a local cooling effect. The residual film left behind gives protection.

   Eg.
   - Ephedrine sulphate jelly is used as vasoconstrictor.
   - Phenyl mercuric nitrate jelly is used as spermicidal contraceptive.

2) **Lubricating jellies:** These jellies are used for lubrication of diagnostic equipments like surgical gloves, catheters, enema and douche nozzles, rectal thermometer. These jellies should be sterile, because they are used as lubricants for articles, which are inserted into sterile regions of the body like urinary bladder.

   Eg.
   - Sodium alginate jelly.
   - Sodium carboxy methyl cellulose lubricating jelly.

3) **Miscellaneous jellies:** Certain jellies are used for special purposes, like patch testing, electro cardiography.

(a) **Patch testing jellies:** These jellies are used as vehicle for allergic agents, which are applied on the skin, to check the sensitivity of the drugs. On drying, the residual film will be formed, which helps to keep the patches separate and avoid confusing results.

(b) **Electro-cardiography jellies:** These jellies are used to reduce electrical resistance, between the patient's skin and the electrodes. These jellies consists sodium chloride, glycerin and pumice powder, where sodium chloride acts as good conductor of electricity and glycerin acts as humectant and pumice powder is used as abrassive.

> **Note:** Pumice powder :- It is a natural product created (obtained) by Volcanos. Due to its abrassive nature, it is used topically in Mechanics soap, Foot soaps, Foot scrubs and house hold cleaners.

Formulation of Jellies

Sr.no	Ingredients	Examples
1.	**Jelling agents (Gelling agents)**	Tragacanth, Sodium alginate, Pectin, Starch, Gelatin, Cellulose derivatives like Methyl cellulose, Carboxy methyl cellulose, Hydroxy propyl methyl cellulose. (HPMC), Carbomers, Polyvinyl alcohol, Bentonite.
2.	**Preservatives**	Methyl paraben (0.2% w/w),Propyl paraben(0.05% w/w), Chlorocresol (0.1% w/w), Benzoic acid (0.2% w/w), Phenyl mercuric nitrate (0.0015% w/w), Benzalkonium chloride (0.02% w/w), Chlorhexidine acetate (0.02% w/w)
3.	**Stabilizers**	Glycerin, Propylene glycol, Sorbitol.
4.	**Chelating agents**	E.D.T.A is used to prevent the sensitivity of bases and medicaments with heavy metals.

Preparation of jellies:

Jellies are generally prepared by dispersing the jelling agent in sufficient quantity of water and allowing it to hydrate for sufficient time. (To prepare jelly, the whole gum or gelling agent is preferred than the powdered gum, because it produces a clear preparation of uniform consistency.)

If medicament is dark coloured, then glass mortar and pastle should be used. Once the gelling agent is hydrated, other ingredients of the preparation, like medicaments, preservatives, humectants, anti oxidants, chelating agents and stabilizers are incorporated, by dissolving in a suitable solvent with continuous stirring. Care should be taken, to avoid high agitation, to prevent excessive entrapment of air.

Note: Since it is difficult to disperse most of gelling agents directly in water, gelling agent is first triturated with small quantity of liquid like wetting (dispersing) agents before the addition of water.

Eg. Glycerin, Propylene glycol, Ethanol.

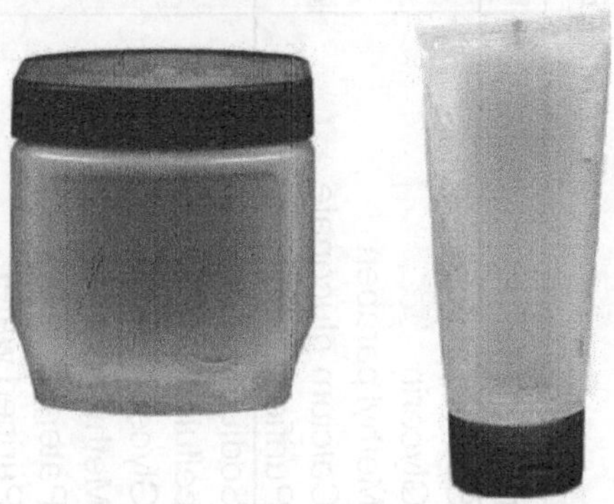

Container for jellies

Dispensing: Jellies consist of a large quantity of water, hence to prevent the loss of water, they should be dispensed in well closed and well filled, wide mouthed, glass containers. Now-a-days, sterile jellies are dispensed in collapsible tubes.

Label: Label should bear all necessary requirements, in addition it should contain auxilliary label like:

- FOR EXTERNAL USE ONLY,
- STORE IN A COOL PLACE.

Storage: Jellies should be stored in a cool place, to prevent their drying.

EXAMPLES FOR JELLIES

S.N	Name of the Jelly	Ingredients (Formulation)	Type and Method of preparation	Uses
1)	Sodium alginate jelly	Sodium alginate Glycerin Methyl paraben Calcium gluconate Purified water	Jelly base made with sodium alginate	◆ Used as dermatological base for other medicated jellies and also used as lubricating jelly.
2)	Sodium carboxy methyl cellulose lubricating jelly	Sodium carboxy methyl-cellulose Glycerin Methyl paraben Patent blue V Purified water	Lubricating jelly with a cellulose ether base	◆ Used for lubricating rubber gloves or finger stalls for rectal examinations.
3)	Ichthammol jelly	Ichthammol Tragacanth (in powder) Alcohol (90%) Glycerin Water	Medicated jelly prepared using, tragacanth as gelling agent.	◆ Used as antiseptic and mild counter irritant
4)	Compound resorcinol and Ichthammol jelly	Resorcinol Ichthammol Starch - glycerin	Medicated jelly prepared using gelatinized starch, as base	◆ Used as antiseptic jelly
5)	Compound zinc-gelatin gel B.P.C. Syn.:Glycero-gelatin jelly	Zinc oxide Gelatin Glycerin Water	Glycero-gelatin jelly	◆ Used as base for preparation for medicated jellies and paste and also used as skin protective.
6)	Ephedrine sulphate jelly	Ephedrine Carbopol - 954 Triethanolamine Purified water (Freshly boiled and cooled)	Carbomer jelly	◆ Used as antiseptic jelly

S.N.	Name of the Jelly	Ingredients (Formulation)	Type and Method of preparation	Uses
7)	Zinc oxide - Bentonite jelly	Zinc oxide Glycerin Bentonite Purified water (Freshly boiled and cooled)	Medicated jelly prepared by using bentonite as gelling agent.	◆ Used as antiseptic and skin protective.
8)	Sulphanilamide jelly	Sulphanilamide Pectin Glycerin Normal saline solution	Medicated jelly prepared by using pectin as gelling agent	◆ Used as antiseptic
9)	Carmellose sodium lubricating jelly	Carmellose sodium Propylene glycol Methyl paraben Purified water (Freshly boiled and cooled)	Lubricating jelly prepared using carmellose sodium - as gelling agent	◆ Used as non-sterile lubricating gel.

SODIUM ALGINATE LUBRICATING JELLY

Rx	
Sodium alginate	3 i sss
Glycerin	fl. 3 i sss
Methyl paraben	gr iii
Calcium gluconate	..q.s..
Purified water... q.s..	fl. 3 xxv
Fiat : Gelatina	Mitte : 3 V
Signa : Utendus, more dicto.	

Conversion :

3 i sss → 1.75 drachms	gr iii → 3 grains
1 drachm = 4 g	15 grains = 1 g
1.75 drachms = 7 g	3 grains = 0.2 g
3 V → 5 drachms = 20 g	fl. 3 xxv → 25 fl. dr = 100 ml

Calculation : 3 v → 5 drachms = 20 g, but calculate for (20 + 2) = 22 g.

Sodium alginate = $\frac{7}{100} \times 22 = 1.54\text{ g}$

Glycerin = $\frac{7}{100} \times 22 = 1.54\text{ml}$

Methyl paraben = $\frac{0.2}{100} \times 22 = 0.044\text{g}$

Calcium glyconate... = q.s.

Purified water........ q.s .... = 22 ml.

Type	Ingredients	Quantity in imperial	Quantity in metric	Quantity taken
Lubricating jelly	Sodium alginate	1.75 dr	7 g	1.54 g
	Glycerin	1.75 fl.dr	7 ml	1.54 ml
	Methyl paraben	3 gr	0.2 g	0.044 g
	Calcium gluconate	q.s	0.05 g (q.s)	..q.s..
	Purified water	25 fl. dr	100 ml	22 ml
	Make: Jelly	Send: 20 g		
	Direction: To be used, as directed.			

Theory:

Sodium alginate jelly is used as lubricant and dermatological vehicle. If sodium alginate is used alone, it gives less viscosity to the preparation, hence traces of calcium gluconate are used, where soluble calcium salts increase the viscosity of sodium alginate jelly.

Glycerin is used as humectant, dispersing agent and also as dehydrating agent, to prevent the drying of jelly. Methyl paraben is used, as preservative.

Procedure:

Since there will be little wastage (loss) during weighing and preparing, to manipulate these practical losses, calculate the ingredients for at least one or two grams extra, than prescribed.

1) Weigh sodium alginate and wet with glycerin in a glass mortar.
2) Freshly boil and cool the water. Dissolve calcium gluconate and methyl paraben in ¾th quantity of freshly boiled and cooled water, by heating on a water bath at 60 °C and stir well.
3) Add sodium alginate and glycerin mixture to it, in small quantities and stir vigorously (use a high speed stirrer), until a homogenous dispersion is obtained.

Dispensing: Weigh the prescribed quantity of gel and transfer to a wide mouthed plastic/ glass jar or collapsible tube, seal and label.

Direction: To be used, as directed.

Storage: Store in a cool place.

Auxilliary label : FOR EXTERNAL USE ONLY.

Uses: It is used as lubricating jelly or as dermatological base (vehicle).

SODIUM CARBOXY METHYL CELLULOSE LUBRICATING JELLY

Rx	
Sodium carboxy methyl cellulose	3 i s
Glycerin	fl. 3 iii sss
Methyl paraben	gr i ss
Patent blue 'V'	..q.s..
Purified water.... q.s....	fl. 3 xxv
Fiat : Gelatina	Mitte : 3 V
Signa : Utendus more dicto.	

Conversion :

3 i s → 1.25 drachms gr i ss → 1.5 grains

1 drachm = 4 g 15 grains = 1 g

1.25 drachms = 5 g 1.5 grains = 0.1 g

fl. 3 iii sss → 3.75 fl. dr = 15 ml

fl. 3 xxv → 25 fl. dr = 100 ml

Calculation : 3 V → 5 drachms = 20 g, but calculate for (20 + 2) = 22 g.

Sodium carboxy methyl cellulose = $\frac{5}{100} \times 22 = 1.1\,g$

Glycerin = $\frac{15}{100} \times 22 = 3.3\,ml$

Methyl paraben = $\frac{0.1}{100} \times 22 = 0.022\,g$

Patent blue V = ..q.s...

Purified water ...q.s.... = 22 ml

Type	Ingredients	Quantity in imperial	Quantity in metric	Quantity taken
Lubricating jelly	Sodium carboxy methyl cellulose	1.25 dr	5 g	1.1 g
	Glycerin	3.75 fl. dr	15 ml	3.3 ml
	Methyl paraben	1.5 gr	0.1 g	0.022 g
	Patent blue 'V'	..q.s..	0.001 g	0.001 g
	Purified water...q.s...	25 fl. dr	100 ml	22 ml
	Make: Jelly	Send: 20 g		
	Direction:To be used, as directed.			

Theory:

Sodium carboxy methyl cellulose is a synthetic gelling agent, which is used for the preparation of lubricating jellies and also for sterile jellies. It is available in different viscosity grades.

Glycerin is used as wetting agent, to disperse sodium carboxy methyl cellulose in water and it also acts dehydrating agent and humectant. Methyl paraben is used as preservative.

Patent blue ' V ' is used as a colouring agent, to warn the user that, it is not suitable to use in sterile regions of the body.

To reduce the risk of microbial contamination, freshly boiled and cooled water should be used.

Procedure:

Since there will be little wastage (loss) during weighing and preparing, to manipulate these practical losses, calculate the ingredients for at least one or two grams extra, than prescribed.

1) Freshly boil and cool the water.
2) Dissolve methyl hydroxyl benzoate (methyl paraben) in $\frac{3}{4}^{th}$ of freshly boiled and cooled water by heating on water bath with stirring.
3) Mix sodium carboxy methyl cellulose with glycerin in a glass mortar.
4) Pour the mixture into methyl paraben solution with continuous stirring, until a clear and homogenous jelly is formed.
5) Dissolve patent blue V in little portion of water, add this colouring solution to the jelly and mix well to distribute uniformly.

Dispensing: Weigh the prescribed quantity of gel and transfer to a wide mouthed, plastic/ glass jar /collapsible tube, seal and label.

Direction: To be used, as directed.

Storage: Store in a cool place

Auxilliary label: FOR EXTERNAL USE ONLY.

Uses: It is used for lubricating rubber gloves or finger stalls for, rectal examinations.

ICHCHTHAMMOL JELLY

Rx	
Ichthammolis	gr xxx
Tragacanth	3 i s
Alcoholis	fl. 3 ii ss
Glycerini	M xxx
Aquam... q.s..	fl. 3 xxv
Fiat : Gelatina	Mitte : 3 v
Signa : Applicandus super dolente parti, more dicto.	

Conversion :

gr xxx → 30 grains

15 grains = 1 g

30 grains = 2 g

3 i s → 1.25 drachms

1 drachm = 4 g

1.25 drachms = 5 g

fl. 3 ii ss→ 2.5 fl. drachms = 10 ml

M xxx → 30 minims = 2 ml

fl. 3 xxv → 25 fl. drachms = 100 ml

Calculation : 3 v → 5 drachms = 20 g, but calculate for (20 + 2) = 22 g.

Ichthammol $= \frac{2}{100} \times 22 = 0.44\,g$

Tragacanth $= \frac{5}{100} \times 22 = 1.1\,g$

Alcohol (90%) $= \frac{10}{100} \times 22 = 2.2\ ml$

Glycerin $= \frac{2}{100} \times 22 = 0.44ml$

Purified water .....q.s.... = 22 ml

Type	Ingredients	Quantity in imperial	Quantity in metric	Quantity taken
Medicated jelly	Ichthammol	30 gr	2 g	0.44 g
	Tragacanth (In powder)	1.25 dr	5 g	1.1 g
	Alcohol (90%)	2.5 fl. dr	10 ml	2.2 ml
	Glycerin	30 minims	2 ml	0.44 ml
	Purified water... q.s...	25 fl. dr	100 ml	22 ml
	Make: Jelly Send: 20 g Direction: Apply over affected part, as directed.			

Theory:

Ichthammol jelly is used as antiseptic and mild counter irritant. It is prepared by using tragacanth, as gelling agent. When tragacanth powder is added to water or vice-versa, a lumpy product will be formed, due to agglomeration of sticky and poorly wettable particles, which are difficult to redisperse. Hence alcohol (90%) is used as a dispersing agent, to disperse tragacanth powder in water, to get a homogenous product.

Glycerin is also used as humectant and also as dehydrating agent, to prevent the evaporation of aqueous portion of the gel.

Procedure:

Since there will be little wastage (loss) during weighing and preparing, to manipulate these practical losses, calculate the ingredients for at least one or two grams extra, than prescribed.

1) In a calibrated wide mouthed glass bottle, take measured quantity of alcohol (90%). To this, add tragacanth powder and shake well to mix uniformly
   (Note: The reverse order of mixing may leads to lump formation).
2) To this, add ¾ th quantity of water and shake immediately.
3) Separately mix ichthamol and glycerin in 5-10 ml of water.
4) Add this mixture to the tragacanth mucilage and shake vigorously.
5) Adjust the final weight by adding remaining portion of purified water and shake well and label.

Direction: Apply over affected part, as directed.

Storage: Store in a cool place.

Auxilliary label: FOR EXTERNAL USE ONLY.

Uses: It is used as antiseptic.

Other examples for Jellies or Gels

1) **Zinc oxide – Bentonite jelly**

Rx

Bentonite	-	10 g
Zinc oxide	-	10 g
Glycerin	-	10 g
Purified water....q.s...	-	100 g

Uses: It is used as astringent and soothing agent.

2) **Zinc gelatin jelly**

Zinc oxide	-	15 g
Gelatin	-	18 g
Glycerin	-	35 g
Purified water	-	35 g

Uses: It is used as astringent.

3) Sulphanilamide jelly

Sulphanilamide	-	6 g
Pectin	-	4.5 g
Glycerin	-	12 g
Normal saline solution	-	42.9 g

Uses: It is used as, antiseptic.

Student's exercise:

1) Define Jellies. Why they are used ?
2) Classify the jellies with examples.
3) What are lubricating jellies ? Why they are used ? Give examples.
4) What type of medicaments used in Medicated jellies?
5) What is the use of Electrocardiography Jelly? Give Examples.
6) Briefly explain the method of preparation of jellies ?
7) What types of containers are used for packing of jellies?
8) What is the purpose of using glycerin in sodium alginate jelly?
9) What is chemical name of methyl paraben and propyl paraben?
10) What is the Latin term for jellies?
11) What is patent blue V.?
12) What for Sodium carboxy methyl cellulose lubricating jelly is used?
13) What is Ichthammol? What is its use?
14) Why tragacanth is used in Ichthammol Jelly?

36 SUPPOSITORIES

Suppositories are medicated, solid dosage forms of various shapes and sizes, meant for insertion into the body cavities like rectum, vagina, urethra, ear, nose, etc. other than mouth, where they melt, dissolve or disperse and exert a local or systemic effect.

Suppositories are prepared by using semisolid bases, which are turned to solid form by treating them under low temperature, because semisolid forms do not have proper shape, consistency and feasibility to introduce into body cavities. Hence they are considered as solid dosage forms eventhough, they are prepared with semi solid bases.

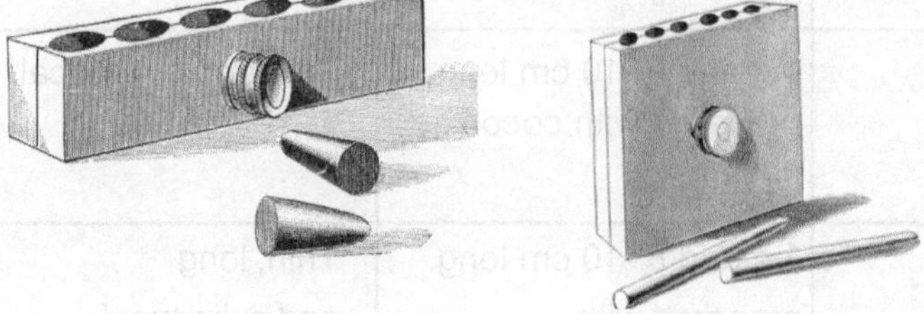

Suppositories mould

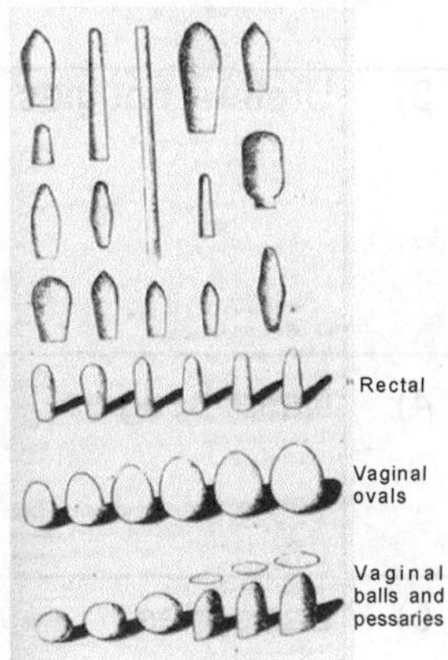

Different shapes of suppositories

Suppositories are used for different purposes such as,

1) For promotion of laxation – during constipation.
2) For soothing of inflamed tissues, to relieve discomfort and pain of haemorrhoids (piles).
3) For promotion of systemic action of the drugs (specially in children and comatose patients).

Types of suppositories:

Suppositories are classified, on the basis of their introduction (insertion) into the different body cavities as,

1) Suppositories : Rectal suppositories
2) Passaries : Vaginal suppositories
3) Bougies : Urethral suppositories
4) Nasal bougies : Nasal suppositories
5) Ear cones : Ear suppositories

Shapes and sizes of suppositories:

Sr.no	Type of suppositories	Weight	Shape
1)	**Rectal suppositories**		
	a) Cocoa butter suppositories	1 – 2 g	Conical
	b) Glycerin suppositories	1 – 4 g Small: 1 g for Infants Medium: 2 g for Children Large: 4 g for adults.	Conical, Rod shaped, Wedge shaped, Tablets or Capsules Oval shaped.
2)	Pessaries (Vaginal suppositories)	4 – 8 g, Prepared with glycero-gelatin base.	Spherical, Oval.
3)	Urethral bougies	2 – 4 g, length about 8 cm, prepared with glycero-gelatin base.	Long, thin and cylindrical forms, rounded in one end
4)	Nasal bougies	1 g and 9 -10 cm long, prepared with cocoa butter	Thin and cylindrical
5)	Ear cones	1 g and 8 -10 cm long, prepared with cocoa butter	Thin, long and cylindrical cone shaped

Advantages of suppositories:

1) Suppositories are easily administered to the children, old persons and to unconscious patients, who cannot swallow the drug, in the form of tablets or capsules easily.
2) Suppositories are convenient mode of administration for drugs, which irritate GIT, cause vomiting and destroyed in acidic pH of the stomach and enzymes of GIT.
3) Suppositories provide faster onset of action as compared to oral administration, because absorption of drug through the rectal mucosa, directly reaches the blood circulation.
4) The suppositories produce local action, at the site of insertion. Hence they are used in the treatment of Haemorrhoids of rectum and infections in vagina.
5) Since they are unit dosage forms, there is no variation in dose of the drug.

Disadvantages:

1) Drugs which are irritant to mucous memberane (rectum), cannot be formulated as suppositories.

2) Suppositories shows problems of melting and their shape may be destroyed above 37 °C. Therefore suppositories should be always stored in freezed condition, throughout their shelf life. Hence their storage is found comparatively difficult, with different climatic conditions.
3) There is leaking problem of material (base) through cavities. Hence suppositories are found uncomfortable to the patient.
4) The administration (insertion) of suppositories is inconvenient and causes embarrassment to the patients.
5) Formulation, manufacturing and even packing, is comparatively difficult.

SUPPOSITORY BASES:

Suppositories are prepared by dissolving or dispersing the medicament in the suppository bases.

Ideal properties of suppository base:

1) It should have good appearance.
2) It should melt or deform at body temperature or dissolve in body fluids.
3) It should retain its shape, when being handled.
4) It should be non-toxic, non-irritant and non-sensitizing to the mucous membrane of the body cavity. It should not have any pharmacological action of its own.
5) It should be compatible with wide range of drugs.
6) It should be easily mouldable, by pouring or cold compression and should not adhere to the mould.
7) It should shrink sufficiently on cooling, to release itself from the mould.
8) It should posses good wetting and emulsifying properties.
9) It should be able to incorporate a high percentage of water in it.
10) It should release the incorporated medicaments, easily and quickly.
11) It should be chemically and physically stable during storage.

Types of suppository bases: Suppository bases are mainly classified into three types:

I. Oily (oleginous or fatty) bases :

1) Theobroma oil (Cocoa butter)
2) Emulsified theobroma oil
3) Hydrogenated oil

II. Aqueous (water soluble or water miscible) bases :

1) Glycero-gelatin base
2) Soap- glycerin base
3) Polyethylene glycol base

III. Emulsifying (synthetic) bases :

1) Witepsol
2) Massa esterinum
3) Massuppol

Preparation of suppositories: Suppositories are prepared by two methods,

1) Hot process (fusion or pouring method)
2) Cold compression method

1) Hot Process (Fusion or pouring method):

This is most commonly used method, for preparation of suppositories. In this method, suppositories are prepared by using "Suppository mould". The suppository base is melted, to this melt medicament is incorporated and is filled (poured) into lubricated mould. After cooling, suppositories will be formed, which are removed from the mould.

Suppository Mould:

Suppositories are prepared by using "Suppository mould" which is made up of stainless steel, brass or plastic. Each mould has six or twelve cavities. Half the part of each cavity is divided in to each halves of the mould, which upon tightening with screw, forms a complete cavity. Moulds are available with different capacities, like 1 g, 2 g, 4 g etc. and their capacities are marked outside of the moulds. Moulds are cleaned by removing the two halves and immersing in hot water containing detergent and then rinsed with water, dried and lubricant is applied, if necessary. Both the halves are joined by tightening the screw and put inverted on the ice.

Lubrication of mould:

Lubrication of mould is necessary, when bases like cocoa butter and glycero-gelatin are used, because they have tendency of sticking to the sides of the metal mould. Therefore to get the suppositories with smooth surface, mould should be lubricated with the lubricants.

But lubrication of mould is not necessary, when macrogols and emulsifying bases are used, because these bases gives the suppositories with polished surface and do not stick to the sides of the mould.

The selected lubricant should have different characteristics, from the suppository base. i.e if the base is oleoginous in nature, lubricant should be aqueous in nature and vice-versa.

Examples for lubricants:

1)	For oily bases (Cocoa butter)	:	Soft soap	-	10 g
			Glycerin	-	10 ml
			Alcohol 90%	-	50 ml
2)	For aqueous bases (Glycero-gelatin base)	:	Liquid paraffin or Arachis oil		

Lubricant should be applied, with the help of a brush or a swab made up of gauze.

Cotton wool should not be used, because the cotton fibers may get detached from it and stick to the mould. Excessive lubrication of mould should be avoided.

Calibration of the mould: The calibration of mould is necessary because, a particular mould gives a same size of suppositories, but their weight may vary. This variation is due to the difference in the density of the medicaments and the base.

A medicament having a density, equal to the base will displace an equal volume of the base, but medicament has a density double than that of the base, will displace half of the volume of the base. Hence the density of the medicament will affect the quantity of base, required for each suppository and it becomes necessary to make an allowance for it. This allowance is called as "displacement value".

Displacement value:

Displacement value is defined as, "the quantity of drug, which displaces one part of the base."

Examples for Displacement value.

Name of the Medicament	Displacement value
Alum	1.8
Aminophylline	1.5
Boric acid	1.5
Choral hydrate	1.5
Cocaine hydrochloride	1.5
Hammamelis dry extract	1.5
Ichthammol	1
Iodoform	4
Phenobarbitone	1
Tannic acid	1= (0.9)
Zinc oxide	5
Phenol	1.1 or 1
Castor oil	1
Resorcinol	1 or 1.5

Calculation of Displacement value :

If the displacement value for a particular drug is not known, it can be calculated by the following steps:

1) Prepare and weigh six suppositories using the base alone = 'a' gram.
2) Prepare and weigh a suppositories containing a known percentage of drug = 'b' gram.
3) Calculate the amount of base, present in the medicated suppositories = 'c' gram.
4) Calculate the amount of medicament, present in the suppositories = 'd' gram.
5) Calculate the amount of base, displaced by'd' gram of medicament = (a-c).

The displacement value of the medicament for the particular base = d/(a-c)

Example: Calculate the displacement value of zinc oxide in theobroma oil suppositories, containing 40 % of zinc oxide and is prepared in a 1 g mould. The weight of 8 suppositories is 11.74 g.

Weight of 8 suppositories containing theobroma oil (a) = 1 x 8 = 8 g

Weight of 8 suppositories containing 40 % of zinc oxide (b) = 11.74 g

Amount of theobroma oil present in 8 suppositories (c)= $\frac{60}{100} \times 11.74 = 7.044 g$

Amount of medicament present in 8 suppositories (d) = $\frac{40}{100} \times 11.74 = 4.696 g$

Amount of theobroma oil displaced by 4.696 g of medicament (a-c)= 8 -7.044 = 0.956 g

$$\text{Displacement value } \frac{d}{(a - c)} = \frac{4.696}{0.956} = 4.912 = \text{Approx. } 5$$

Packing of suppositories :

Extemporaneously prepared suppositories and pessaries are generally wrapped individually in metal foil or waxed (butter) paper.

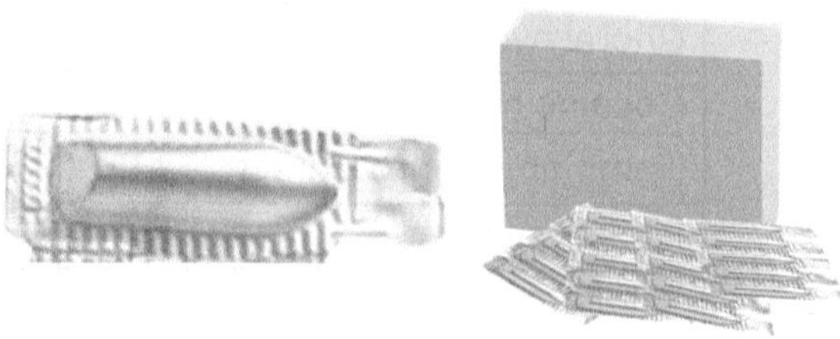

Suppositories

They are also packed in shallow, partitioned, cardboard or plastic boxes, which hold the suppositories in upright position and donot allow them, to come in contact with each other. But these boxes do not provide sufficient protection from the atmosphere, hence this type of packing cannot be used for suppositories, which contain drugs and bases which are sensitive to atmospheric conditions.

Suppositories which are hygroscopic in nature, Eg-Glycero-gelatin suppositories should be packed in tightly closed glass or plastic containers (jars).

Many commercial suppositories are packed separately in aluminium foil or polyvinyl chloride or polyethylene strip. Now-a-days, suppositories are directly moulded into primary packaging, made up of plastic material or aluminium foils, moulds are sealed and finally packed in cartons.

Storage: Since suppositories are sensitive to the heat, they will melt at higher temperature and loose their consistency. Hence they should be stored in a cool or cold place ,so that they can retain their shape, through out their self life.

Label: Label should bear all necessary information. In addition, it should contain auxilliary label like,

1) FOR RECTAL USE ONLY or FOR VAGINAL USE ONLY. (to indicate type of suppository).
2) The recommended storage condition like STORE IN A COOL PLACE or STORE AT COLD CONDITION or STORE IN REFRIGERATOR.

Direction: Label should give information (direction) to the patients about, insertion of suppository and how many times to be inserted.

BORIC ACID SUPPOSITORY

Rx	
Acidi borici	gr ii
Cacaonis butyri...q.s	gr xv
Fiat: Suppositorium	Mitte:Tales octo
Signa: Insert unus suppositorium recto, more dicto.	

Conversion :

gr ii → 2 grains

1 grain = 60 mg

2 grains = 120 mg

15 grains = 1 g

Calculation : For (8+2) = 10 Suppositories

Boric acid, per Suppository = 120 mg

For 10 Suppositories = 120 X 10 = 1200 mg

= 1.2 g

Cocoa butter q.s... to 10 Suppository= 1 X 10 = 10 g

Displacement value of Boric acid = 1.5

i.e. 1.2 g boric acid displaces $= \frac{1.2}{1.5}$ = 0.8 g of Cocoa butter

∴ The quantity of cocoa butter required = 10 - 0.8 g

= 9.2 g

Revised formula for 10 suppositories

Boric acid --- 1.2 g

Cocoa butter --- 9.2 g

Formula for lubricant

Soft soap --- 1 g

Glycerin --- 1 ml

Alcohol (90%) --- 5 ml

Type	Ingredients	Quantity in imperial	Quantity in metric	Quantity taken
Cocoa butter suppositories, containing insoluble solid.	Boric acid	2 gr	120 mg	1.2 g
	Cocoa butter q.s....	15 gr	1 g	9.2 g
	Make: Suppository	Send: Such 8		
	Direction: Insert one suppository to rectum, as directed.			

Theory :

These suppositories contain an insoluble solid like boric acid, which acts as anti-infective. In this preparation cocoa butter is used as base, in which boric acid is insoluble. Therefore suppositories are prepared by dispersing boric acid in the melted base, by fusion method.

In this preparation, heating of cocoa butter is very important because, it solidifies in to different polymorphic (crystalline) forms, when melted and cooled. These polymorphs may exist as stable and metastable forms, depending upon the temperature of melting and rate of cooling.

Polymorphic form	Nature	Melting point
Gamma (γ) form	Meta stable	18 °C
Alpha (α) form	Meta stable	22 °C
Beta (β^{I}) form	Meta stable	28 °C
Beta (β) form	Stable	34.5 °C

If cocoa butter is melted at less than 36°C and slowly cooled, it forms stable (β) form, which melts at body temperature. If cocoa butter is overheated above 36° C, after cooling, it forms meta stable polymorphs, which melts at lower temperature 15-22°C. These meta stable forms return to stable form after several days, but these suppositories become unsuitable for use.

Therefore cocoa butter is melted, on a water bath only 2/3rd of its quantity and then immediately removed from the heat and remaining base is melted with constant stirring. This avoids over heating of cocoa butter.

Lubrication of mould is necessary because, cocoa butter has the tendency of sticking to the sides of the mould. Hence lubricant containing combination of soft soap, glycerin and alcohol is used.

Since cocoa butter contracts after cooling, it leads to formation of hallow depression at the centre top of the suppositories. Hence to avoid this problem, mould is over filled and excess of base is trimmed off horizontally after setting, using a sharp knife or blade.

Warmed slab (tile) is used for levigation of boric acid and cocoa butter, to prevent rapid cooling and solidification of the base during mixing.

Procedure:

1) Calculate the quantities of ingredients required, by taking displacement value of the medicament into account. To manipulate the practical losses during preparation and for over filling of the mould, calculate the quantities of ingredients for two extra suppositories, than prescribed numbers.
2) Clean the suppository mould with hot water and detergent, finally rinse with water. Dry it thoroughly, lubricate and invert on the ice, to drain the excess of lubricant and cool the mould.

3) Grate (shred) the cocoa butter into small pieces and transfer to a china dish, and heat over a water bath, until only 2/3rd of the base has melted and then remove it from the heat. Melt remaining portion of the base, with constant stirring by spatula.

4) Heat the cleaned slab (tile), until it becomes warm to the hand. Place the weighed amount of boric acid on warmed tile and pour the half of the portion of melted cocoa butter and levigate (mix) them as quickly as possible, using flexible spatula and then transfer to the dish. Stirr to form a homogenous mixture and cool, until it just becomes thick to pourable.

5) Pour the dispersion into each cavity to overflowing. Care must be taken to stir the mass continuously, to ensure the even distribution of the medicament, otherwise it leads to sedimentation of insoluble solids in melted mass, after softing.

6) Leave for two to three minutes, until the mass has just set, trim off the excess from the mould horizontally, using sharp knife or razer blade (Trimming at this stage produces a clean cut, which cannot be obtained when the mass has become hard.)

7) After trimming, keep the mould for ½ an hour in a refrigerator or on ice, then open the mould, remove the suppositories.

8) Blot (wipe) the excess lubricant if present, by rolling suppositories on a cellulose tissue paper or clean cloth.

Dispensing: Wrap individual suppository in wax paper and put in partitioned box, or in wide mouthed container, close it tightly with plastic screw cap and label.

Direction: Insert one suppository to rectum, as directed.

Storage: Store in a cool place or store in referigerator or store in a cold temperature.

Auxillary label:
- FOR RECTAL USE ONLY.
- STORE IN A COOL PLACE. OR STORE IN REFERIGERATOR.

Uses: Boric acid suppositories are used, as local anti-infective.

Other similar examples for suppositories

1. **Bismuth subgallate suppositories BPC**

   Rx

Bismuth subgallate	-	2.4 g
Cocoa butter	-	7.2 g

   Uses: These suppositories are used, as mild astringent and soothing preparation for the treatment of haemorrhoids.

2. **Alum powder suppositories**

Alum powder	-	180 mg
Menthol	-	30 mg
Cocoa butter...q.s...	-	1 g

   Uses: These suppositories are used as antiseptic in the treatment of rectal infections.

COCOA BUTTER SUPPOSITORIES CONTAINING SOLUBLE SOLIDS

When a soluble substance is added to the cocoa butter base, it causes depression in melting point so that, suppositories become too soft to use (handle). Because soluble solid and cocoa butter acts as "eutectic" (impurities) to each other, hence leads to lowering of melting point.

To overcome this problem, a hardening agent like white bees wax is incorporated, which has high melting point (62°C - 64°C). Hence it raises the melting point of cocoa butter, so that its melting point does not exceed 37°C and gives a solid consistency, to the suppositories.

Examples for the substances, which causes lowering of melting point of cocoa butter are,

- Phenol
- Chloral hydrate
- Thymol
- Crestone
- Salol

Disadvantages of bees wax, as hardening agent in suppositories:

The melting point of cocoa butter is 35 °C, but melting point of beeswax is 62 °C to 64°C. Therefore, to prepare a mixture of cocoa butter and bees wax, temperature must be raised to 15 °C to 20 °C, more than the melting point of cocoa butter. This may cause over heating and delays its solidifying point.

Remedy: Instead of adding soluble solid to the base at initial stage, add at the end when base turns to thick creamy form, with continuous stirring until solid powder completely dissolves in the base. This method avoids the addition of bees wax. But this method is suitable (applicable), when the concentration of soluble solid presents in a lower concentration.

Eg. 1) Phenol: Upto 15% of the suppository

2) Chloral hydrate: Upto 25% of the suppository

If suppositories are prepared with soluble solid, without using hardening agent, then fusion method should be used and suppositories should be stored under refrigeration (cold temperature), to maintain the shape, until their use.

CHLORAL HYDRATE SUPPOSITORY

Rx	
Chloral hydrate	gr ii
Cocaonis butyri...q.s..	gr xv
Fiat:Suppositorium	Mitte:Tales sex
Signa:Insert unus suppositorium recto apud nocte.	

Conversion :

gr ii → 2 grains

1 grain = 60 mg

2 grains = 120 mg

15 grains = 1 g

Calculation : For (6+2) = 8 Suppositories

Chloral hydrate for one Suppository = 120 mg

For 8 Suppositories = 120 X 8 = 960 mg (0.96 g)

Cocoa butter for 8 Suppositories = 1 X 8 = 8 g

The displacement value of Chloral hydrate = 1.5

i.e. 0.96 g of Chloral hydrate displaces = $\frac{0.96}{1.5}$ = 0.64 g of Cocoa butter

∴ The quantity of Cocoa butter required = 8 – 0.64 g

= 7.36 g

Revised formula for 8 suppositories

Chloral hydrate --- 0.96 g

Cocoa butter --- 7.36 g

Formula for lubricant

Soft soap --- 1 g

Glycerin --- 1 ml

Alcohol (90%) --- 5 ml

Type	Ingredients	Quantity in imperial	Quantity in metric	Quantity taken
Cocoa butter suppositories, containing soluble solid	Chloral hydrate	2 gr	120 mg	0.96 g
	Cocoa butter....q.s....	15 gr	1 g	7.36 g
	Make: Suppository for a child of 6 months			Send: Such 6
	Direction: Insert one suppository to rectum, at night.			

Theory:

These are cocoa butter suppositories, containing soluble solid like- chloral hydrate. When chloral hydrate dissolves in cocoa butter, it lowers the melting point of cocoa butter so that, it becomes too soft, to use (handle) and finally gives unsatisfactory suppositories. Because both chloral hydrate and cocoa butter acts as 'eutectic' or 'impurities' to each other and form a mixture, with a lowering of melting point.

Hence bees wax can be incorporated as a hardening agent. It has melting point 62°C to 64°C, which nullifies the depression of melting point and makes the cocoa butter base hard and helps in making of suppositories, whose melting point does not exceed 37°C. But heating of the mixture of cocoa butter and bees wax, 15 °C to 20 °C more than that of cocoa butter, may causes overheating and ultimately delays the solidifying (setting) point of cocoa butter.

In this prescription, the concentration of chloral hydrate is less than 25% of the suppository, therefore it does not affect largely the depression of melting point of cocoa butter. Hence incorporation of bees wax is found to be not necessary.

The chloral hydrate suppositories are prepared by adding chloral hydrate to the cocoa butter at the end, when it turns to thick creamy form, with continuous stirring until it completely dissolves.

Procedure:

1) Calculate the quantities of ingredients required by taking displacement value of the medicament into account. To manipulate the practical losses, during preparation and for over filling of mould, calculate the quantities of ingredients for two extra suppositories, than prescribed numbers.
2) Clean the suppository mould with hot water and detergent, finally rinse with water. Dry it thoroughly, lubricate and invert on the ice, to drain excess lubricant and cool the mould.
3) Grate (shred) the cocoa butter into small pieces and transfer to a china dish, and heat over a water bath, until only 2/3rd of the base has melted and then remove it from the heat. Melt the remaining base with constant stirring with spatula.
4) Cool and stir the melted cocoa butter, to get consistency of thick cream. Add chloral hydrate and dissolve it completely by continuous stirring.
5) When chloral hydrate dissolves completely, pour the mixture into each cavity of the mould, sufficiently to over flowing.
6) Leave for two to three minutes, until the mass has just set, trim off the excess from the mould horizontally, using sharp knife or razor blade (Trimming at this stage produces a clean cut, which cannot be obtained when the mass has become hard).
7) After trimming, keep the mould for ½ an hour in a refrigerator or on ice, then open the mould, remove the suppositories.
8) Blot (wipe) the excess lubricant, if present, by rolling the suppositories on a cellulose tissue paper or clean cloth.

Dispensing: Wrap individual suppository in wax paper and put in partitioned box, or in wide mouthed container, close it tightly with plastic screw cap and label.

Direction: Insert one suppository to rectum, at night.

Storage: Store in refrigerator or store in a cold temperature.

Auxilliary label:
- FOR RECTAL USE ONLY.
- STORE IN REFRIGERATOR

Uses: Chloral hydrate acts as hypnotic and sedative. Hence these suppositories are used to induce sleep, in infants and children.

PHENOL SUPPOSITORY

Rx	
Phenolis	gr iii
Cocaonis butyri...q.s	gr xv
Fiat:Suppositorium	Mitte: Tales sex
Signa: Insert unus suppositorium recto, more dicto	

Conversion :

gr iii → 3 grains — 3 grains = 180 mg

1 grain = 60 mg — 15 grains = 1 g

Calculation : For (6+2) = 8 Suppositories

Phenol for one Suppository = 180 mg

For 8 Suppositories = 180 X 8 = 1440 mg = 1.44 g

Cocoa butter for 8 Suppositories = 1 X 8 = 8 g

The displacement value of Phenol = 1

i.e. 1.44 g of Phenol displaces = $\frac{1.44}{1}$ = 1.44 g of cocoa butter

Calculation for Bees wax

For 100 g of base = 20% of Bees wax is required.

But for '8' g base = $\frac{8 \times 20}{100}$ = 1.6 g Bess wax is required.

∴ For preparation of '8' suppositories cocoa butter required is,

Cocoa butter - (Phenol + Bees wax)

8 g - (1.44 g + 1.6 g) = 4.96 g Cocoa butter required.

Revised formula for 8 suppositories

Phenol = 1.44 g

Bees wax = 1.6 g

Cocoa butter = 4.96 g

8 g

Formula for lubricant

Soft soap = 1 g

Glycerin = 1 ml

Alcohol (90%) = 5 ml

Type	Ingredients	Quantity in imperial	Quantity in metric	Quantity taken
Cocoa butter suppository, containing soluble solid. Bees wax is used as hardening agent	Phenol	3 gr	180 mg	1.44 g
	Cocoa butter ..... q.s....	15 gr	1 g	6.56 g
	Make: Suppository Send: Such 6 Direction: Insert one suppository to rectum, as directed.			

Theory:

These are cocoa butter suppositories containing a soluble solid like phenol. When phenol is dissolved in cocoa butter, it leads to lowering of melting point of cocoa butter so that, it is difficult to handle (use) and hence gives unsatisfactory suppositories.

The lowering of melting point is, due to the eutectic phenomenon. Because cocoa butter and phenol acts as impurities to each other and form a mixture, with a lowering of melting point.

Therefore the depression of melting point is nullified by adding a hardening agent like white bees wax, which has higher melting point (62-64 ºC). Hence gives the hardness to the cocoa butter base and helps in making of suppositories, whose melting point does not exceed 37 ºC.

If the concentration of phenol is less than 15% of the suppository, then there is no need of adding bees wax. But in this prescription the concentration of phenol is 18%. Hence bees wax is used as hardening agent.

Procedure:

1) Calculate the quantities of ingredients required by taking displacement value of medicament into account. To manipulate the practical losses during preparation and for over filling of the mould, calculate the quantities of ingredients for two extra suppositories, than prescribed numbers.
2) Clean the suppository mould with hot water and detergent, finally rinse with water. Dry it thoroughly, lubricate and invert on the ice, to drain excess lubricant and cool the mould.
3) Grate (shread) cocoa butter and bees wax and melt in a china dish on water bath. To the melted mass, add phenol with continuous stirring.
4) Pour the mixture into each cavity of the mould, sufficiently to overflowing.
5) Leave for two to three minutes until the mass has just set, trim off the excess from the mould horizontally, using sharp knife or razor blade (Trimming at this stage produces a clean cut, which cannot be obtained when the mass has become hard).
6) After trimming, keep the mould for ½ an hour in a refrigerator or on ice, then open the mould, remove the suppositories.
7) Blot (wipe) the excess lubricant, if present, by rolling the suppositories on a cellulose tissue paper or clean cloth.

Dispensing: Wrap individual suppository in wax paper and put in partitioned box, or in wide mouthed container, close it tightly with plastic screw cap and label.

Direction: Insert one suppository to rectum, as directed.

Auxilliary label:
- FOR RECTAL USE ONLY.
- STORE IN REFRIGERATOR OR COLD PLACE.

Storage: Store in refrigerator or cold place.

Similar example

Tannic acid	-	180 mg
Cocoa butter q.s.	-	1 g

Solution: Tannic acid does not affect the melting point of cocoa butter. But if suppositories are made with cocoa butter, using fusion method, they cannot retain proper shape. Therefore a hardening agent like, bees wax (1/3rd the amount of cocoa butter) is used.

Uses: Tannic acid suppositories are used, as astringent.

COCOA BUTTER SUPPOSITORIES, CONTAINING SEMISOLIDS

Certain suppositories are also prepared by incorporating medicaments in the form of semisolids, because medicaments are available in the form of their extracts or tinctures.

Ex. Belladonna soft extract

Belladonna green extract BPC

Ichthamol are commonly used as semisolids.

Method: Semisolid extracts are very viscous (thick) in nature. Therefore for the preparation of suppositories with semisolids, following steps are used.

1) First reduce the viscosity of the semisolid extract, by triturating it with enough water on a warm tile, to form a homogenous liquid, which has consistency similar to glycerin or lesser than that.
2) Transfer this dilution to a tared dish and add sufficient quantity of the melted cocoa butter, to produce a weight equal to the nominal capacity of the mould (i.e. amount equivalent to the capacity of mould with plain cocoa butter) and the number of suppositories, including excess being made.

   For example, assume 120 mg Belladonna green extract is present in 1 g of suppository.

   Then, the quantity of Belladonna green extract for '8' suppositories = 8 x 120 mg
   = 960 mg

   After dilution of Belladonna green extract with water, if it weighs 1.5 g, the amount of base required is = (8x1) – 1.5 = 6.5 g.
3) After transferring the dilution to tared dish, stir the mass vigorously, to form a "Mechanical emulsion" and prepare the suppositories in a normal way.

Note:

Mechanical emulsion: Mechanical emulsion is one type of emulsion, prepared by using solid fat, like cocoa butter.

If immiscible liquid is distributed throughout a solid fat, by trituration on a tile or in a mortar, an emulsion will be formed, that cannot readily separate into its components, because the continuous phase is a solid fat, which prevents the coalescence of the distributed globules of liquid, such a type of dispersion is called as "Mechanical emulsion".

For the preparation of suppositories, formation of a stable mechanical emulsion (satisfactory dispersion) is necessary, therefore,

1) The fluid mixture must be stirred vigorously, to produce a perfect dispersion.
2) Pouring of this dispersion to the mould should be delayed to the last possible moment so that, the globules of aqueous liquid are enclosed in a solid film of fat.

   For the preparation of these types of suppositories, synthetic bases like Whitepsol, Massa estarinum are found to be more suitable than cocoa butter, because synthetic bases contain emulsifying agents, which can absorb 30% of its own weight of water. But due to the presence of high percentage of water in these suppositories, they are more susceptible to microbial attack, hence preservatives should be incorporated, for their long storage.

SUPPOSITORY OF BELLADONNA GREEN EXTRACT BPC.

Rx	
Extracti belladona viridis	gr ii
Cocaonis butyri…q.s..	gr xv
Fiat:Suppositorium	Mitte:Tales sex
Signa: Insert unus suppositorium recto, more dicto.	

Conversion :

gr ii → 2 grains

1 grain = 60 mg

2 grains = 120 mg

15 grains = 1 g

Calculation : For (6+2) = 8 Suppositories

Belladona liquid extra required for one suppository = 120 mg

Belladona liquid extra required for 8 suppositories = 120 X 8 = 960 mg

Belladona green extract is diluted with water to get consistency of glycerin. It has been observed that 1.8 ml water added, which is obtained by weighing the dilution.

The Displacesment value of water = 1

∴ 1.8 ml of water displaces 1.8 g of cocoa butter

∴ Cocoa butter required = [8 - (0.96+1.8)]

= 8 - 2.76 g

= 5.24 g

Revised formula for 8 suppositories

Belladonna green extract --- 0.96 g

Water --- 1.8 ml

Cocoa butter --- 5.24 g

Type	Ingredients	Quantity in imperial	Quantity in metric	Quantity taken
Cocoa butter suppository, containing semisolid	Belladonna green extract	2 gr	120 mg	0.96 g
	Cocoa butter ….. q.s….	15 gr	1 g	5.24 g
	Make: Suppository	Send: Such 6		
	Direction: Insert one suppository to rectum, as directed.			

Theory:

It is a cocoa butter suppository containing semisolid like Belladonna green extract, which helps in relieving the pain of haemorrhoids and anal fistula.

Belladonna green extract is highly viscous in nature, therefore it is diluted with water to get a homogenous mixture, which has consistency, similar to the glycerin or less than that.

This dilution is mixed with cocoa butter, so as to obtain nominal capacity of the mould. (i.e. amount equivalent to the capacity of mould with plain cocoa butter.)

Stable mechanical emulsion is prepared by vigorous stirring and pouring of this dispersion to the mould should be delayed to the last possible moment, so that globules of Belladonna green extract are enclosed in a solid film of cocoa butter.

Over heating of Belladonna green extract should be avoided, because it leads to the formation of irreversible precipitate.

Procedure:

1) Calculate the quantities of ingredients required by taking displacement value of medicament into account. To manipulate the practical losses during preparation and for over filling of the mould, calculate the quantities of ingredients for two extra suppositories, than prescribed numbers.
2) Take measured quantity of belladonna green extract on a warmed tile, gradually add sufficient water and mix (levigate) uniformly with ointment spatula until, it gets consistency similar to glycerin.
3) Transfer the above dilution to a china dish and add calculated amount of melted cocoa butter and triturate vigorously to form a stable mechanical emulsion.
4) Pour this dispersion to the each cavity of the mould, over flowing.
5) Leave for two to three minutes until the mass has just set, trim off the excess base from the mould horizontally, using sharp knife or razor blade (Trimming at this stage produces a clean cut, which cannot be obtained when the mass has become hard.)
6) After trimming, keep the mould for ½ an hour in a refrigerator or on ice, then open the mould, remove the suppositories.
7) Blot (wipe) the excess lubricant, if present, by rolling the suppositories on a cellulose tissue paper or clean cloth.

Dispensing: Wrap individual suppository in wax paper and put in partitioned box, or in wide mouthed container, close it tightly with plastic screw cap and label.

Direction: Insert one suppository to rectum, as directed.

Storage: Store in a cool place.

Auxilliary label:
- FOR RECTAL USE ONLY.
- STORE IN A COOL PLACE.

Uses: These suppositories are used, in relieving of the pain of haemorrhoids and anal fistula.

Similar example of suppository

Ichthammol	---	300 mg
Cocoa butter...q.s..	---	1 g

Uses: These suppositories are used as, antiseptic in the treatment of rectal infections.

COCOA BUTTER SUPPOSITORIES CONTAINING LIQUIDS

The liquids, incorporated in suppositories are divided into two groups,

1) **Liquid which are volatile in nature:** Volatile oils – like eucalyptus oil or liquids whose medicinal property depends on their volatile constituents (Eg. Peru balsam) are used for preparation of suppositories. While preparing suppositories, these liquids should not be lost by evaporation.

2) **Aqueous or hydro-alcoholic liquids:** The medicinal property of these substances depends on their non-volatile constituents. (Eg. Liquid extract of Belladonna, Liquid extract of Hamamelis). While preparing suppositories, these liquids can be concentrated by evaporation (i.e. removal of solvent from these liquids is permissible.)

The addition of volatile oils to the cocoa butter, lowers the melting point and makes the base too soft, then hardening agent like white bees wax is required to be added, to raise the melting point.

If the concentration of volatile oil is less than 10%, then there is no need of adding bees wax and the such suppositories should be storred preferabally in refrigerator (cold place), to maintain shape, until their use.

Better solution to over come this problem is, use high melting point, synthetic fatty bases like Whitepsol and Massa estarinum.

About 20% of aqueous or hydroalcoholic liquids can be incorporated in cocoa butter as mechanical emulsion. Otherwise synthetic bases capable of absorbing upto 30% of aqueous or 20% of alcoholic liquids can be used for preparation of suppositories.

In case, if these proportions exceed, liquids are concentrated by evaporation or suppositories are prepared in large sizes.

SUPPOSITORY OF EUCALYPTUS OIL

Rx	
Olei eucalypti	M i ss
Cocaonis butyri...q.s..	gr xv
Fiat:Suppositorium	Mitt:Tales sex
Sgna: Utendus, more dicto.	

Conversion :

M i ss → 1.5 minims   gr xv → 15 grains

15 minims = 1 ml   15 grains = 1 g

1.5 minims = 0.1 ml

Calculation : Calculate for (6+2) = 8 Suppositories

Eucalyptus oil required = 0.1 ml X 8 = 0.8 ml

Cocoa butter for 8 Suppositories = 1 X 8 = 8 g

Displacement value of Eucalyptus oil = 1

i.e. 1 ml of Eucalyptus oil displaces 1 g of cocoa butter

∴ 0.8 ml will displace 0.8 g of cocoa butter

∴ Cocoa butter base required = 8 - 0.8

= 7.2 g

Revised formula for 8 suppositories

Eucalyptus oil ---- 0.8 ml

Cocoa butter ---- 7.2 g

Type	Ingredients	Quantity in imperial	Quantity in metric	Quantity taken
Cocoa butter suppository, containing liquid.	Eucalyptus oil	1.5 minims	0.1 ml	0.8 ml
	Cocoa butter..... q.s...	15 gr	1 g	7.2 g
	Make: Suppository Send: Such 6 Direction: To be used, as directed.			

Theory :

It is a cocoa butter suppository containing volatile liquid, which acts as antiseptic. Generally when volatile liquid (oil) is incorporated to cocoa butter, causes depression of melting point, due to eutectic mechanism i.e. both volatile oil and cocoa butter acts as impurities to each other and hence cause lowering of melting point. In that case, melting point is raised by incorporating a hardening agent like bees wax, which gives stiffness to the base and raises the melting point of suppositories, not exceeding 37°C.

But in this prescription, concentration of eucalyptus oil does not exceed 10% of suppository. Hence there is no need of adding bees wax to the base. If these suppositories are prepared without adding bees wax, they must be stored in refrigerator to maintain their shape, until their use.

Procedure :

1) Calculate the quantities of ingredients required, by taking displacement value of the medicament into account. To manipulate the practical losses during preparation and for over filling of the mould, calculate the quantities of ingredients for two extra suppositories, than prescribed numbers.
2) Clean the suppository mould with hot water and detergent, finally rinse with water. Dry it thoroughly, lubricate and invert on the ice to drain excess lubricant and cool the mould.
3) Grate (shred) the cocoa butter into small pieces and transfer to a china dish, and heat over a water bath, until only 2/3rd of the base has melted and then remove it from the heat. Melt the remaining portion or base with constant stirring with spatula.
4) Cool and stir the melted cocoa butter, to get consistency of thick cream. Add eucalyptus oil and dissolve it completely by continuous stirring.
5) When eucalyptus oil dissolves completely, pour the mixture into each cavity of the mould, sufficiently to over flowing.
6) Leave for two to three minutes, until the mass has just set. After setting, trim off the excess from the mould horizontally, using sharp knife or razor blade (Trimming at this stage produces a clean cut, which cannot be obtained when the mass has become hard.)
7) After trimming keep the mould for ½ an hour in a refrigerator or on ice, then open the mould, remove suppositories. Blot (wipe) excess lubricant if present, by rolling them on a cellulose tissue paper or clean cloth.

Dispensing: Wrap individual suppository in wax paper and put in partitioned box, or in wide mouthed container, close it tightly with plastic screw cap and label.

Direction: To be used, as directed.

Storage : Store in a cold temperature (in refrigerator).

Auxillary label:
- FOR RECTAL USE ONLY.
- STORE IN A COOL PLACE.

Uses : Eucalyptus oil suppositories are used as, pessaries (vaginal suppositories) for antiseptic action.

GLYCERO – GELATIN SUPPOSITORY B.P.

Rx

Gelatin	3 iv
Glyerini	fl. 3 xvii ss
Aquam...q.s....	fl. 3 xxv
Fiat:Suppositorium for infant	Mitte:Tales sex

Signa: After unwrapping, moisten the suppository with a little water and insert into the rectum.

Conversion :

3 iv → 4 drachms	fl. 3 xvii ss → 17.5 fl. drachms
1 drachm = 4 g	1 fl. drachm = 4 ml
4 drachms = 16 g	17.5 fl. drachms = 70 ml
	fl. 3 xxv → 25 fl. drachms = 100 ml

Calculation : For (6 + 4) = 10 Suppositories.

The specific gravity of the glycero - gelatin base = 1.2

Weight of one Suppository = 1 g

Total weight of 10 Suppositories = 1 X 10 X 1.2

= 12 g

So, calculate for 12 g

Gelatin = $\frac{16}{100} \times 12 = 1.92$ g

Glycerin = $\frac{70}{100} \times 12 = 8.4$ g

(Since, 1 ml of glycerin = 1.254 g

$\therefore$ 8.4 g of glycerin = $\frac{8.4}{1.254} = 6.7$ ml)

Water ...q.s..... = 12 ml

Revised formula for 10 suppositories

Gelatin --- 1.92 g

Glycerin --- 6.7 ml

Water..q.s.. --- 12 ml

Type	Ingredients	Quantity in imperial	Quantity in metric	Quantity taken
Suppository	Gelatin	4 dr	16 g	1.92 g
containing, water	Glycerin	17.5 fl. dr	70 ml	6.7 ml
soluble base	Purified water...q.s...	25 fl. dr	100 ml	12 ml
glycero-gelatin.	Make: Suppository for an infant Send: Such 6 Direction: After unwrapping, moisten the suppository with a little water and insert into the rectum.			

Theory:

This suppository is prepared by using a water soluble base – Glycero-gelatin, which is a combination of glycerin and gelatin.

Gelatin dissolves in hot water and forms a solution, which sets as a jelly after cooling. This characteristic of gelatin is utilized to convert glycerin into solid form, to use as suppository base.

Since glycerin is hygroscopic in nature, when it comes in contact with rectal mucous membrane, it absorbs (withdraws) moisture and causes temporary irritation to the rectal mucosa. Hence promotes peristaltic movement and evacuation of feacal discharge.

Because of its non-volatile and emollient nature, it is also used as non-dehydrating agent, to prevent the suppositories from drying off quickly.

Glycerin also used as a preservative to prevent putrefaction of the gelatin, because glycerin exerts high osmotic pressure, which helps in killing of microorganisms by withdrawing the water from their cells.

For the preparation of suppositories, weight of base is very important, because the specific gravity of cocoa butter is 1, but specific gravity of glycero-gelatin is 1.2. Generally displacement values of the medicaments are calculated with reference to the cocoa butter. Therefore calculate the amount of base, displaced by medicament in normal way as like cocoa butter and multiply that value by the density factor 1.2.

After preparation of glycero-gelatin suppositories, they should be lubricated lightly with liquid paraffin, to prevent sticking to each other and to the container.

Procedure:

> **Note:** The usual size of Glycero-gelatin suppository for a child and infants is 2 g, but incase of unavailability of 2 g capacity mould, prepare the suppositories using 1 g capacity suppository mould.

Prepare sufficient base for 10 g to manipulate the heavy loss during preparation due to the sticky nature of the base. In this preparation, over filling of mould is not necessary because glycero-gelatin base contracts very little on cooling. But if the cavities are unavoidably over filled the excess may be trimmed off, after setting, with the help of sharp knife or blade.

1) Lubricate the mould with liquid paraffin or arachis oil and keep the mould inverted on the ice.
2) Heat the glycerin to 100 °C, in a china dish on a water bath.
3) Heat purified water to boiling, remove it from heat and add weighed quantity of gelatin and stir gently to dissolve.
4) Add the hot glycerin, to the aqueous solution of gelatin and take the weight of the dish and content. Stir the mixture gently, to avoid entrapment of air bubbles, until gelatin dissolves completely and gel is formed.
5) Maintain the base at 100 °C for 1 hour, to make it sterilized.
6) After this, take the weight of dish and content. If necessary, add the hot purified water to adjust the loss of weight, due to evaporation of water during heating.

7) Pour the hot mass into each cavity of the chilled mould sufficiently, leave for two to three minutes, until the mass has just set.

8) After setting, trim off any excess base with a sharp knife or razor blade.

9) Place the mould on ice or keep in refrigerator for about half an hour.

8) On a cleaned tile, spread liquid paraffin. Remove the suppositories from the mould and place on the tile, roll each suppository to provide a slight coating of lubricant, to prevent sticking of suppositories to each other and packing material.

Dispensing: Glycerin is very hygroscopic in nature, therefore transfer these suppositories in to air tight glass container and close tightly and label.

Direction: Glycero-gelatin suppositories should be moistened with water, before inserting into rectum to enhance the lubrication, which also prevents excessive withdrawing of water from rectal mucosa and decreases irritation. Therefore label should contain direction like 'After unwrapping, moisten the suppository with a little water and insert into rectum'.

Storage: Store in a cool place.

Auxilliary label:
- FOR RECTAL USE ONLY.
- STORE IN A COOL PLACE.

Uses: Gelatin gives stiffness to the suppositories. Due to hygroscopic nature of glycerin, it absorbs the water from rectal mucosa and causes temporary irritation and hence promotes the peristalsis, which helps in easy evacuation of the bowel. Hence glycero-gelatin suppositories are used, as mild laxative in infants and children for constipation problems.

ZINC OXIDE – GLYCERO GELATIN SUPPOSITORY

Rx	
Zinci oxidi	gr i
Glycero-gelatin base…q.s...	gr xv
Fait:Suppositorium	Mitte:Tales sex
Signa: After unwrapping, moisten the suppository with a little water and insert into the rectum.	

Conversion :

gr i → 1 grain

1 grain = 60 mg

gr xv →15 grains = 1 g

Calculation : For (6+2) = 8 Suppositories

Zinc oxide for one suppository = 60 mg

∴ For 8 suppositories = 60 X 8 = 480 mg = (0.48 g)

Amount of base required for 8 Suppositories = 8 X 1 X 1.2 g

= 9.6 g

Displacement value of zinc oxide = 5

i.e. 5 g of zinc oxide displaces = 1 g of cocoa butter

∴ 0.48 g of zinc oxide displaces = $\frac{0.48}{5}$

= 0.096 g of cocoa butter

Specific gravity of glycero gelatin base = 1.2

Amount of glycero gelatin base required = 0.096 X 1.2

= 0.1152 g

Total base required = 9.6 - 0.1152

= 9.4848 g ≡ 9.5 g

Formula for glycero-gelatin base B.P

Gelatin	---	14 parts
Glycerin	---	70 parts
Water	---	16 parts
Total base		100 parts

According to formula, calculate the ingredients for 9.5 g of base,

(1) When 100 g base requires 14 g of gelatin,

9.5 g of base will requires = $\frac{14}{100}$ X 9.5 = 1.33 g

(2) When 100 g base requires 70 g of Glycerin

9.5 g of base will requires = $\frac{70}{100}$ X 9.5 = 6.65 g ≡ 5.30 ml

(Since, 1 ml of glycerin = 1.254 g

∴ 6.65 g glycerin= $\frac{6.5}{1.254}$ = 5.3 ml)

(3) When 100 g base requires 16 ml of water

9.5 g of base will requires = $\frac{16}{100}$ X 9.5 = 1.52 ml

Revised formula for 8 Suppositories

Zinc oxide = 0.48 g

Gelatin = 1.33 g

Glycerin = 6.65 g (5.30 ml)

Water = 1.52 ml

Type	Ingredients	Quantity in imperial	Quantity in metric	Quantity taken
Suppository, with glycero-gelatin base.	Zinc oxide	1 gr	60 mg	0.48 g
	Glycero gelatine base..q.s..	15 gr	1 g	9.5 g
	Make: Suppositories Send: Such 6 Direction: After unwrapping, moisten the suppository with a little water and insert into the rectum.			

Theory :

It is a medicated suppository of zinc oxide, prepared by using glycero-gelatin as a base. Zinc oxide acts as astringent and soothing agent. Glycerin promotes the peristaltic movement and evacuation of lower bowel. It also acts as preservative, to prevent "putrifaction" of gelatin. It also acts as a humectant and dehydrating agent, to prevent the suppositories from drying off. Gelatin gives stiffness to the suppositories.

Glycero-gelatin base is 1.2 times denser than the cocoa butter, hence this factor is to be taken into account, during calculation of the amount of base. Because the displacement value is given in accordance with cocoa butter. Therefore calculate the amount of base displaced by medicament, in normal way as like cocoa butter and multiply that value by the density factor 1.2.

Procedure :

1) Consider the density of the base for calculation and calculate all the ingredients for more extra suppositories than prescribed, to manipulate the heavy loss during preparation, because of sticky nature of base.
2) Lubricate the mould with liquid paraffin or arachis oil and put inverted on the ice.
3) Heat the glycerin to 100 °C, in china dish on a water bath.
4) Heat purified water to boiling, remove it from heat and add weighed quantity of gelatin and stir gently to dissolve.
5) Add the hot glycerin to the aqueous solution of gelatin and take the weight of the dish and content. Stir the mixture gently, to avoid entrapment of air bubbles until gelatin dissolves completely and gel is formed.
6) Maintain the base at 100 °C for 1 hour, to make it sterilized.
7) After this, take the weight of dish and content. If necessary, add the hot purified water to adjust the loss of weight, due to evaporation of water during heating.
8) Weigh finely powdered zinc oxide (# 120) and add in small amount to the molten base with stirring. Continue the stirring until the preparation becomes viscous enough to be pourable.
9) Pour the hot mass into each cavity of the chilled mould sufficiently, leave for two to three minutes, until the mass has just set.
10) Place the mould on ice or keep in refrigerator for about half an hour and trim off any excess with a sharp knife or razor blade.
11) On a cleaned tile, spread liquid paraffin. Remove the suppositories from mould and place on the tile, roll each suppository, to provide a slight coating of lubricant to prevent sticking of suppositories to each other and to the packing container.

Dispensing: Glycerin is very hygroscopic in nature, therefore transfer these suppositories in to air tight glass container and close tightly and label

Direction: After unwrapping, moisten the suppository with a little water and insert into rectum.

Storage: Store in a cool place.

Auxilliary label:
- FOR RECTAL USE ONLY.
- STORE IN A COOL PLACE.

Uses: Zinc oxide acts as mild astringent and soothing agent. Glycerin promotes peristalsis, which helps in easy evacuation of bowel. Therefore these suppositories are used, in the treatment of constipation and piles.

SOAP-GLYCERIN SUPPOSITORY

Rx	
Glyerini	3 xxii ss
Sodii carbonatis	3 i
Stearic acid	3 ii
Fait:Suppositorium	Mitte:Tales quinque

Signa: After unwrapping, moisten the suppository with a little water and insert into rectum.

Conversion :

3 xxii ss → 22.5 drachms

1 drachm = 4 g

22.5 drachms = 90 g

3 i → 1 drachm = 4 g

3 ii → 2 drachms = 8 g

Calculation : For (5+3) = 8 Suppositories

The specific gravity of the soap glycerin is = 1.25

∴ The base required will be 1.25 times of cocoa butter, to fill the same number of suppositories.

∴ Total weight for 8 suppositories = 8 X 1 X 1.25 g = 10 g

But the formula is given for 102 g

∴ Calculate for 10.2 g to get weighable quantities.

Glycerin $= \frac{90}{102} \times 10.2 = 9$ g

(Since, 1 ml of glycerin = 1.254 g

∴ 9 g glycerin $= \frac{9}{1.254} = 7.2$ ml)

Sodium carbonate $= \frac{4}{102} \times 10.2 = 0.4$ g

Stearic acid $= \frac{8}{102} \times 10.2 = 0.8$ g

Revised formula for 8 Suppositories

Glycerin	--- 7.2 ml
Sodium carbonate	--- 0.4 g
Stearic acid	--- 0.8 g

Type	Ingredients	Quantity in imperial	Quantity in metric	Quantity taken
Soap glycerin suppositories.	Glycerin	22.5 gr	90 g	7.2 ml
	Sodium carbonate	1 dr	4 g	0.4 g
	Stearic acid	2 dr	8 g	0.8 g
	Make: Suppository of 1 g Send: Such 5 Direction: After unwrapping, moisten the suppository with a little water and insert into rectum.			

Theory: Soap glycerin suppositories are prepared by using glycerin as a base, which promotes peristalsis and evacuation of bowel.

In this preparation, saponification reaction takes place, between free fatty acids of stearic acid and alkali like -sodium carbonate and produces soap (Sodium stearate). This soap is irritant in nature, hence promotes the peristaltis.

When soap glycerin base is cooled, it contracts and forms hallow depression at the top of suppositories. Hence to avoid this problem, mould is over filled and excess of base is trimmed off horizontally after setting, with the help of sharp knife or blade.

In this prescription, the standard formula is given for 102 g instead of 100 g, because when stearic acid is added to the mixture of glycerin and sodium carbonate, frothing takes place at the top of the mixture due to saponification reaction. This froth is considered as waste and should be removed off from the base, before pouring in to the mould. Therefore to compensate this loss, ingredients are taken 2 g extra.

During preparation, stearic acid should be added slowly in to the mixture of glycerin and sodium carbonate, with continuous stirring to avoid excessive froathing and hence expelling of the froath from the dish and to prevent the entrapment of the air bubbles, in the base.

Procedure:

1) Calculate the quantities of ingredients required, by taking displacement value of the medicament into account. To manipulate the practical losses during preparation and for over filling of the mould, calculate the quantities of ingredients for three extra suppositories, than prescribed numbers.
2) Dissolve calculated amount of sodium carbonate, in glycerin on a water bath with stirring.
3) To the above content, slowly add stearic acid, heat carefully with continuous stirring, until effervescence ceases completely and solution is complete.
4) Confirm that, the solution is free from air bubbles and add the hot solution in to the mould, to overflow and allow to cool.
5) Allow the mass to set. After setting, trimmed off the excess of base with the help of sharp blade or knife.
6) Place the mould on ice or in refrigerator for half an hour.

7) Open the mould and remove the suppositories, blot off excess lubricant, if present, by rolling them on a cellulose tissue paper.
8) From these suppositories, select best five and wrap each suppository in a butter paper separately.

Dispensing: Glycerin is very hygroscopic in nature, therefore transfer these suppositories into an air tight glass container and close tightly and label.

Direction: After unwrapping, moisten the suppository with a little water and insert into the rectum.

Storage: Store in a cool place.

Auxilliary label:
- FOR RECTAL USE ONLY
- STORE IN A COOL PLACE.

Uses: Soap–glycerin suppositories are used, for easy evacuation of bowel during constipation.

SUPPOSITORIES WITH MACROGOL BASE

Macrogol bases consist of the mixture of polyethylene glycols of different molecular weights. (Carbopols or Macrogol bases).

1) Macrogol suppositories are prepared by fusion method i.e. Macrogols are melted together in a china dish. If base consists water or water soluble ingredients, they are heated separately to the same temperature as macrogol base and then added to the melted mass, with continuous stirring to get a stable emulsion.
2) If insoluble ingredients are there, they are incorporated in the same manner of cocoa butter suppositories, containing insoluble solids.
3) The mixture is poured to the moulds overflowing, because macrogols contract significantly on cooling. After setting, excess of base is trimmed off, using a sharp knife or blade.

Eg. **ICHTHAMMOL SUPPOSITORY WITH MACROGOL BASE.**

Rx	
Ichthammolis	2 %
Macrogol base…q.s	1 g
Fiat: Suppositorium	Mitte:Tales octo
Signa: Insert unus suppositorium recto, more dicto.	

Calculation : For (8+2) = 10 Suppositories

For 10 Suppositories, total macrogol base required = 10 X 1 = 10 g

Ichthammol requires is 2 %

i.e..100 g base consists = 2 g Ichthammol

But, for 10 g base = $\frac{2}{100}$ X 10 = 0.2 g of Ichthammol is required

Displacement value of Ichthammol is = 1

i.e. 1 g Ichthammol disaplaces, 1 g of base

∴ 0.2 g of Ichthammol displaces, 0.2 g of base

∴ The amount of base required = (10 - 0.2) = 9.8 g

Formula for macrogol base :

PEG - 600	---	50 g
PEG - 1540	---	30 g
PEG - 400	---	20 g

Total base		100 g

100 g of Macrogol base requires, 50 g of PEG 600

But, 9.8 g of Macrogol base requires = $\frac{9.8}{100}$ X 50 = 4.9 g

100 g of macrogol base requires, 30 g of PEG 1540

But, 9.8 g of macrogol base requires = $\frac{9.8}{100}$ X 30 = 2.94 g

100 g of macrogol base requires - 20 g of PEG 400

9.8 g of macrogol base requires = $\frac{9.8}{100}$ X 20 = 1.96 g

Ichthammol is soluble in water, hence use water to mix Ichthammol with base

i.e out of 1.96 g of PEG 400, replace 1 g by 1 g (1 ml) of water (Since density of water is 0.98 g/ cc)

Then (1.96 g - 1 g) = 0.96 g PEG 400 is required.

Revised formula for 10 Suppositories

Ichthammol	0.2 g
Macrogol base	
PEG 600	4.9 g
PEG 1540	2.94 g
PEG 400	0.96 g
Water	1 ml

Type	Ingredients	Quantity in imperial	Quantity in metric	Quantity taken
Suppository with macrogol base.	Ichthammol	2 %	2 %	0.2 g
	Macrogol base ...q.s..	15 gr	1 g	1 g
	Make: Suppository Send: Such 6 Direction: Insert a suppository to rectum, as directed.			

Theory :

This is a suppository, containing macrogol base. This macrogol base consists a blend of different PEGs, having different molecular weight such as PEG-6000, PEG-1540 and PEG-400 in suitable proportions.

Ichthammol acts as antiseptic, which is soluble in macrogol base. These suppositories are prepared by fusion method.

The Displacement value of Ichthammol is 1 and specific gravity of PEG base is 1. Therefore calculations are done similar to the cocoa butter suppositories.

Note: During preparation of Macrogol suppositories, mould should not be lubricated and should not be chilled. Because macrogol do not stick to the sides of mould, and cooling causes brittleness, if water is present in the base.

Procedure :

1) Melt all the PEGs together in a china dish, with stirring upto 60 ºC.
2) Dissolve Ichthammol in water, and heat to the same temperature of the melt (60 ºC).
3) Add Ichthammol solution to the melted PEG base and stir well, until it mixture becomes pourable.
4) Pour the mass into each cavity of the mould, to overflowing.
5) After filling, allow to cool at room temperature, when mass just set, trimmed off the excess mass, with the help of sharp knife or blade.
6) After 30 to 40 minutes, open the mould and remove the suppositories.

Dispensing: Wrap individual suppository in wax paper and put in partitioned box, or in wide mouthed container, close it tightly with plastic screw cap and label.

Direction: Insert a suppository to rectum, as directed.

Storage : Store in a cool place.

Auxillary label:
- FOR RECTAL USE ONLY.
- STORE IN A COOL PLACE.

Uses : Ichthammol suppositories are used, as antiseptic in the treatment of rectal infections.

Student's exercise:

1) What are suppositories? Explain their advantages.
2) Give different types of suppositories.
3) What are the advantages and dis-advantages of suppositories?
4) What should be the ideal properties of suppository base?
5) Classify the different types of suppository bases with examples.
6) Why lubrication of mould is essential for preparation of suppositories ?
7) Give the examples for lubricants used in lubrication of mould.
8) Comments : Calibration of mould is necessary before preparing the suppositories.
9) What is displacement value? Give examples for displacement value.
10) Briefly explain how to determine displacement value of the medicament.
11) Classify the cocoa butter suppositories with examples.
12) How will pack the suppositories?
13) Comment : Glycero-gelatin suppositories should be always stored in air tight containers.
14) What should be the auxilliary label for suppositories?
15) Comment : Suppositories should be stored in a cool or cold place.

16) Write displacement value of Boric acid, phenol, chloral hydrate and water.
17) Comment : For preparation of suppositories, cocoa butter should not be heated more than 30 ºC.
18) What is the alternate technique to prevent polymorphism of cocoa butter?
19) Define Haemorrhoids and Anal fistura.
20) How suppositories are administered (introduced)?
21) What is melting point for suppositories?
22) How to prepare suppositories containing phenol ? What are different shapes and sizes of suppositories?
23) Is there any importance of shape and size for suppositories and why?
24) What is mould capacity and nominal capacity of the mould?
25) Why bees wax is required for preparation of suppositories?
26) What is polymorphism? Which are the different polymorphs of cocoa butter?
27) Which lubricant is necessary for preparation of cocoa butter suppositories?
28) What is alum? What is use of alum suppositories?
29) Why glycerin is used in the Glycero-gelatin suppositories ?
30) Comment : Gelatin is used for preparation suppository base.
31) Comment : For the preparation of Glycero-gelatin Suppositories - specific gravity of Glycero-gelatin is very essential.
32) Why Glycero-gelatin suppositories should be lubricated by liquid paraffin, after their preparation?
33) What is putrefaction? How it is done for gelatin?
34) How will you dispense the Glycero-gelatin suppositories?
35) What are the different sizes of Glycero-gelatin suppositories?
36) Write the formula for Glycero-gelatin base BP.
37) What is the use of Zinc oxide – Glycero-gelatin suppositories?
38) Define constipation and piles.
39) Comment : Soap glycerin suppositories are prepared using sodium carbonate and stearic acid.
40) Comment : For preparation of cocoa butter and Glycero-gelatin suppositories, over filling of mould is necessary.
41) Incase of soap-glycerin suppositories, why standard formula is given for 102 g instead of 100 g?
42) Give the examples for substances causing lowering of melting point of cocoa butter.
43) What are Disadvantages of bees wax as a hardening agent in suppositories?
44) Incorporation of bees wax is not necessary in case of phenol and chloral hydrate suppositories if their concentration is _____ and ___
45) How will you store the cocoa butter suppositories containing phenol and chloral hydrate?

46) What is the use of chloral hydrate suppositories?
47) How the phenol suppositories are prepared if, concentration of phenol is more than 15%?
48) How will you prepare chloral hydrate suppositories containing less than 25% of chloral hydrate?
49) What is "Mechanical emulsion"? What are its advantages?
50) Why synthetic bases are preferred over cocoa butter suppositories?
51) Give the examples for semisolids used for preparation of suppositories.
52) Give the examples for synthetic bases for suppositories.
53) Briefly explain the procedure followed for preparation of suppositories containing Belladonna green extract.
54) Briefly explain the method used for preparation of Soap-Glycerin Suppositories.
55) What type of liquids can be incorporated for the preparation of suppositories? Give Examples.
56) Comment : Addition of Volatile oils to the Cocoa butter lowers the melting point.
57) How will your prepare suppositories containing liquids?
58) What are the alternate methods used for preparation of suppositories containing liquids.
59) What is the use of Eucalyptus oil suppositories?
60) Brief explain the preparation of Eucalyptus oil suppositories.
61) Give the different formulas for macrogol bases.
62) How will you pack the Ichthammol suppositories?
63) Why combinations of different macrogols (PEGs) are used for preparation of macrogol base?

37 PESSARIES (VAGINAL SUPPOSITORIES)

Latin term : Pessus

Vaginal suppositories are also called as "pessaries", which are larger than rectal suppositories and varies in weight from 4 to 8 grams. They are available in different shapes like, oval, ball, conical wedge shaped or rod shaped. Special shapes of pessaries are manufactured and are supplied with applicator, to facilitate insertion into the vagina.

Now-a-days, pessaries are also available as tablets (Vaginal tablets) and Capsules (Vaginal capsules).

Pessaries are mainly used for their local action on the vagina. Pessaries are prepared using glycero-gelatin, as base.

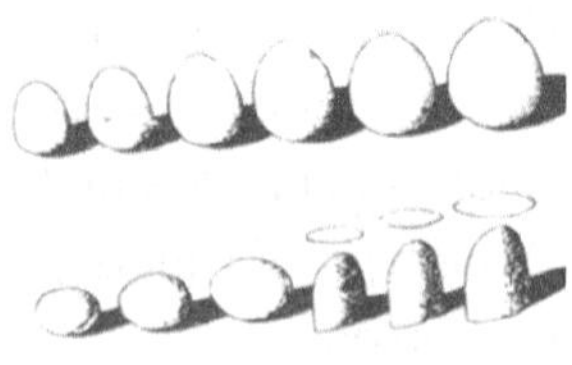

Different shape of pessaries

Eg. For pessaries.

- Lactic acid pessaries
- Crystal violet pessaries
- Stilboestrol pessaries

Heat treatment of pessary's base: Gelatin may be contaminated with pathogenic microorganisms including strains of Escherichia colli, which can cause urinary tract infection. Therefore pharmaceutical gelatin should be free from pathogens. Hence as a precaution, the base for glycero-gelatin pessary is heated at 100°C for one hour. Heating process and osmotic effect (pressure) of the high concentration of glycerin destroys most of the contaminant pathogens.

While preparing pessaries, medicaments should not be incorporated until the heating process completes, to avoid the degradation of medicament and base.

Eg:

1) If lactic acid is heated with glycero-gelatin, it hydrolysis the gelatin and the product will not set properly.
2) If glycero-gelatin bases, containing Ichhthamol are over heated, they may become insoluble.
3) Gelatin base is incompatible with many of the substances like,

eg. Tannic acid, Ferric chloride, Gallic acid

Dispensing: Due to hygroscopic nature of glycerin, it absorbs moisture. Therefore moulded pessaries should be dispensed in tightly closed glass containers.

For compressed type pessaries, tablet containers are used.

Storage: Pessaries should be stored in a cool or cold place.

Label: Label of pessaries should bear all necessary informations. In addition it should contain auxiliary label like,

- FOR VAGINAL USE ONLY,
- STORE IN A COOL PLACE.

Direction: Usually the label of pessaries consist, of instruction (direction) for patients, to "Moisten pessary with water before insertion into vagina, to reduce the stinging caused by osmotic withdrawal of the water, from the tissues during dissolution in the vagina".

eg. Di-iodohydroxy-quinoline and Nystain pessaries should compulsory bears this direction on their label.

LACTIC ACID PESSARY B.P.C.

Rx.	
Lactic acid	5%
Glycero-gelatin base ....q.s...	1 g
Fiat : Pessus	Mitte : Tales sex
Signa : After unwrapping, moisten the pessary with a little water and insert into vagina.	

Conversion: 5% of lactic acid means 5 g of lactic acid in 100 g of glycero-gelatin base. (The usual size of lactic acid pessary is 8 g. In case of unavailability of the mould of 8 g capacity, prepare pessaries of 1 g each).

Calculation: For 6+2 = 8 Pessaries

Specific gravity of glycero-gelatin base = 1.2

The quantity of glycero-gelatin base required for 8 pessaries = 8 x 1x 1.2 = 9.6 g

Displacment value of lactic acid is = 1

$\therefore$ Amount of lactic acid required to medicate 9.6 g base = $\frac{9.6}{100} \times 5 = 0.48\text{g}$

Formula for Glycero-gelatin base BP

Gelatin	---	14 g
Glycerin	---	70 g
Water	---	16 ml
Total base	---	100 g

According to formula, calculate the ingredients for 9.6 g of base.

1) 100 g of base requires 14 g of gelatin

9.6 g base requires = $\frac{14}{100} \times 9.6 = 1.344\text{g}$

2) 100 g of base requires 70 g of glycerin

9.6 g base requires = $\frac{70}{100} \times 9.6 = 6.7\text{ g} = 5.35\text{ ml}$

(Since 1 ml glycerin = 1.254 g, so 6.72 g = $\frac{6.72}{1.254} = 5.35\text{ ml}$)

3) 100 g of base requires 16 ml of water

9.6g of base requires = $\frac{16}{100} \times 9.6 = 1.536\text{ml}$

Revised formula for 8 pessaries

Lactic acid	---	0.48 g
Gelatin	---	1.344 g
Glycerin	---	5.35 ml
Water	---	1.536 ml

Type	Ingredients	Quantity in imperial	Quantity in metric	Quantity taken
Pessaries.	Lactic acid	5 %	5 %	0.48 g
	Glycero-Gelatin base	1 g	1 g	9.6 g
	Prepare: Pessaries Send: such 6 Direction: After unwrapping, moisten the pessary with a little water and insert into vagina.			

Theory:

Lactic acid pessaries are prepared by using glycero-gelatin base. Lactic acid is used in the preparation of pessaries, because the vaginal flora of healthy women is usually composed of rod shaped bacteria- Lacto bacillis acidophilis.

These bacteria produces lactic acid, which gives acidic nature to the vaginal area and prevents the penetration and prolifiration of pathogenic bacteria, which can cause infectious infertility in the vagina as well as the upper regions of the genital organs.

Therefore in the absence of lacto bacillis bacteria, lactic acid is required (administered) in the form of pessaries.

Procedure:

1) Consider the density of the base for calculation and calculate all the ingredients for more extra (two) pessaries, than prescribed to manipulate the heavy loss during preparation, because of sticky nature of the glycero-gelatin base.
2) Lubricate the mould with liquid paraffin or arachis oil and put inverted on the ice.
3) Heat the glycerin to 100 °C in china dish, on a water bath.
4) Heat purified water to boiling, remove it from heat and add weighed quantity of gelatin and stir gently to dissolve.
5) Add the hot glycerin to the aqueous solution of gelatin and take the weight of the dish and content. Stir the mixture gently to avoid entrapment of air bubbles until gelatin dissolves completely and gel is formed.
6) Maintain the base at 100 °C for 1 hour to remove (kill) contaminant microorganisms.
7) When solution completes, take the weight of dish and content. If necessary add the hot purified water to adjust the loss of weight, due to evaporation of water during heating.
8) Weigh required amount of lactic acid and add in small amount to the molten base with stirring. Continue the stirring, until the preparation is viscous enough to pourable.

9) Pour the hot mass into each cavity of the chilled mould sufficiently. Leave for 2-3 minutes, until the mass has just set.
10) After setting, trim off, any excess with a sharp knife or razor blade. Place the mould on ice or keep in refrigerator, for about half an hour.
11) On a cleaned tile, spread liquid paraffin. Remove the pessaries form mould and place on the tile, roll each pessary to provide a slight coating of lubricant, to prevent sticking of pessaries to each other and to the packing container.

Dispensing: Glycerin is very hygroscopic in nature, therefore transfer these pessaries in to air tight glass container and close tightly and label

Direction: After unwrapping, moisten the pessary with a little water and insert into vagina.

Storage: Store in a cool place.

Auxiliary label:
- FOR VAGINAL USE ONLY.
- STORE IN A COOL PLACE.

Uses: Lactic acid pessaries are used as antiseptic in the treatment of vaginal infections.

Similar example for Pessaries

Ichthammol	10%
Glycero-gelatin base ....q.s......	4 g

Prepare: Pessaries containing 10% Ichthammol of 4 g each

Uses: This pessaries are used as antiseptic in the treatment of vaginal infections.

Student's exercise:
1) Define pessaries? In which shapes and sizes they are available?
2) Give the examples for pessaries.
3) Explain about the heat treatment of pessaries base.
4) What will be the auxilliary label for pessaries?
5) What direction should be there on the label of pessary's and why?
6) Give the formula for Glycero-gelatin base B.P.
7) What are the Lactic acid pessaries?
8) What is the meaning of slinging?
9) How the pessaries are administered ?
10) What are the advantages and disadvantages of Glycero-gelatin suppository bases?

38 POULTICE

Poultice are also called as "Cataplasms". These are ancient class of semisolid preparations, meant for external application.

Poultices are soft, viscous, paste like wet masses of medicament and other solid ingredients applied to the skin, while they are hot, to reduce the inflammation, pain or to acts as counter irritant.

Poultices were used in ancient times, to drain infectious material from the diseased tissues. They are applied when they are hot, because poultice stimulates body surface or alleviate an inflammed area by supplying medicament in the presence of heat. Heavy kaolin is commonly used in the preparation of poultice because, it acts as a carrier of heat. Poultices contain antiseptics, anti-inflammatory and counter irritant agents.

Only two poultices are official in B.P.C.

1) Kaolin poultice B.P.C
2) Magnesium sulphate poultice (paste) B.P.C

Kaolin poultice contains more than 50% of heavy kaolin and about 40% of glycerin. Therefore they form very thick paste, with good heat retaining capacity.

Kaolin is good adsorbent, which absorbs infectious and water material. Since glycerin is hygroscopic in nature, it withdraws exudate from the infected tissues.

Due to their absorptive and hygroscopic nature, kaolin and glycerin are used in poultice, for the treatment of boils and similar infections.

Application: For application, poultice is heated along with container or in a china dish with occasional stirring, until it can only just be tolerated on the back of the hand. Then hot mass is spread thickly, on dressing material or lint and applied to the affected part (area), as hot as the patient can bear.

Dispensing:

1) To prevent the absorption of moisture by glycerin and loss of volatile constituents, poultices are usually dispensed in tightly closed, small wide mouthed containers made up of tin or thermo resistant, soda lime glass and closed with plastic screw calp, lined with an imperineable layer or closed with ship on lids.
2) If poultice are supplied in tin container, then on the label caution should be given to the patients as, "Loosen the lid before heating".
3) If poultices are supplied in glass container then, caution is given as "Transfer the required amount of poultice to a small kitchenware (or china dish) and heat to avoid breaking of glass container from direct heating.

Directions: Poultices should bear direction on the label that "Heat the preparation and spread thickly on lint or dressing material and apply to the applied part as hot as the patient can bear".

Label: Along with general requirements of label, poultice should bear auxillary label as

- FOR EXTERNAL USE ONLY
- STORE IN COOL PLACE

Storage: Store in cool place to prevent the evaporation of volatile ingredients.

KAOLIN POULTICE B.P.C.

Rx.	
Heavy kaolin (finely sifted and dried)	3 Xiii
Boric acid (finely sifted)	gr LXVii ss
Methyl salicylate	M iV
Thymol	gr i
Peppermint oil	M i
Glycerin	fl. 3 x ss
Fiat : Poultice	Mitte : 3 Vii ss

Signa : Spread the warm poultice on a lint (dressing material) and apply on the affected part as hot as the patient can bear.

Conversions:

3 xiii → 13 dr	gr LXVii ss→ 67.5 grains
1 dr = 4 g	15 gr = 1 g
13 dr = 52 g	67.5 gr = 4.5 g
M iv → 4 minims	gr i → 1 gr = 60 mg
1M = 0.06 ml	fl. 3 x ss = 10.5 fl. dr = 42 ml
4 M = 0.24 ml	

Calculation: For 3 Vii ss → 7.5 dr = 30 g, but calculate for (30+2) = 32 g

Heavy kaolin $= \frac{52}{100} \times 32 = 16.64\text{g}$

Boric acid $= \frac{4.5}{100} \times 32 = 1.44\text{ g}$

Methyl salicylate $= \frac{0.24}{100} \times 32 = 0.0768\text{ ml(q.s)}$

Thymol $= \frac{60}{100} \times 32 = 19.2\text{mg (q.s)}$

Peppermint oil $= \frac{0.06}{100} \times 32 = 0.0192\text{ml (q.s)}$

Glycerin $= \frac{42}{100} \times 32 = 13.44\text{ml}$

Type	Ingredients	Quantity in imperial	Quantity in metric	Quantity taken
Semisolid preparation for external use	Heavy kaolin (finely sifted)	13 dr	52 g	16.64 g
	Boric acid (finely sifted)	67.5 gr	4.5 g	1.44 g
	Methyl salicylate	4 Minims	0.24 ml	0.0768 ml
	Thymol	1 gr	60 mg	19.2 mg
	Peppermint oil	1 Minim	0.06 ml	0.0192 ml
	Glycerin	10.5 fl. dr	42 ml	13.44 ml
	Make : Poultice Send: 30g Direction: Spread the warm poultice on a lint (dressing material) and apply on the affected part as hot as the patient can bear.			

Theory:

This is an only one official poultice in B.P.C., which mainly consists more than 50% of heavy kaolin and 40% of glycerin. Kaolin can acts as carrier of heat. Glycerin, because of its hygroscopic nature, withdraws the infectious material from the tissues of boils or similar infections. (Glycerin also acts as humectant). Boric acid acts as an antiseptic. Methyl salicylate and thymol acts as counter irritant. Peppermint oil is used, as perfume.

Since, kaolin is liable to be contaminated with bacterial spores of Clostridium tetanii, it is necessary to heat up to 120 °C for one hour to kill these spores, but kaolin should not be heated above 120 °C, because it may leads to decomposition of glycerin.

Procedure:

1) Accurately weigh required amount of heavy kaolin and spread as a thin layer, on a sheet of paper or tray of aluminium foil and dry at 100 °C in hot air oven, for 10 -15 minutes. Allow to cool and pass through sieve no.180, to get freshly sifted powder.
2) Sift the required amount of boric acid. Mix both kaolin and boric acid uniformly, in a mortar.
3) To this powder mixture, gradually add measured amount of glycerin and triturate, to get a smooth paste.
4) Transfer this paste to a suitable sized china dish or thermo resistant glass jars. Cover with aluminium foil and heat on sand bath, at 120°C for 1 hour with occasionally stirring and allow it to cool.
5) Dissolve thymol, in methyl salicylate and also add peppermint oil. Add this mixture to a cooled mass and mix thoroughly.

Dispensing: Since thymol, methyl salicylate and peppermint oil are volatile in nature and glycerin absorbs moisture from atmosphere, transfer the kaolin poultice to a thermo resistant soda lime glass bottle or container made up of tin and tightly close with metallic screw cap, lined with impermeable layer.

Direction: Spread the warm poultice on a lint (dressing material) and apply on the affected part, as hot as the patient can bear.

Storage: Store in a cool place, to prevent the evaporation of volatile ingredients like thymol, methyl salicylate and peppermint oil.

Auxillary label: FOR EXTERNAL USE ONLY.

Uses: Kaolin poultice is used to reduce inflammation, pain and drain out the infectious material, from the diseased tissues. It is also used as counter irritant.

39 POWDERS

Latin term: Pulvis

Pharmaceutical powders are solid dosage forms of medicament, in which one or more drugs are dispensed in a finely divided state, with or without excipients. Powders are available in crystalline or amorphous form and they can be used either internaly or externaly.

Advantages of powders:

1) Powders are generally more stable than liquid dosage forms, because chemical reactions like hydrolysis and oxidation takes place more slowly in solid dosage forms, compared to liquid dosage forms.
2) Large quantities of bulky drugs can be easily administered in the powder form.
3) It is convenient for the physician, to prescribe a specific amount of powdered drug, depending upon the need of the patients.
4) Powders can be easily taken up by children and elderly patients, compared to the tablets and capsules.
5) The chances of incompatibilities are less in powders, compared to liquid dosage forms.
6) Due to small particle size of powders they offer rapid dissolution, absorption hence enhanced bioavailability and rapid onset of action, compared to the other solid dosage forms like tablets, capsules and pills.
7) Powders are easy to carry and transport, than liquid dosage forms.
8) Powder dosage form is most economical, because it does not require large number of machinery or special techniques, for their preparation.

Disadvantages of powders:

1) Drugs which are hygroscopic and deliquescent in nature, cannot be dispensed in powder form.
2) Accurate measurement of dose is difficult, specially in case of bulk powder.
3) Highly volatile drugs are not suitable for dispensing in powder form.
4) Drugs having bitter saline, nauseous and unpleasant taste, cannot be dispensed in powder form.
5) The drugs, which will get inactivated in the stomach or cause irritation in stomach, can not be administered in powder dosage form.
6) Powder preparation includes number of steps like, milling, sieving, mixing, drying etc. Hence its preparation and dispensing is, time consuming.

Classification of powders:

Depending on their physical form and intended use, powders are classified as,

1) Simple powders for internal use.
2) Compound powders for internal use.
3) Bulk powders for internal use.
4) Bulk powders for external use.

5) Powders enclosed in Cachets and Hard gelatin capsules.
6) Compressed powders (Tablet triturates or Moulded tablets).
7) Powders requiring special dispensing.

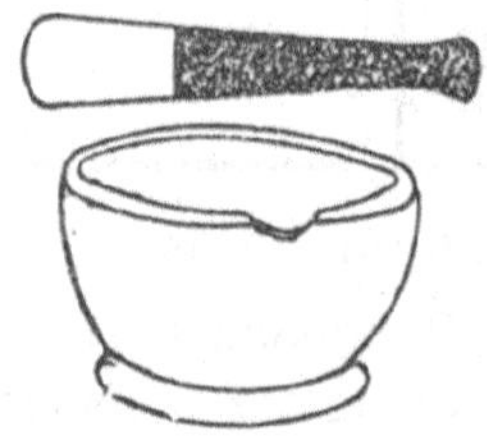

Mortar and pestle

1) Simple powders (Simple divided powders):

Simple powders consist of only one active ingredient either in crystalline or amorphous form. If the powder is in crystalline form, it is reduced to fine powder and they are weighed and generally wrapped as individual (divided) doses and dispensed.

Therefore simple powders are also called as, simple divided powders.

The medicament dispensed as simple powder has large doses, so that it can be dispensed alone without adding excipients (diluents).

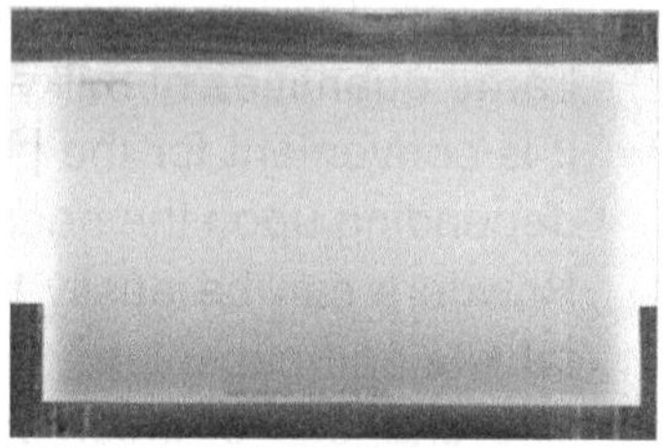

Eg: Aspirin podwer contains 600 mg of aspirin

Paracetamol podwer contains 500 mg of paracetamol

2) Compound powders for internal use (Compound divided powders):

Compound powders contain two or more than two active ingredients, which are mixed together and then dispensed as individual doses. Therefore these powders are also called as compound divided powders.

Eg. 1) Powder containing combination of Aspirin, paracetamol and caffiene powder.

2) Aspirin and caffiene powder.

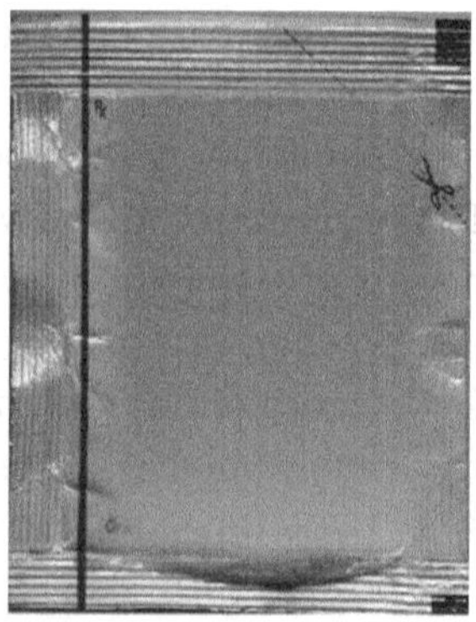

Advantages of divided powders :

1) Divided powders have the advantage of accurate dosage, where the accuracy of dose is extremely important / essential.
2) Divided powders are suitable for children or older patients, since they are administered by dispersing in water and swallowed.

Disadvantage : The unpleasant taste of drug can not be masked in divided doses.

Dispensing :Divided powders are supplied or dispensed by wrapping in suitable paper. Special papers are available for enclosing powders with or without lining.

The paper used for packing of powder should have following ideal properties,

1) It should fold easily (readily).
2) It should provide protection to the contents, without cracking at the folds or springing back in its position on folding.
3) It should be impermeable to atmospheric conditions like moisture, air and light.
4) It should be water repellent.
5) It should be light in weight and look elegant.

Powder papers of special grades are available readily in different sizes, otherwise pharmacist may cut the sheets in suitable sizes and preserve them or cut to a desired size, whenever needed.

Generally for wrapping of powder, white demy (glazed) paper is used.

The shape of the paper should be rectangular. The size of paper depends upon the quantity of powder to be enclosed and the size of the powder box, in which the powder packets are to be packed.

The wrapping of powders may be done by single wrapping or double wrapping.

1) If the drug is resistant to atmospheric conditions, it can be dispensed in single wrapping.
2) If the drug is sensitive to the atmospheric conditions like, the drug and ingredients are too volatile or hygroscopic in nature, then the powder should be dispensed in double wrapping (lined with waxed paper). Eg. : Menthol, Thymol, Citric acid.
3) These individual doses (packets) are stacked and then packed in paper board box. But these provide little protection against the atmospheric conditions. Hence wide mouthed, screw capped glass or plastic containers are used, which provide air tight seal.
4) Proprietary powders are dispensed in moisture proof, individual sachets, with outer paper board carton.

Folding of the powders in powder paper:

Cut the paper of suitable size depending upon the quantity of powder, to be packed and size of the box, which is used for packing.

Generally paper is cut for the size of 12 cm x 10 cm and folded as shown in figure below,

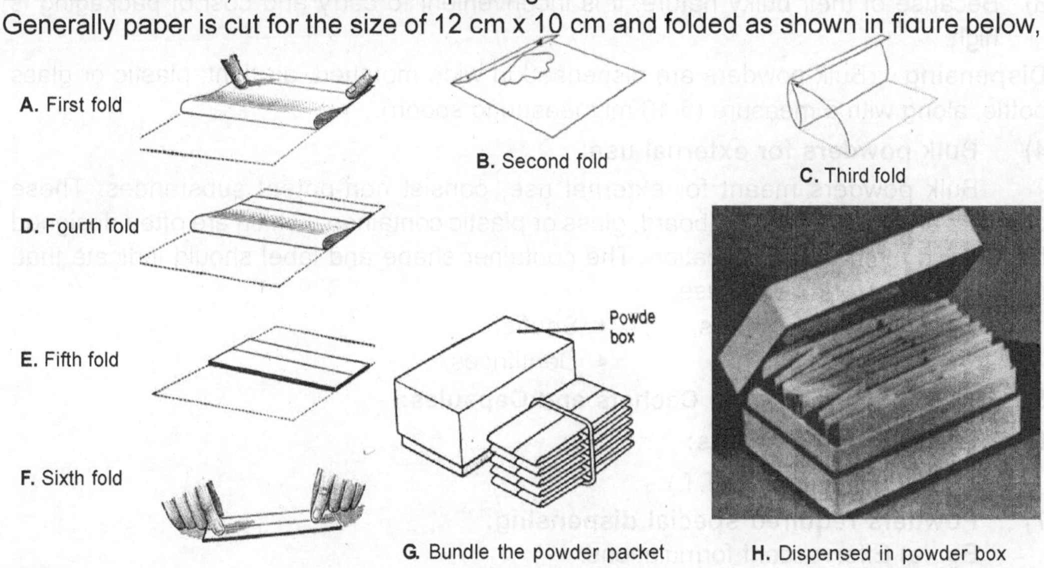

Steps involved in powder dispensing

Advice for patients (Label directions) : Patients should be directed that individual powder is dispersed in little water and swallowed or placed on the back of the tongue, before swallowing.

3) Bulk powders for internal use (Undivided powders)

Bulk powder consists of two or more than two active ingredients with or without additional ingredients, in several doses. Powders are dispensed in bulk, when the accuracy of dose is not important.

Generally antacids, laxatives, indigestion powders and nutritional powders containing, multivitamins and minerals are formulated as bulk powders for internal use.

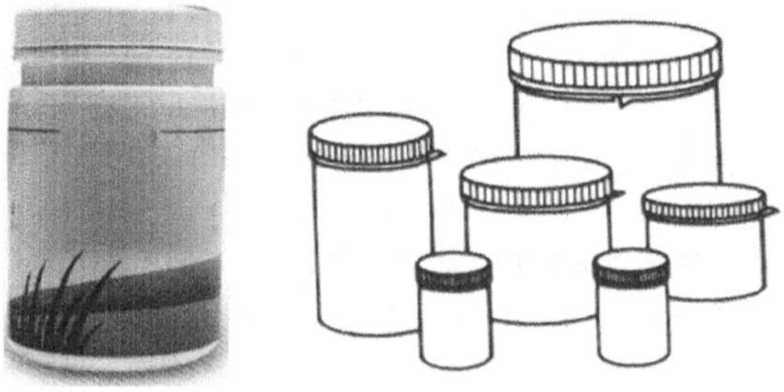

Wide mouthed containers for bulk powder

Eg. :
- Compound Rhubarb powder B.P.C. (Gregory's powder)
- Compound Magnesium trisilicate oral powder.

Advantages of undivided powders :

1) Useful for drugs, having bulky nature, with a large dose.
   Eg. Light magnesium carbonate.
2) Absorption rate is faster, than compressed tablets or capsules.
3) Certain drugs are more stable in the form of dry powder, than liquid preparations.

Disadvantages :

1) Measurement of dose may not be accurate.
2) Difficult to mask unpleasant taste of the drugs.
3) Because of their bulky nature, it is inconvenient to carry and cost of packaging is high.

Dispensing : Bulk powders are dispensed in wide mouthed, air tight, plastic or glass bottle, along with a measure (5-10 ml measuring spoon).

4) Bulk powders for external use:

Bulk powders meant for external use, consist non-potent substances. These powders are supplied in cardboard, glass or plastic containers, which are often designed for specific method of application. The container shape and label should indicate that, they are meant for external use.

Eg.
- Dusting powders,
- Snuffs,
- Insufflations,
- Dentifrices.

5) Powders enclosed in Cachets and Capsules:

6) Compressed powders:

Eg. Tablets triturates (T.T.)

7) Powders required special dispensing:

Eg. a) Effervescent formulations.

b) Eutectic powders.

c) Powders containing potent medicaments.

d) Explosive powders.

e) Powders containing Hygroscopic and deliquicent substances.

f) Powders containing efflroscent substances.

8) Lozenges
9) Pastilles

Note: Lozenges and Pastilles are disccused in detail individualy in coming chapters. Students are required to see individual chapters.

Rules for dispensing of powders: The rules which are followed for the dispensing of powders are,

1) There will be loss of powder during weighing, mixing, dividing. To manipulate these un-avoidable practical losses, always weigh the ingredients for one extra powder, than prescribed. eg. if we have to send five powders, weighing should be done for six.
2) After calculation, if the quantities of ingredients obtained are in fraction of weight, then weigh for sufficient extra powder, to produce directly weighable quantities.
3) If the weight of material is less than 100 mg (2 gr.) it is difficult to weigh on dispensing balance. Therefore enough quantity of a suitable diluent should be mixed, to raise the total weight of powder, at least 100 mg (2gr.). Lactose is generally used as diluent, because it is colourless, odourless, inert and soluble in nature.
4) If the formula of powder contains a liquid, that should be added by triturating with a suitable diluent, where liquid will adsorb on the diluent (adsorbent). The quantity of the diluent taken should be such that, the total weight of each divided powder comes in a range of directly weighable amount.

Minimum weighable amount:

On a dispensing balance, the minimum weighable quantity should not be less than 100 mg or 2 grains (120 mg) to maintain an error of + 5%. This means that any substance which is to be supplied as 100 mg, then it must not be less than 95 mg and not more than 105 mg. But efforts should be made to weigh, near to 100 mg to get high degree of accuracy.

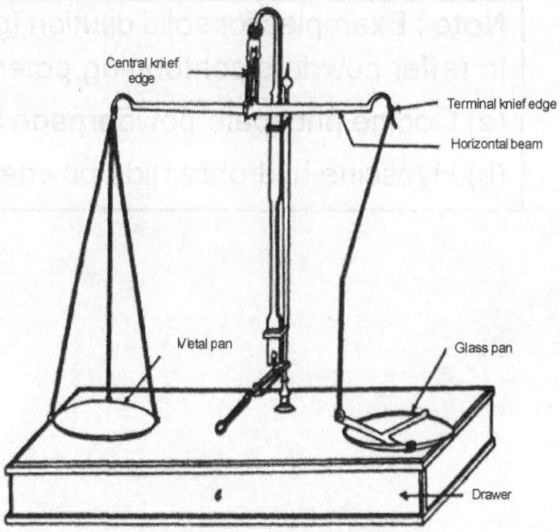

Dispensing balance

On dispensing balance, the minimum weighable quantity,

a) For potent medicaments is 300 mg.

b) For non-potent medicaments or substances, is 100 mg.

Substances which are having smaller doses, containing a potent or non-potent medicaments should be weighed on a high quality analytical/digital balance or by trituration (dilution) with an inert substance.

Following procedure (methods) should be used for dispensing of substances having dose less than minimum weighable amount.

Solid dilutions: Take minimum weighable quantity of drug or substance (i.e. 100 mg) on a dispensing balance and triturate it with a inert solid substance such as lactose, starch, sugar, dextrose or tri-calcium phosphate. Then dispense the triturated powder containing the required dose of the drug.

Geometric dilution: Geometric dilution is generally used to increase the bulk of very small quantity of the drug for weighing purpose or to mix it uniformly to make a bulk mixture.

1) In this method, a small quantity of active ingredient (drug) is mixed with an equal quantity of diluent (lactose).
2) Total weight of this powder mixture is again mixed with the same weight of the diluent (1:1).
3) This process is repeated for several times as possible until all the powder is mixed. This process is also called as "doubling method."

Triturate:

1) 100 mg of drug + 100 mg of lactose = total weight of triturate is 200 mg.
2) 200 mg of triturate + 200 mg of lactose = 400 mg of triturate.
3) 400 mg of triturate + 400 mg of lactose = 800 mg of triturate.

Now the final mixture of 800 mg contains 100 mg of drug.

From this triturate, weigh out a quantity, which is equal to the prescribed dose of the drug.

eg. If the dose is 25 mg, weigh 200 mg of this mixture, it will contain active drug dose as 25 mg.

Note : Examples for solid dilution (geometric dilution), students are required to reffer powders contenning potent medicaments.

(a) Codine phospate powderpage no : 513

(b) Hyoscine hydrobromide powder page no : 515

ASPIRIN POWDER

Rx	
Acidi acitylsalicylici	gr X
Fiat : Pulvis	Mitte : Tales sex
Signa : Capiendus unum dolore urgente.	

Conversion :

gr X → 10 grains

1 grain = 60 mg

10 grains = 600 mg

Calculation : For (6+1) = 7 powders

∴ Aspirin = 600 x 7 = 4200 mg = 4.2 g

Weight for each powder = $\frac{4.2}{7} = 0.6$ g

Type	Ingredients	Quantity in imperial	Quantity in metric	Quantity taken
Simple powder, for oral use.	Aspirin	10 gr	600 mg	4.2 g
	Make: Powder Send: Such 6 Direction: One powder to be taken whenever pain is there.			

Theory:

This is a simple powder, containing only one ingredient (medicament) for internal use. Aspirin is acetyl salicylic acid, which is a non-steroidal anti-inflammatory analgesic and anti-pyretic drug (NSAID).

The dose of aspirin is large enough so that, the drug itself can be dispensed without adding any diluents. Aspirin (acetyl salicylic acid) is in crystalline form, therefore it should finely grounded to dispense as single dose.

Procedure:

Since there will be little wastage (loss) during weighing, mixing and dividing, to manipulate these practical losses, calculate the quantity of the ingredients for at least one extra powder, than prescribed.

1) Finely powder the aspirin in a dry mortar.
2) Weigh the required amount of aspirin.
3) Divide the above powder into six equal parts so that, each weighing accurately 600 mg, and discard the rest of (remaining) powder.

Dispensing: Pack each powder in demy (butter) paper, according to the pharmaceutical art. Transfer these packed powders, in to a suitable container or envelop and label.

Direction: One powder to be taken whenever pain is there.

Storage: Store in a dry place (or at room temperature).

Uses: Aspirin powder is used as analgesic and antipyretic.

Similar examples for simple powder:

1) Rx

Calcium gluconate 1 g

Make: Powder Send: Such 4

2) Rx

Paracetamol 500 mg

Make: Powder Send: Such 8

COMPOUND MERCUROUS CHLORIDE POWDER

Rx	
Hydrargyri subchloridi	gr i
Sodii bicarbonatis	gr ii
Rhei pulverati	gr ss
Fiat : Pulvis	Mitte : Tales Sex
Signa : Unus ter in die, inter cibos sumendum.	

Conversion:

gr i → 1 grain gr ss → $\frac{1}{2}$ grain = 30 mg

1 grain = 60 mg

gr ii → 2 grains = 120 mg

Calculation: For (6+1) = 7 powders

Mercurous chloride	=	60 mg	X	7	=	420 mg
Sodium bicarbonate	=	120 mg	X	7	=	840 mg
Rhubarb powder	=	30 mg	X	7	=	210 mg
Total for seven powders	=					1470 mg

Weight for each powder = $\frac{1470}{7}$ = 210 mg

Type	Ingredients	Quantity in imperial	Quantity in metric	Quantity taken
Compounded divided powder, containing more than one ingredient, for internal use	Mercurous chloride	1 gr	60 mg	420 mg
	Sodium bicarbonate	2 gr	120 mg	840 mg
	Rhubarb powder	0.5 gr	30 mg	210 mg
	Make: Powder Send: Such 6 Direction: One powder to be taken three times a day, in between meals.			

Theory:

This is a compound divided powder, containing more than one drug in various proportions. Hence it is dispensed by mixing mercurous chloride, sodium bicarbonate and rhubarb powder together, and then divided into individual dose.

In dispensing this type of powder, mixing technique is very important, which is done by dilution method i.e. by mixing the ingredients in the order of increasing weights and then divided into individual doses according to weight specified in prescription.

Procedure:

There will be little wastage (loss) during weighing, mixing and dividing, hence to manipulate these practical losses, calculate the quantity of the ingredients for at least one extra powder, than prescribed.

1) Finely powder mercurous chloride, sodium bicarbonate and rhubarb powder separately, using mortar and pestle.
2) Weigh accurately the required amount of each ingredient separately. Mix them in ascending order of weights (in the order of increasing weights) by trituration.
3) Divide this powder mixture into 6 parts, of each weighing 210 mg and discard rest of the powder.

Dispensing: Sodium bicarbonate is a hygroscopic substance and rhubarb powder contains volatile constituents, therefore pack each powder in double wrapper, lined with butter paper, according to the pharmaceutical art. Tie these packets, with a paper ribben and transfer into a suitable container or envelop and label.

Direction: One powder to be taken three times a day, in between meals.

Storage: Store in a dry place.

Uses: This powder is used as purgative and antacid, because

Mercurous chloride act as cathartic,

Rhubarb powder act as purgative,

Sodium bicarbonate act as antacid.

COMPOUND SODIUM BICARBONATE POWDER

Rx	
Sodii bicarbonatis	gr i
Heavy Magnesii oxidi	gr ii
Sicci aluminium hydroxide gel	gr iii
Fiat : Pulvis	Mitte : Tales octo
Signa : Unus pulvis. b.i.d sumendum.	

Conversion:

gr i → 1 grain = 60 mg

gr ii → 2 grains = 120 mg

gr iii → 3 grains = 180 mg

Calculation: For (8+1) = 9 powders

Sodium bicarbonate = 60 mg X 9 = 540 mg

Heavy magnesium oxide = 120 mg X 9 = 1080 mg

Dried aluminium hydroxide gel = 180 mg X 9 = 1620 mg

Total for nine powders = 3240 mg

Weight for each powder = $\frac{3240}{9}$ = 360 mg

Type	Ingredients	Quantity in imperial	Quantity in metric	Quantity taken
Compounded divided powder, for internal use.	Sodium bicarbonate	1 gr	60 mg	540 mg
	Heavy magnesium oxide	2 gr	120 mg	1080 mg
	Dried aluminium hydroxide gel	3 gr	180 mg	1620 mg
	Make: Powder Send: Such eight. Direction: One powder to be taken, two times a day.			

Theory:

This is a compound powder, containing more than one ingredient in various proportions. All the ingredients are act as antacids. This antacid powder mixture can be prepared by dilution method i.e. by mixing the ingredients in the order of increasing weights and then divided into individual doses according to weight specified in prescription.

Procedure:

There will be little wastage (loss) during weighing, mixing and dividing, hence to manipulate these practical losses, calculate the quantity of the ingredients for at least one extra powder, than prescribed.

1) Finely powder all the three ingredients, sodium bicarbonate, heavy magnesium oxide and dried aluminium hydroxide gel, separately.
2) Weigh each ingredient and mix them uniformly in increasing order of their weight, in a mortar by trituration.
3) Divide the mixture into eight equal parts, each weighing 360 mg and discard the remaining powder.

Dispensing: Sodium bicarbonate is hygroscopic in nature, therefore pack each powder in double wrapper, lined with butter paper, according to the pharmaceutical art. Stack these packets, with a rubber band and transfer into a air tight container or envelop and label.

Storage: Store in a dry place.

Uses: This powder is used as antacid because,

Sodium bicarbonate is a fast acting antacid	---	Dose = 5 g
Heavy magnesium oxide acts as antacid	---	Dose = 500 mg
Dried aluminium hydroxide gel also acts as an antacid	---	Dose = 1 g

Similar example for Compound divided powder:

1) Rx

Aspirin	300 mg
Paracetamol	150 mg
Caffeine	50 mg
Make: Powder	Send: Such 4

Uses: This powder is used as analgesic and antipyretic.

COMPOUND RHUBARB POWDER B.P.C.

Synonym: Gregory's powder

Rx	
Rhei pulverati	3 Vi s
Magnesii carbonatis levis	3 Viii
Magnesii carbonatis heavy	3 Viii
Ginger	3 ii ss
Fiat : Pulvis	Mitte : 3 ii ss
Signa: Cochleare minimum pulvis, more dicto capindus.	

Conversion:

3 Vi s → 6.25 drachms   3 Viii → 8 drachms = 32 g

1 drachm = 4 g   3 ii ss → 2.5 drachms = 10 g

6.25 drachms = 25 g

Calculation: 3 ii ss → 2.5 dr = 10 g, but calculate for (10 + 2) = 12 g powders

Rhubarb powder $= \frac{25}{100} \times 12 = 3$ g

Light magnesium carbonate $= \frac{32}{100} \times 12 = 3.9$ g

Heavy magnesium carbonate $= \frac{32}{100} \times 12 = 3.9$ g

Ginger (Finely powdered) $= \frac{10}{100} \times 12 = 1.2$ g

Type	Ingredients	Quantity in imperial	Quantity in metric	Quantity taken
Bulk powder, for internal use	Rhubarb powder	6.25 dr	25 g	3 g
	Light magnesium carbonate	8 dr	32 g	3.9 g
	Heavy magnesium carbonate	8 dr	32 g	3.9 g
	Ginger (Finely powdered)	2.5 dr	10 g	1.2 g
	Make: Powder	Send: 10 g.		
	Direction: 5 ml spoonful powder to be taken, as directed.			

Theory:

Compound rhubarb powder is also called as Gregory's powder. In this preparation, both light and heavy magnesium carbonates are used, because light magnesium carbonate disperses easily and remains for longer time in the suspension, when it is dispersed in a liquid, but it is more bulky in nature. Heavy magnesium carbonate is less bulky in nature. Hence to reduce bulkiness of the powder, heavy magnesium carbonate is used.

Rhubarb powder acts as purgative (laxative). Both light and heavy magnesium carbonate acts as antacids. Ginger powder acts as flavouring agent and prevents the gripping action, produced by rhubarb. Ginger also acts as carminative.

It is very difficult to get fine powder of vegetable drugs, in mortar and pestle for laboratory scale, therefore such powders should be used, which are already available in fine powder form

Procedure:

There will be little wastage (loss) during weighing and mixing, hence to manipulate these practical losses, calculate the quantity of the ingredients for at least 1 or 2 grams extra powder, than prescribed.

1) Weigh the each ingredient according to calculation.
2) Select a suitable mortar so that, it should holds comfortably all the powder ingredients (because light magnesium carbonate is very bulky in nature, it occupies more area).
3) Mix the ginger and rhubarb powder by light trituration in the mortar. Then mix light magnesium carbonate and heavy magnesium carbonate by light trituration

> **Note:** Do not triturate (grind) the powder too vigorously, because heavily rubbed powder becomes compacted mass and this compacted mass will not miscible in water.

4) After light trituration, occasionally loosen the powder from the bottom of the mortar and scrap it from the sides, with the help of spatula.
5) Pass this powder through sieve no. 120, to break the lumps, if any formed and to get fine powder, then remix uniformly with the help of spatula.

Dispensing: Rhubarb powder is sensitive to the light, hence it undergoes discolouration. Rhubarb and ginger powders contain volatile constituents. Therefore to prevent their discolouration and volatalisation, transfer the prescribed amount of powder in to a airtight, wide mouthed, light resistant container, close it tightly with screw cap and label. Supply with 5 ml measuring spoon.

Direction: 5 ml spoonful powder to be taken, as directed.

Storage Store in a dark place.

Uses: This powder is used as laxative, antacid and carminative.

COMPOUND MAGNESIUM TRISILICATE ORAL POWDER B.P.

Rx	
Magnessi trisilicatis	3 vi s
Cretae pulverati	3 vi s
Heavy magnessi carbonatis	3 vi s
Sodii carbonatis	3 vi s
Fiat : Pulvis	Mitte : 3 v
Signa: Cochleare minimum pulvis t.i.d., more dicto sumendum.	

Conversion :

3 vi s → 6.25 drachms

1 drachm = 4 g

6.25 drachms = 25 g

Calculation : 3 v → 5 drachms = 20 g, but calculate for (20 + 2) = 22 g.

Magnesium trisilicate = $\frac{25}{100} \times 22 = 5.5\text{g}$

Chalk powder = $\frac{25}{100} \times 22 = 5.5\text{g}$

Heavy magnesium carbonate= $\frac{25}{100} \times 22 = 5.5\text{g}$

Sodium carbonate = $\frac{25}{100} \times 22 = 5.5\text{g}$

Type	Ingredients	Quantity in imperial	Quantity in metric	Quantity taken
Bulk powder, for internal use.	Magnesium trisilicate	6.25 dr	25 g	5.5 g
	Chalk powder	6.25 dr	25 g	5.5 g
	Heavy magnesium carbonate	6.25 dr	25 g	5.5 g
	Sodium carbonate	6.25 dr	25 g	5.5 g
	Make: Powder	Send: 20 g.		
	Direction: 5 ml spoonful powder to be taken, three times a day, as directed.			

Theory:

This is a bulk powder containing the active ingredients like magnesium trisilicate, heavy magnesium carbonate, and sodium bicarbonate, which all are acts as antacid. Chalk powder acts as adsorbent and also as antacid.

This powder is used as an antacid, when the accuracy of dose is not important. This powder is prepared by method of dilution i.e. the mixing of the ingredients are done in the order of their increasing weight.

Procedure:

There will be little wastage (loss) during weighing and mixing, hence to manipulate these practical losses, calculate the quantity of the ingredients for at least 1 or 2 grams extra powder, than prescribed.

1) Weigh sodium bicarbonate, magnesium trisilicate, heavy magnesium carbonate chalk powder, according to calculation.
2) Mix all the ingredients in suitable size mortar in ascending order of their weights.
3) After mixing pass this powder through sieve no.120, then lightly remix the powder.

Dispensing: Transfer the prescribed amount of powder in to a airtight, wide mouthed container, close it tightly with screw cap and label. Supply with 5 ml measuring spoon.

Direction: 5 ml spoonful powder to be taken three times a day, as directed.

Storage: Store in a dry place.

Uses: This powder is used as antacid and adsorbent, in the treatment of dyspepsia.

Student's exercise:

1) Define powders and classify with example.
2) What is the difference between simple and compound divided powder ?
3) How will you dispense bulk powders, meant for internal use?
4) What are the advantages and disadvantages of compound divided powders?
5) What are the advantages and disadvantages of undivided powders meant for internal use?
6) Classify the powders meant for external use.
7) What are the advantages of powders over liquid dosage forms?
8) What type of drugs cannot be formulated as powders? Give examples.
9) What is the minimum weighable quantity of powder on dispensing balance and why ?
10) Enumerate the methods of mixing of powders.
11) What is geometric ratio?
12) Define: Dyspepsia, laxative, cathertic and purgative.
13) What is the difference between cathertic and purgative?
14) What is the chemical name of calomel?
15) What is the use of Mercurous chloride?
16) Give the ideal properties of powder paper.
17) Comment : Double wrapping is required for hygroscopic powders.

40 DUSTING POWDERS

Latin term : Pulvis conspersus

Dusting powders are bulk powders meant for external application to the skin for antiseptic, antipyretic, protective, lubricant, adsorbent, astringent and antiperspirant purposes.

Dusting powders should be homogenous and in a very fine state of sub division, to enhance the effectiveness of the medicament and minimize the local irritation. Hence dusting powder should be passed through a sieve no. 120 or 180, to get very fine powder.

In additional, dusting powder should have,

1) Free flowability.
2) Easy spreadability.
3) Non-irritability.
4) Non-grittiness.
5) Good absorption and adsorption capacities.
6) Compatable with skin secretions.

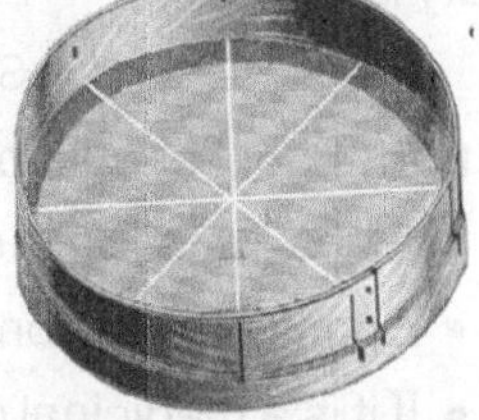

Sieve

Dusting powders must be able to protect the skin from irritation, caused by friction, moisture and chemical irritants.

In dusting powders along with medicament, other ingredients like adsorbents and lubricants are also incorporated, to adsorb the watery portion of the wound and get stuck on the applied part of the body and enhance the spreadability or flow property, so as to make powder to flow easily, on the affected part.

Classification of dusting powders:

They are of two types,

1) Medicinal dusting powders:

Medicinal dusting powders are used mainly for superficial skin conditions. These must be free from pathogenic microorganisms and spores. These should not be applied to cuts and open wounds, therefore sterility of powders is rarely essential.

Eg.
- Compound zinc oxide dusting powder,
- Chlorhexidine dusting powder,
- Hexa-chlorophene dusting powder.

2) Surgical dusting powders:

Surgical dusting powders are used in body cavities and major wounds, on burns and on the umbilical cord of the infants. Hence these powders must be sterilized, before their use. They usually contain antibacterial, anti-infective agents or adsorbents.

Eg.
- Boric acid dusting powder
- Salicylic acid dusting powder.

Dusting powders are mixed with one or more inert substances like starch, kaolin, zinc oxide and talc. Starch and kaolin are included for their absorptive properties. Talc is used for its lubricant property. But starch and talc are liable to contamination with pathogenic microorganisms, hence they should be sterilized by dry heat method at 160°C for 1 hour, before incorporating in the powder. This procedure is not necessary, if the final product is being subjected to sterilization process.

Dispensing: Dusting powders are dispensed in perforated or shifter top containers or in aerosol containers. They are applied by sprinkling directly on to the affected area or applied by using powder puff or a sterile gauze pad.

Label : In addition to general label requirements, label of dusting powder should bear the auxillary label like,

- FOR EXTERNAL USE ONLY.
- STORE IN A DRY PLACE.

Direction: Label should bear suitable direction about its application like,

Eg.
- Lightly dust on the affected area as directed.
- Sprinkle lightly on the affected area two or three times a day.
- If it is a medicinal dusting powder, then label should bear – "Do not apply on open wound and broken skin".

Storage: Dusting powders should be stored at room temperature or in a dry place.

COMPOUND ZINC OXIDE - SALICYLIC ACID DUSTING POWDER

Rx	
Zinci oxidi	ʒ V
Acidi salicylici	ʒ i s
Amyli pulverati	ʒ X Viii sss
Fiat : Pulvis conspersus	Mitte : ʒ ii ss
Signa: Consperge dolenti parti more dicto.	

Conversion:

ʒ V → 5 drachms ʒ i s → 1.25 drachms = 5 g

1 drachm → 4 g ʒ XViii sss → 18.75 drachms = 75 g

5 drachms → 20 g ʒ ii ss → 2.5 drachms = 10 g

Calculation: ʒ ii ss → 2.5 dr = 10 g, but calculate for (10 + 2) = 12 g

Zinc oxide $= \frac{20}{100} \times 12 = 2.4\,g$

Salicylic acid $= \frac{5}{100} \times 12 = 0.6\,g$

Starch powder $= \frac{75}{100} \times 12 = 9.0\,g$

Type	Ingredients	Quantity in imperial	Quantity in metric	Quantity taken
Bulk powder, for external use.	Zinc oxide	5 dr	20 g	2.4 g
	Salicylic acid	1.25 dr	5 g	0.6 g
	Starch powder	18.75 dr	75 g	9.0 g
Dusting powder	Make: Dusting powder	Send: 10 g.		
	Direction: Lightly dust on the affected part, as directed.			

Theory:

This is a medicinal dusting powder. It contains medicinally active ingredients like, salicylic acid and zinc oxide. Salicylic acid has bacteriostatic and fungicidal properties and also acts as keratolytic agent. Zinc oxide acts as an antiseptic, astringent, protective and adsorbent.

In this preparation starch is used, which acts as a excellent adsorbent by adsorbing watery portion of the wound and get stuck on the affected part for longer time and it also enhances the spreadability of the powder.

This medicated powder is applied to the open wounds. Therefore it should be sterilized in hot air oven at 160ºC for one hour, by spreading as thin layer over a sheet of paper.

After sterilization, pass the powder through a sieve no. 120 to get homogenous and very fine powder, to enhance effectiveness and minimize the local irritation and friction on the affected part. Since sieving may cause segregation of the ingredients, powder is lightly remixed with spatula and then packed.

Procedure:

There will be little wastage (loss) during weighing and mixing, hence to manipulate these practical losses, calculate the quantity of the ingredients for at least 1 or 2 grams extra powder, than prescribed.

1) Weigh separately zinc oxide, salicylic acid and starch powder, according to the calculation.
2) In a suitable mortar, mix all the three powders in the ascending order of their weights, with light trituration.
3) After uniform mixing, transfer this powders on a sheet of paper and spread as a thin layer with spatula, sterilize by keeping in hot air oven at 160°C for one hour.
4) After sterilization, cool the powder to room temperature and pass through sieve no. 120 to remove gritty particles and to get very fine powder.
5) After sieving, once again mix the powder, lightly with spatula.

Dispensing: Transfer the prescribed quantity of powder into a shifter top or re-closable, perforated plastic container and label.

Direction: Lightly dust on the affected part, as directed.

Storage: Store in a dry place.

Auxilliary label: FOR EXTERNAL USE ONLY.

Uses: Zinc oxide has antiseptic and astringent action. Salicylic acid has bacteriostatic and fungicidal properties. It also acts as a keratolytic agent. Therefore these two ingredients are used together, as a dusting powder, to prevent skin infections by lessening and absorbing exudate from the lessions and inhibit the skin microbial flora by the virtue of bacteriostatic properties. Hence this powder is used as antiseptic and keratolytic.

ZINC STARCH AND TALC DUSTING POWDER B.P.C.

Rx	
Zinci oxidi	3 vi s
Amyli pulverati	3 vi s
Talcum	3 xii ss
Fiat : Pulvis conspersus	Mitte : 3 vii ss
Signa: Cosperge dolenti parti si opus sit b.i.d - t.i.d.	

Conversion:

3 vi s → 6.25 drachms = 25 g

3 xii ss → 12.5 drachms = 50 g

Calculation: 3 vii ss → 7.5 drachms = 30 g, but calculate for (30+2) = 32 g

Zinc oxide $= \frac{25}{100} \times 32 = 8\text{ g}$

Starch powder $= \frac{25}{100} \times 32 = 8\text{ g}$

Purified talc sterilized $= \frac{50}{100} \times 32 = 16\text{ g}$

Type	Ingredients	Quantity in imperial	Quantity in metric	Quantity taken
Bulk powder, for external use. Dusting powder	Zinc oxide	6.25 dr	25 g	8 g
	Starch powder	6.25 dr	25 g	8 g
	Purified talc sterilized	12.5 dr	50 g	16 g
	Make: Dusting powder	Send: 30 g.		
	Direction: Sprinkle lightly onto the affected area two - three times a day.			

Theory:

This powder is used as an adsorbent – antiseptic dusting powder. It contains zinc oxide, which acts as antiseptic and good adsorbent. Starch is used as adsorbent, to adsorb watery portion of wounds, which also get stuck on to the affected part, for longer time.

In this powder, talc is used because of its good adsorbing and excellent flow (lubricant) properties. But talc is a mineral ingredient and it will be easily contaminated by pathogenic bacteria and spores of Clostridium titani and Anthrax. Therefore talc should be sterilized, in hot air oven at 160ºC for at least one hour, before use.

In this prescription, sterilized talc is used. Hence there is no need of sterilizing the powder, once again.

Procedure:

There will be little wastage (loss) during weighing and mixing, hence to manipulate these practical losses, calculate the quantity of the ingredients for at least 1 or 2 grams extra powder, than prescribed.

1) Separately weigh zinc oxide, starch and talc according to calculation.
2) In a suitable mortar, mix all three ingredients in the increasing order of their weights i.e. first mix zinc oxide and starch by trituration and then add sterilized talc– mix uniformly.
3) Pass this powder mixture through the sieve no. 120 to get a homogenous and very fine powder.
4) After sieving, lightly remix the powder, by spatulation on a sheet of paper.

Dispensing: Transfer the prescribed quantity of powder into a shifter top or re-closable perforated plastic container and label.

Direction: Sprinkle lightly on the affected area, two - three times a day.

Storage: Store in a dry place.

Auxillary label: FOR EXTERNAL USE ONLY.

Uses: This powder is used as excellent adsorbent and antiseptic dusting powder.

Student's exercise:

1) Define dusting powders. Give examples.
2) What are the ideal properties of dusting powders?
3) What should be the particle size of dusting powder? Give reason.
4) How will you classify the dusting powders?
5) Why adsorbents and lubricants are necessary in dusting powders ?.
6) What is talc? Why it is used in dusting powder ?
7) What are the basic ingredients used in dusting powders ?
8) Give the examples for medicinal and surgical dusting powders.
9) Comment : Medicinal dusting powders should not be applied on cuts and open wounds.
10) Why sterilization of talc or starch is necessary in surgical dusting powder ?
11) How will you dispense dusting powder?
12) How the dusting powders can be applied ?
13) What direction (caution) will you give on the label of medicinal dusting powder?
14) Why zinc oxide and salicylic acids are used in the preparation of dusting powders?

41 INSUFFLATIONS

Latin term : Insufflatio.

Insufflations are medicated dusting powders meant for introduction into body cavities such as nose, throat, ears and vagina, with the help of an apparatus known as "Insufflator".

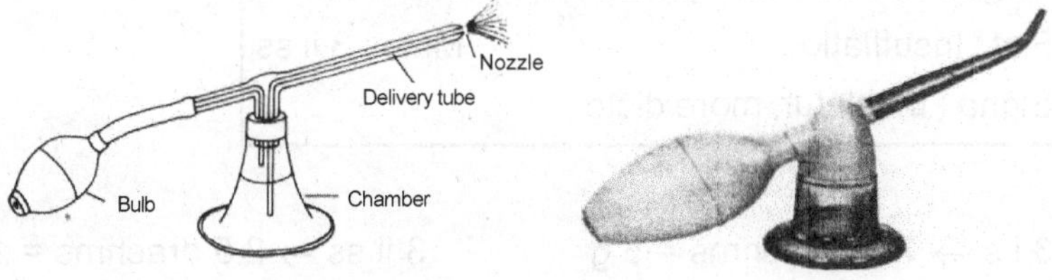

Insufflator

Insufflator is a simple apparatus, which sprays the powder in a stream of finely divided particles, all over the site of application. Insufflations are used to produce a local effect, as in the treatment of ear, nose and throat infections, with antibiotics or to produce a systemic effect from a drug, which is destroyed in GIT.

The particle size of material included in insufflation, should be very fine and these should be free from irritant and sensitizing effects.

Example for insufflations:

- Camphor, menthol, ammonium chloride insufflation.
- Boric acid insufflation.

Disadvantages of insufflations:

1) It is difficult to obtain a measured quantity of drug, as a uniform dose.
2) Insufflator gets blocked, when it is slightly wet or the powder becomes wet.

Hence this drawback can overcome, by the use of pressurized (metered) aerosol, which provides excellent control of dose through metered valves and protects the product from external environment (moisture air and light). Hence these containers are used for administration of potent drugs.

Snuffs: If insufflations are intended to be used only in nasal cavity, then they are called as "snuffs", which are inhaled into nostril for their antiseptic, decongestion and bronchodilator action. Snuffs are dispensed in small, flat metal boxes, with a hinged lid. But now-a-days they are dispensed in pressurized aerosol containers.

Label: In addition to general label requirements, label of insufflation should indicate, the type of insufflation i.e, if insufflation is meant for particular body cavities like nose, ear or vaginal then label should bear,

- FOR NASAL USE ONLY
- FOR EAR USE ONLY
- FOR VAGINAL USE ONLY

Storage: Insufflations should be stored in a dry place or at room temperature.

CAMPHOR - MENTHOL INSUFFLATION

Rx	
Mentholis	3 i s
Camphorae	3 i s
Ammonil chloridi	3 vii ss
Magnessi carbonatis pulverati	3 xv
Fiat : Insufflatio	Mitte : 3 ii ss
Signa : Inhaletur, more dicto.	

Conversion :

3 i s → 1.25 drachms = 5 g   3 ii ss → 2.5 drachms = 10 g

3 vii ss → 7.5 drachms = 30 g   3 xv → 15 drachms = 60 g

Calculation : 3 ii ss → 2.5 dr = 10 g, but calculate for (10 + 2) = 12 g

$$\text{Menthol} = \frac{5}{100} \times 12 = 0.6 \text{ g}$$

$$\text{Camphor} = \frac{5}{100} \times 12 = 0.6 \text{ g}$$

$$\text{Ammonium chloride} = \frac{30}{100} \times 12 = 3.6 \text{ g}$$

$$\text{Magnesium carbonate powder} = \frac{60}{100} \times 12 = 7.2 \text{ g}$$

Type	Ingredients	Quantity in imperial	Quantity in metric	Quantity taken
Bulk powder, for external use for nose.	Menthol	1.25 dr	5 g	0.6 g
	Camphor	1.25 dr	5 g	0.6 g
	Ammonium chloride	7.5 dr	30 g	3.6 g
	Magnesium carbonate powder	15 dr	60 g	7.2 g
	Make: Insufflation	Send: 10 g.		
Eutectic mixture.	Direction: To be inhaled, as directed.			

Theory:

This is a bulk powder meant for external use, which is used as insufflation for the treatment of nasal congestion (bronchitis and sinusitis).

In this prescription, menthol and camphor get liquefied on mixing with each other and form a eutectic mixture, because each of them acts as impurity, to one another. Therefore melting points of both camphor and menthol decreases and mixture of them also shows lower melting point, than room temperature. Due to lowering of melting points, powder will convert into liquid or semisolid.

Ammonium chloride is not a eutectic substance, but it is a deliquescent substance. Therefore when it is mixed with mixture of camphor and menthol, due to the formation of liquid, it also converts into liquid.

To overcome this problem magnesium carbonate is used as adsorbent, which adsorbs the liquid, which is liberated by eutectic reaction, between camphor and menthol and makes the powder dry and free flowable.

In this case, powder is prepared by mixing both camphor and menthol by trituration and allowed to form liquid (eutectic formation). Then to this mixture, sufficient quantity of magnesium carbonate is added to adsorb liquid formed (liberated). After complete adsorption of liquid from magnesium carbonate, ammonium chloride is mixed uniformly on a sheet of paper, by light spatulation.

Larger particles will irritate the sensitive tissues of the nose. Hence this powder should be passed through sieve no. 120, to get very fine powder.

Procedure:

There will be little wastage (loss) during weighing and mixing, hence to manipulate these practical losses, calculate the quantity of the ingredients for at least 1 or 2 grams extra powder, than prescribed.

1) Weigh separately camphor, menthol, aluminium chloride and magnesium carbonate, according to calculation.
2) Dissolve camphor in little portion of alcohol, in a chaina-dish and allow to evaporate. When alcohol evaporates, camphor will subdivide into fine particles.
3) Convert menthol crystals into fine powder, by triturating in a mortar.
4) In a mortar, triturate both camphor and menthol together. When they convert into liquid completely, add magnesium carbonate and mix well with spatula so that, powder becomes completely dried and free flowing.
5) Transfer the powder mixture on a butter paper and uniformly mix aluminium chloride lightly, with the help of spatula.
6) Pass this powder through sieve no. 120 to remove gritty particles, if present and to get a homogenous and very fine powder.

Dispensing: Weigh prescribed amount of powder and transfer into a small, wide mouthed, shifter top, plastic container and label.

Direction: To be inhaled, as directed.

Storage: Store in a cool place

Auxilliary label:
- FOR NASAL USE ONLY.
- STORE IN A COOL PLACE.

Uses: Mixture of camphor and menthol relieves the symptoms of bronchitis and sinusitis. Aluminium chloride acts as expectorant. Therefore this insufflation is used in the treatment of bronchitis and sinusitis (nasal congestion) and also as expectorant.

Student's exercise:

1) Define insufflations. Give examples.
2) What is insufflator?
3) What types of drugs are formulated as insufflations, give examples?
4) Comment : Particle size of insuffulation should be very fine.
5) What are advantages and disadvantages of insufflations?
6) What types of containers are used for dispensing of insufflations?
7) What is snuff?
8) What is the difference between snuff and insufflation?
9) Write the storage condition for insufflations.
10) Why menthol and camphor are used in insufflation.
11) Briefly explain how will you prepare camphor menthol insufflation.
12) Comment : Ammonium chloride is a deliquescent substance.
13) What is benzoin and prepared storax. What are their uses?

42 DENTIFRICES (TOOTH POWDERS)

Latin term: Dentifricium

Dentifrices are bulk powders, used to clean the surface of the teeth, with the help of tooth brush. Dentifrices should have following properties.

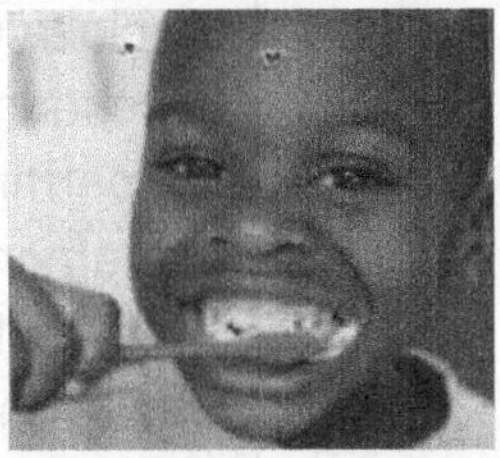

1) It should be finely powdered.
2) It should have cleansing action.
3) It should have mild degree of abrasiveness.
4) It should have good flavour.

To fulfil above characteristics of dentifrice, various types of ingredients are used such as,

1)	Detergents (cleansing agents)	Sodium lauryl sulphate, Hard soap.
2)	Abrassives	Calcium carbonate, Calcium sulphate, Dibasic calcium carbonate, Sodium chloride, Sodium bicarbonate, Pumice stone(powder)
3)	Sweetening agents	Saccharine sodium
4)	Flavouring agents	Volatile oils like Peppermint oil, Clove oil

The strong abrasive substance should not be used, because it may damage the smooth structure of the tooth.

Dispensing: Dentifrices are dispensed in perforated or shifter top containers, which should give protection to the powder from contamination by air, light, moisture and microorganisms.

Label:

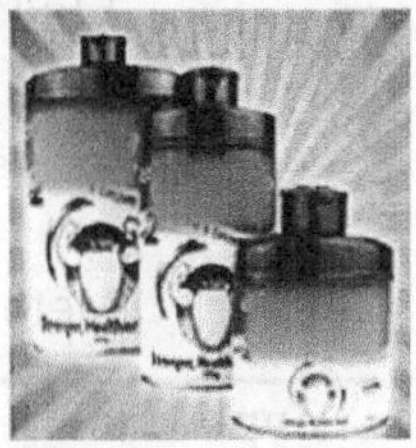

In addition to general label requirements, label of dentifrice should contain auxilliary label like,

- FOR EXTERNAL USE ONLY,
- STORE IN A DRY PLACE.
- Brush throughly, at least twice a day, as directed by a dentist or physician.
- Children of 6 years age and under should have adult supervision and use only a small amount.
- Do not swallow, children should spit and rinse throughly after brushing.

DENTIFRICE N.F.

Rx	
Hard soap (Finely powdered)	3 i s
Precipitated calcium carbonate	3 xxiii s
Saccharin sodium	gr iii
Peppermint oil	M Vi
Cinnamon oil	M iii
Methyl salicylate	M Xii
Fiat : Dentifricium	Mitte : 3 vii ss
Signa : Clean the surface of the teeth with the help of tooth brush.	

Conversion :

3 i s → 1.25 drachms
1 drachm = 4 g
1.25 drachms = 5 g
3 xxiii s → 23.25 drachms = 93 g
M iii → 3 minims = 0.2 ml

gr iii → 3 grains
15 grains = 1 g
3 grains = 0.2 g
M Vi → 6 minims = 0.4 ml
M Xii →12 minims = 0.8 ml

Calculation : 3 vii ss → 7.5 drachms = 30 g, but calculate for (30+2) = 32 g.

Hard soap (Finely powdered) = $\frac{5}{100} \times 32 = 1.6$ g

Precipitated calcium carbonate = $\frac{93}{100} \times 32 = 30$ g

Sodium saccharin = $\frac{0.2}{100} \times 32 = 0.064$ g

Peppermint oil = $\frac{0.4}{100} \times 32 = 0.128$ml

Cinnamon oil = $\frac{0.2}{100} \times 32 = 0.064$ml

Methyl salcicylate = $\frac{0.8}{100} \times 32 = 0.256$ml

Type	Ingredients	Quantity in imperial	Quantity in metric	Quantity taken
Bulk powder, for external use	Hard soap in fine powder	1.25 gr	5 g	1.6 g
	Precipitated calcium carbonate	23.25 dr	93 g	30 g
	Saccharin sodium	3 gr	0.2 g	0.064 g
	Peppermint oil	6 minims	0.4 ml	0.128 ml
	Cinnamon oil	3 minims	0.2 ml	0.064 ml
	Methyl salicylate	12 minims	0.8 ml	0.256 ml
	Make: Dentifrice	Send: 30 g.		
	Direction: Clean the surface of the teeth with the help of tooth brush.			

Theory:

Dentifrice is a bulk powder used externally, for cleaning the surface of the tooth, with the help of tooth brush. Hard soap acts as detergent, which helps in cleansing of the surfaces of tooth.

Precipitated calcium carbonate gives mild abrasiveness for polishing the teeth. Saccharin sodium is synthetic a sweetening agent, used to give an agreeable sweetening taste to the tooth powder. Peppermint oil, cinnamon oil and methyl salicylate are used as flavouring agents, to give a pleasant flavour to the dentifrice.

Gritty particles may damage (irritate) the smooth mucous membrane of the gum. Therefore, to get very fine powder, it should be passed through the sieve no. 120.

Procedure:

There will be little wastage (loss) during weighing and mixing, hence to manipulate these practical losses, calculate the quantity of the ingredients for at least 1 or 2 grams extra powder, than prescribed.

1) Accurately weigh precipitated calcium carbonate and divide into two equal portions.
2) Take one portion of precipitated calcium carbonate and mix with hard soap, by light trituration.
3) Triturate the saccharin sodium, to give fine powder in a mortar. To this powder add cinnamon oil, peppermint oil and methyl salicylate and mix them uniformly, by light spatulation. To this powder, add second portion of precipitated calcium carbonate and mix uniformly.
4) Mix the two powders thoroughly and then pass through sieve number 120, to get very fine powder. After sieving, once again remix the powder lightly, on a sheet of paper.

Dispensing: Weigh prescribed amount of powder and transfer to a perforated or shifter top plastic or metallic container and label.

Direction: Clean the surface of the teeth, with the help of tooth brush.

Storage: Store in a dry place.

Auxilliary label:
- FOR EXTERNAL USE ONLY.
- STORE IN A DRY PLACE.

Uses: It is used for cleansing of tooth surface.

Student's exercise:

1) Define dentifrices? What are the ideal requirements of dentifrices?
2) What are the basic ingredients required for dentifrices?
3) How abrasive material works in dentifrices? Give examples for abrasives.
4) Which flavouring agents are used in dentifrices?
5) Which types of containers are used for dispensing of dentifrices?

43 EFFERVESCENT FORMULATIONS

(Effervescent Powders and Granules)

Effervescent formulations are specially formulated solid dosage forms of medicament, intended to be taken internally. They are formulated (dispensed) in two types.

1) Effervescent powders: Eg. Seidlitz powder B.P.C.
2) Effervescent granules: Eg. Sodium phosphate - effervescent granule NP

The basic requirements of effervescent formulations are,

1) Medicament : Sodium phosphate, Sodium bromide
   Potassium iodide, Potassium citrate
   Piperazine, Quinine salicylate.
2) Acid : Citric acid, Tartaric acid
3) Base : Sodium bicarbonate

When effervescent formulation (may be powder or granules) is added to the water, acid-base reaction takes place between citric acid, tartaric acid and sodium bicarbonate and produces effervescence, due to the liberation of CO_2. The solution remaining after effervescence is called as "carbonated water".

1) This carbonated water serves, to mask the bitter, saline or nauseous taste of the medicament.
2) The liberated CO_2 stimulates the flow of gastric juice, which helps in the quick absorption of the medicament.

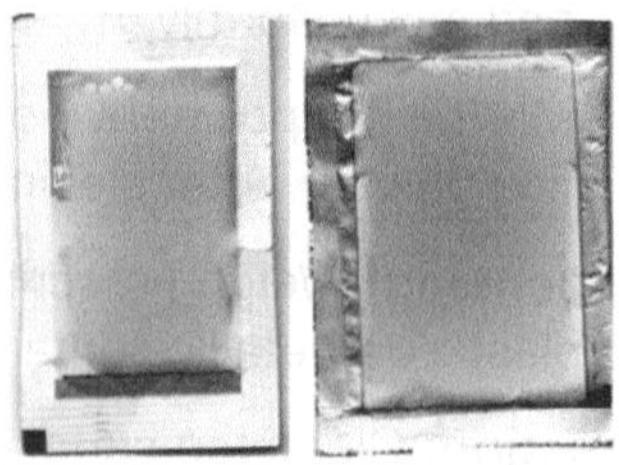

Example for effervescent powder

Hence patients are advised to, mix the powder (granules) in water and take the preparation, while effervescing.

Effervescent preparations are more palatable, if they are slightly acidic in taste. Therefore in efferesent formulations, the quantity of acid is slightly more than that is required, to neutralize the base.

In certain formulations sucrose or saccharine is used as sweetening agent, to mask the disagreeable bitter or nauseous taste of the medicaments.

Note: Effervescent powder is dispensed in very fine state (powder). Due to increased surface area, powder dissolves very fast in water. This leads to violent and uncontrollable effervescence, with consequent loss of solution and the medicament, due to their overflowing from the container. This also leads to loss of carbon dioxide, due to the reduced carbonation of the solution.

Therefore care must be taken, while using effervescent powder i.e. first the content of blue paper is added to the water, then content of white paper is added slowly with stirring. Then liquid should be to be taken, while effervescing.

EFFERVESCENT COMPOUND POWDER B.P.C.

Synonym- Seidlitz powder (Effervescent citro-tartrate of soda powder)

Rx	
No. 1 Powder	
Sodii potassii tartratis	gr CX ii ss
Sodii bicarbonatis	gr XXXVii ss
No. 2 Powder	
Acidi tartraci	gr XXXVii ss
Fiat : Pulvis	Mitte : Tales quatuor
Signa : Mix one pair of powder in water slowly and to be taken, while effervescing.	

Conversion :

gr CX ii ss → 112.5 grains

15 grains = 1 g

112.5 grains = 7.5 g

gr XXXVii ss → 37.5 grains = 2.5 g

Calculation : For (4+1) = 5 powders.

No. 1 Powder

Sodium potassium tartrate = 7.5 g X 5 = 37.5 g

Sodium bicarbonate = 2.5 g X 5 = 12.5 g

Total for 5 powders = 50.0 g

Weight for each powder = $\frac{50}{5}$ = 10 g

No. 2 Powder

Tartaric acid = 2.5 X 5 = 12.5 g

Weight for each powder = $\frac{12.5}{5}$ = 2.5 g

Type	Ingredients	Quantity in imperial	Quantity in metric	Quantity taken
Compound divided powder. Effervescent powder for internal use.	No. 1 Powder :			
	Sodium potassium tartrate	112.5 gr	7.5 g	37.5 g
	Sodium bicarbonate	37.5 gr	2.5 g	12.5 g
	No. 2 Powder :			
	Tartaric acid	37.5 gr	2.5 g	12.5 g
	Make: Powder Send: Such 4			
	Direction: Slowly mix one pair of powder in water and to be taken, while effervescing.			

Theory:

Seidlitz powder is one of the effervescent formulation. It contains the medicament – sodium potassium tartrate, which acts as a saline purgative. When this powder is added to the water, an acid base reaction takes place between, tartaric acid and sodium bicarbonate and produces effervescence, due to the liberation of carbon dioxide.

The solution remaining after effervescing, is called as "carbonated water". This carbonated water helps in dissolving of drug, sodium potassium tartarate and masking of its unpleasant saline taste. The liberated carbon dioxide also stimulates the flow of gastric juice and helps in the quick absorption of sodium potassium tartrate.

$$2NaHCO_3 + C_4H_4O_6 \longrightarrow C_4H_2Na_2O_6 + 2CO_2\uparrow + 2H_2O$$

Sodium bicarbonate   Tartaric acid   Sodium tartrate

This formulation is dispensed by packing the ingredients in two different packets, as powder no 1 and powder no 2.

Powder no. 1 consists of sodium potassium tartrate and sodium bicarbonate, it is wrapped in **blue colour paper.**

Powder no. 2 consists of tartaric acid and it is wrapped in **white paper.**

Seidlitz powder is used as an effervescent draught.i.e In a tumbelerful of cold or warm water, the contents of powder no.1 is dissolved, to this slowly add the content of powder no.2, mix well and that mixture is to be taken immediately, while effervescening.

Procedure:

There will be little wastage (loss) during weighing, mixing and dividing, hence to manipulate these practical losses, calculate the quantity of the ingredients for at least one extra powder, than prescribed.

1) Weigh separately tartaric acid, sodium potassium tartrate and sodium bicarbonate according to calculation.
2) Triturate each powder separately.
3) Mix sodium bicarbonate and sodium potassium tartrate in a mortar, with light trituration. From this triturate, weigh accurately 10 g of powder and pack (wrap) in blue coloured, paper lined with butter paper. Prepare five such powders.
4) Weigh 2.5 g of finely powdered tartaric acid and pack (wrap) in white paper lined with butter paper. Prepare such 5 powders.

Dispensing: Sodium bicarbonate and tartaric acid are hygroscopic in nature, at high humidity. Therefore dispense this powder in double wrapper, lined with butter (wax) paper, tie of packets (No.1 and 2) with paper ribbon. Transfer these packets into a wide mouthed container, close it tightly with screw cap and label.

Direction: Slowly mix one pair of powder in water and to be taken, while effervescing.

Storage: Store in a dry place.

Auxilliary label: STORE IN A DRY PLACE.

Uses: This powder is used as an 'effervescent draught', as saline purgative.

44 EFFERVESCENT GRANULES

Effervescent granules are the specially prepared solid dosage form of the medicament for internal use. They usually contain:

1) Medicament
2) Acid - Eg. Citric acid, Tartaric acid
3) Base - Eg. Sodium bicarbonate

Before administration, effervescent granules are intended to be dissolved or dispersed in the prescribed quantity of water. After mixing with water, acid-base reaction takes place and effervescence will be produced, due to the liberation of CO_2.

The solution remaining after effervescence (after release of CO_2) is called as carbonated water. This carbonated water serves (helps) to mask the bitter and saline or nauseous taste of medicament and liberated CO_2 stimulates the flow of gastric juice, which influences the quick absorption of medicament. Sometimes sucrose or saccharin is used as sweetening agent along with acids and base, to mask unpleasant bitter and nauseous taste of the medicaments.

Reason: Effervescent powder dissolves very fast in water, due to increased surface area. This leads to violent and uncontrollable effervescence with loss of CO_2 and ultimately the carbonation of solution may decrease, to a great extent.

Therefore effervescent granules are preferred than effervescent powder since, granules dissolves slowly in water than powder due to decrease in surface area. Therefore carbonation of solution can be sustained (controlled), to avoid complete loss of CO_2.

Eg. Sodium phosphate effervescence granules USP

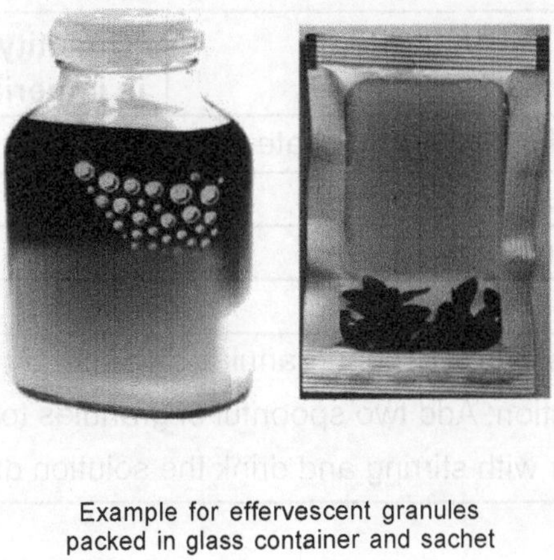

Example for effervescent granules packed in glass container and sachet

SODIUM PHOSPHATE EFFERVESCENT GRANULES USP

Rx

Sodii phosphatis sicci	3 L
Sodii bicarbonatis	3 CX iX s
Acidi tartraci	3 LXiii
Acidi citratis	3 XL ss
Fiat : Granules	Mitte : 3 vii ss

Signa : Add two spoonful of granules to a tumblerful of water with stirring and drink the solution during effervescing.

Conversion :

3 L → 50 drachms
1 drachm = 4 g
50 drachms = 200 g

3 CX iX s → 119.25 drachms = 477 g
3 LXiii → 63 drachms = 252 g
3 XL ss → 40.5 drachms = 162 g
3 vii ss → 7.5 drachms = 30 g

Calculation : 3 vii ss → 7.5 drachms = 30 g, but calculate for (30+2) = 32 g.

Dried sodium phosphate $= \frac{200}{1000} \times 32 = 6.4$ g

Sodium bicarbonate $= \frac{477}{1000} \times 32 = 15.264$ g

Tartaric acid $= \frac{252}{1000} \times 32 = 8.064$ g

Citric acid $= \frac{162}{1000} \times 32 = 5.184$ g

Type	Ingredients	Quantity in imperial	Quantity in metric	Quantity taken
Bulk powder, for internal use.	Dried sodium phosphate	50 dr	200 g	6.4 g
	Sodium bicarbonate	119.25 dr	477 g	15.264 g
	Tartaric acid	63 dr	252 g	8.064 g
Effervescent granules.	Citric acid	40.5 dr	162 g	5.184 g
	Make: Effervescent granules Send: 30 g Direction: Add two spoonful of granules to a tumblerful of water with stirring and drink the solution during effervescing.			

Theory:

It is one of the effervescent formulation, in granular form. It consists the medicament-sodium phosphate, which acts as cathartic. The unpleasant saline taste of sodium phosphate, is masked by using effervescent forming ingredients like tartaric acid, citric acid and sodium bicarbonate.

It is formulated in the granular form, to avoid violent and uncontrollable effervescence and to get controlled dissolution rate, as compared to the effervescent powder.

Effervescent granules are prepared by "**fusion (heat) method**". Tartaric acid is anhydrous in nature, but citric acid contains one molecule of water of crystallization, which is liberated during heating. This water is used as a moistening (granulating) agent, for the preparation of granules. All the ingredients are powdered and mixed together. The mixed blend is then placed, over a pre-heated porcellin or metallic dish and mixed till a coherent mass is formed.

In this method, the water required for granulation, is obtained from two sources.

1) **From water of crystallization of citric acid i.e. citric acid contains one molecule of water of crystallization, which is liberated during heating.**

$3\ NaHCO_3 + C_6H_8O_7.H_2O \rightarrow C_6H_5Na_3O_7 + 3CO_2\uparrow + 3H_2O$

Sodium bicarbonate, Citric acid, Sodium citrate

2) **The water produced from the reaction between, tartaric acid and sodium bicarbonate.**

$2\ NaHCO_3 + C_4H_6O_6 \rightarrow C_4H_2Na_2O_6 + 2CO_2\uparrow + 2H_2O$

Sodium bicarbonate, Tartaric acid, Sodium tartrate

- In the preparation of effervescent granules, pre-heating of the dish is important before transfering the powder in to it, to ensure the liberation of water of crystallization, from the citric acid.
- If dish is heated after the addition of powder blend, water will liberate slowly and it will evaporates simultaneously. As a result, sufficient water will not be available, to make a coherent mass to prepare granules. Generally heating is done, up to 1-5 minutes.
- The damp mass produced is passed through a suitable sieve and the granules produced are dried in an oven, at a temperature not exceeding 60 ºC and then packed in air tight container.

Granulation by fusion method usually results in loss of weight, due to:

1) Loss of moisture from the damp mass, by evaporation.
2) Loss of CO_2 in the chemical reaction, between acids and base.

The loss in weight is approximately equal to one seventh of the total weight of powder. Hence it must be taken into consideration during calculating the quantity of ingredients is more than 1000 g. (Hence this prescription consist ingredients of weight, nearly 1090 g).

Procedure:

There will be little wastage (loss) during weighing, mixing and granulation, hence to manipulate these practical losses, calculate the quantity of ingredients for at least 1 or 2 grams extra, than prescribed.

1) Accurately weigh sodium phosphate, tartaric acid, citric acid and sodium bicarbonate, according to calculation.
2) Mix all the ingredients in ascending order of their weights, by trituration.
3) Place a porcelin dish on a water bath and heat the water bath, to boiling point.
4) Place the powder mixture in to the hot porcelain dish, which is kept on a boiling water bath.
5) Stir the powder mixture with the help of spatula, for 1-5 minutes i.e. until a damp (coherent) mass is formed.
6) Remove the damp mass from the dish and immediately pass through the sieve number 20, by placing on a damy (butter) paper.
7) Dry the granules by spreading on a sheet of paper, in hot air oven at temperature not exceeding 60 °C.

Dispensing: Weigh the prescribed quantity of granules and transfer in to wide mouthed container, close it tightly with screw cap and label. Supply with 5 ml measuring spoon.

Direction: Add two spoonfuls of granules, to a tumblerful of water with stirring and drink the solution, during while effervescing.

Storage: Store in a dry place.

Auxilliary label: STORE IN A DRY PLACE.

Uses: Sodium phosphate effervescent granules are used as saline cathartic.

Student's exercise:

1) Define effervescent formulations and give examples
2) What are the basic requirements of effervescent formulations?
3) What are the advantages of effervescent formulations?
4) What is carbonated water?
5) Comment : Effervescent formulations are slightly acidic in taste
6) What is scidlitz powder? Write its ingredients.
7) Why sodium potassium tartarate is formulated as effervescent powder?
8) Briefly enumerate the principle behind the preparation of effervescent powder (Scidlitz powder).
9) Why Scidlitz's powder is dispensed in two different paper packets?
10) Which label direction will you write for effervescent powder?
11) What is the disadvantage of effervescent powder?

12) Define effervescent granules.
13) Why effervescent granules are preferred than effervescent powder?
14) Comment : For the preparation of effervescent granules, both citric acid and tartaric acids are used.
15) Why pre-heating of petridish is necessary for the preparation of effervescent granules?
16) Briefly enumerate the principle involved in the preparation of effervescent granules.
17) Why granulation by fusion method leads to loss of weight and how will you compensate this loss?
18) What is the use of sodium phosphate effervescent granules?
19) What direction will you write on the label of effervescent granules?

45 EUTECTIC POWDER OR EUTECTIC MIXTURE

In Greek 'eutectic' means easy melting. When two or more low melting point substances are mixed together they liquefy due the formation of a new compound, which has a lower melting point, than the room temperature. Such substances are called as "eutectic substances" and mixture is called as "eutectic mixture" or eutectic powder.

Examples for Eutectic substances:

- Camphor
- Menthol
- Thymol
- Phenol
- Salol
- Chloral hydrate
- Aminopyrine
- Antipyrine
- Phenacitin
- Acetonilide
- Aspirin

Any of these substances if, mixed together, turn to liquid form (eutectic mixture) due to depression in melting point of the mixture, below room temperature. The reason is that, each ingredient becomes the impurity for another one. Therefore melting point of each of the ingredient is further lowered, to below the room temperature and ultimately the mixture becomes liquid. Hence it is considered that, the formation of eutectic mixture is, due to physical change than the chemical change.

Procedure for dispensing Eutectic substances:

Practically eutectic substances are dispensed as a powder mixture, by two methods by using some adsorbents, which should be inert in nature.

Eg.
- Magnesium carbonate
- Kaolin
- Light magnesium oxide
- Bentonite

Method-1:

The principle involved in this method is, keeping away the particles of one eutectic substance from the particles of other eutectic substance. This is achieved by mixing each eutectic substance separately, with sufficient quantity of adsorbent. Then both mixtures are mixed together on a sheet of paper, by light spatulation (do not triturate). Usually the amount of adsorbent should be equal to the amount of the components of the eutectic mixture.

Eg. Camphor, Menthol, Kaolin - Eutectic powder.

Method-2:

In this method, eutectic substances are first triturated together, in order to force them to liquefy. To this liquid an adsorbent is added, it adsorbs the liquid which is liberated and makes the powder free flowing.

Eg. Insufflation of Camphor, menthol and ammonium chloride.

Dispensing: Eutectic mixtures (powders) consists volatile substances like camphor menthol, thymol etc. Hence to prevent their volatalization, they are dispensed as follows,

1. If eutectic powder is meant for internal use, it should be dispensed in double wrapped paper packets and these packets are then placed in airtight, wide mouthed plastic or glass container.
2. If the eutectic powder is for external use (Eg. Insufflation) that should be dispensed in small shifter top plastic boxes.

Storage: Eutectic powders (mixtures) should be stored in a cool place in an air tight container, to prevent the volatalization of ingredients, at higher temperature.

CAMPHOR - MENTHOL EUTECTIC POWDER

Rx	
Camphorae	gr xx
Mentholis	gr x
Kaolin	gr xxx
Fiat : Pulvis	Mitte : Tales quatuor
Signa : Unus pulvis, b.i.d sumendum.	

Conversion :

gr xx → 20 grains   gr x → 10 grains = 0.6 g

1 grains = 60 mg   gr xxx → 30 grains = 1800 mg (1.8 g)

20 grains = 1200 mg (1.2 g)

Calculation : For (4+1) = 5 powders.

Camphor = 1.2 g X 5 = 6 g

Menthol = 0.6 g X 5 = 3 g

Kaolin = 1.8 g X 5 = 9 g

Total for 5 powders = 18 g

Weight for each powder = $\frac{18}{5}$ = 3.6 g

Type	Ingredients	Quantity in imperial	Quantity in metric	Quantity taken
Compound divided powder, for internal use.	Camphor	20 gr	1.2 g	6 g
	Menthol	10 gr	0.6 g	3 g
	Kaolin	30 gr	1.8 g	9 g
	Make: Powder	Send: Such 4		
	Direction: One powder to be taken, two times a day.			

Theory:

This is a compound divided powder containing eutectic substances like camphor and menthol, which are acts as carminative. Since each of them acts as impurity to each other, when they are mixed together, the melting point of camphor and menthol lowers and also their mixture shows low melting point, than room temperature. Due to lowering of melting point, powder will convert into liquid or semisolid.

To overcome this problem, kaolin is used as adsorbent, which makes the eutectic mixture dry and free flowing. In this case, eutectic powder is prepared, by mixing camphor and menthol with equal quantities of kaolin separately and then both are combined together on a sheet of paper, by light spatulation.

To subdivide the camphor into fine particles, camphor has to dissolve in small portion of alcohol. When alcohol evaporates, camphor will get converted into fine particles.

Procedure:

Since there will be little wastage (loss) during weighing, mixing and dividing, to manipulate these practical losses, calculate the quantity of ingredients for at least one extra powder, than prescribed.

1) Weigh separately camphor, menthol and kaolin, according to the calculation.
2) Dissolve camphor in small quantity of alcohol and allow the alcohol to evaporate, at room temperature.
3) After evaporation of alcohol, camphor gets precipitated as fine powder (sub divided state).
4) Mix this fine powder of camphor, with half of the portion of kaolin by light spatulation separately.
5) Mix menthol with remaining half of the portion of kaolin, by light spatulation, separately.
6) Mix the above two powder blends uniformly with the help of spatula, on a sheet of butter paper (to avoid trituration).
7) Weigh the prescribed amount of powder and enclose in a double wrapper, lined with butter paper. Prepare such four powders (Packets).

Dispensing:

Both camphor and menthol are volatile in nature. Therefore to prevent their volatalization the powder is packed in double wrapper, which is lined with butter paper and transfer these packets into a wide mouthed, air tight plastic or glass container, close tightly with plastic screw cap and label.

Direction: One powder to be taken, two times a day.

Storage: Store in a cool place.

Auxilliary label: STORE IN A COOL PLACE.

Uses: Camphor-menthol eutectic powder is used as, carminative.

Student's exercise:

(1) What is the meaning of Eutectic?
(2) Define eutectic substances. Give examples.
(3) What types of substances are used for dispensing of eutectic substances?
(4) Briefly enumerate the different methods used for preparation of eutectic powders.
(5) How will you dispense the eutectic powders?

46 EXPLOSIVE POWDER

When an oxidizing agent is triturated with a reducing agent, there are chances of violent explosion, due to the pressure applied, which may leads to serious consequences because both acts as incompatible to each other.

Examples for,

Oxidising agents	**Reducing agents**
• Potassium chlorate	• Tannic acid
• Potassium permanganate	• Charcoal
• Potassium nitrate	• Sulphur
• Potassium dichromate	• Sulphides
• Potassium citrate	
• Silver nitrate	

Now-a-days, prescription of such incompatible substances in powder form, is very rare as far as possible. Such prescription should not be dispensed. But in case it is required to be dispensed, then they are dispensed by two methods.

Method-1:

In this method, each ingredient is powdered separately, in separate mortars and then mixed them together lightly, with other ingredients of prescription and dispensed in double wrapped powder packet or in a tightly closed wide mouthed container.

Method-2:

In this method, each ingredient is powdered separately and also dispensed them separately by wrapping in powder packets, with suitable directions to the patients regarding its use.

Eg. Compound powder containing potassium citrate, tannic acid and sucrose powder.

Storage: Explosive powders should be stored in a dry place.

POTASSIUM CITRATE AND TANNIC ACID POWDER

Rx	
Potassi citratis	gr x
Acidi tannici	gr v
Sacchari	gr v
Fiat : Pulvis	Mitte : Tales quatuor
Signa : Solve unus pulvis, cyanthus amplus aqua, utendus gargarisma.	

Conversion :

gr x → 10 grains   gr v → 5 grains = 300 mg (0.3 g)

1 grain = 60 mg

10 grains = 600 mg (0.6 g)

Calculation : For (4+1) = 5 powders.

Potassium citrate	=	0.6 g	X	5	=	3 g
Tannic acid	=	0.3 g	X	5	=	1.5 g
Sucrose	=	0.3 g	X	5	=	1.5 g

Total for five powders					=	6 g
Weight for each powder	=	$\frac{6}{5}$			=	1.2 g

Type	Ingredients	Quantity in imperial	Quantity in metric	Quantity taken
Compound divided powder, for internal use.	Potassium citrate	10 gr	0.66 g	3.3 g
	Tannic acid	5 gr	0.33 g	1.65 g
	Sucrose	5 gr	0.33 g	1.65 g
	Make : Powder Send: Such 4 Direction: Dissolve one powder in a tumblerful of water and to be used as gargle.			

Theory:

This is a compound divided powder for oral use, it contains an oxidizing agent like potassium citrate and reducing agent like tannic acid. As both potassium citrate and tannic acid are incompatible to each other, when they are triturated together, it may result in a violent explosion due to pressure applied.

Hence this powder is dispensed by powdering potassium citrate and tannic acid separately, in separate mortars and then both powders are mixed, lightly with sucrose on a sheet of paper by light spatulation.

Sucrose is used as sweetening agent, to mask the unpleasant (salty) taste of potassium citrate.

Procedure:

There will be little wastage (loss) during weighing, mixing and dividing, hence to manipulate these practical losses, calculate the quantity of ingredients for at least 1 or 2 extra powder, than prescribed.

1) Weigh separately potassium citrate, tannic acid and sucrose, according to calculation.
2) Triturate potassium citrate in a dry mortar, to get fine powder.
3) In a separate mortar triturate tannic acid.
4) On a sheet of butter paper, mix sucrose and tannic acid lightly with spatula, then add potassium citrate powder and mix uniformly.

Dispensing:

Both tannic acid and sucrose are hygroscopic substances. If tannic acid absorbs the moisture, it forms the lumps. Therefore accurately weigh the prescribed amount of powder and enclose in double wrapper, lined with butter paper. Prepare such 4 powders and discard the remaining powder. Transfer these packets into a wide mouthed plastic or glass container, close it tightly and label.

Direction: Dissolve one powder in a tumblerful of water and to be used as gargle.

Storage: Store in a dry place.

Auxilliary label: STORE IN A DRY PLACE.

Uses: Both tannic acid and potassium citrate acts as astringents. Hence this powder is used as astringent.

Student's exercise:

1) Define oxidising and reducing agents and give examples.
2) Define explosive powder.
3) How will you dispense explosive powders?
4) How will you store the explosive powders?

47 POWDERS CONTAINING POTENT MEDICAMENTS

The substances (drugs) having a maximum dose of less than one grain (60 mg) are called as "potent drugs" or " potent medicaments".

Examples for potent drugs,

Drugs		Maximum dose
Hyoscine hydrobromide	---	0.5 mg (0.3 to 0.6 mg)
Codeine phosphate	---	10 – 60 mg
Propranolol	---	10 - 40 mg
Prednisone	---	8 – 10 mg
Phenobarbitone sodium	---	15 mg

Dispensing of such a small dose (quantity) of drug is very difficult, because minimum weighable quantity for potent drugs on dispensing balance is 300 mg. Hence such potent drugs are dispensed by dilution method i.e. the potent drug is triturated with some diluent, like lactose in a definite proportion, to make a weighable quantity.

Generally for dispensing of potent drugs, lactose is used as a diluent because it is white, inert, economical, easily available in market and compatible with large number of drugs.

Method:

1) Reduce the potent powder into fine state, by triturating in a mortar.
2) To this fine powder, add equal quantity of diluent by trituration.
3) To this triturate, incorporate the remaining amount of diluent in successive portion with through trituration each time, until whole of the diluent has been added.

Note: The whole amount of the diluent should never be added to the drug at once, because the potent drug will not be mixed uniformly and thoroughly in the diluent. This results in uneven dose in divided powders.

Dispensing:

Powders containing – potent medicaments are dispensed as individual doses, by wrapping in paper packets (if the drug is hygroscopic in nature, it should be dispensed in double wrapped powder packets) and finally these packets are stored in wide mouthed tightly closed, plastic or glass containers.

Now-a-days, these type of powders are dispensed as sachets or as capsules.

Storage: These powders should be stored at room temperature.

CODEINE PHOSPHATE POWDER

Rx	
Codeine phosphate	$\frac{1}{4}$ gr
Fiat : Pulvis	Mitte : Tales octe
Signa : Unus pulvis nocte sumendum.	

Conversion and Calculation : For (8 + 2) = 10 powders

1 grain = 60 mg

$\frac{1}{4}$ grain = $\frac{1}{4}$ X 60 = 15 mg

For 1 powder, Codeine phosphate = 15 mg

For 10 powder, Codeine phosphate = 15 mg X 10 = 150 mg

The minimum dispensable quantity for a powder is 100 mg

Therefore, the quantity of powder is increased by triturating Codeine phosphate with lactose as,

Lactose = (100 mg X 10 powders - 150 mg Codeine phosphate)
= 1000 - 150
= 850 mg is required

Revised formula for 10 powders :

Codeine phosphate --- 150 mg
Lactose ...q.s.. --- 850 mg

Total weight of powder --- 1000 mg

Therefore weight for each powder = $\frac{1000}{10}$ = 100 mg

100 mg of powder contains = $\frac{150}{1000}$ X 100 = 15 mg

Divide the 1000 mg of final powder mixer into 10 parts (powders), so that each powder weighing 100 mg containing "15 mg" of codeine phosphate.

Type	Ingredients	Quantity in imperial	Quantity in metric	Quantity taken for each powder (packet)
Simple divided powder, containing potent drug.	Codeine phosphate	¼ gr	15 mg	100 mg
	Make: Powder Send: Such 8 Direction: One powder to be taken, at night.			

Theory:

This is a powder containing single potent drug in very small dose, because codeine phosphate is a potent drug having small dose of (10 – 40 mg). In this preparation, the prescribed dose is 15 mg.

This dose is so small that, drug cannot be weighed individually on dispensing balance. Hence it is dispensed using diluent – lactose by dilution method.

Procedure:

Since there will be little wastage (loss) during weighing, mixing and dividing, to manipulate these practical losses, calculate the quantity of ingredients for at least one extra, powder than prescribed.

1) Weigh the required quantity of codeine phosphate and lactose.
2) Triturate both of them in a mortar to get even distribution.
3) From this triturate, weigh the 100 mg of powder and enclose in paper packet. Prepare such 8 packets and discard the remaining powder.

Dispensing: Tie the powder packets by paper ribbon and transfer these packets in a envelope or in tightly closed wide mouthed plastic or glass container.

Storage: Store in a cool place.

Direction: One powder to be taken, at night.

Uses: Codeine phosphate is an alkaloidal salt, which acts as analgesic and antitussive.

HYOSCINE HYDROBROMIDE POWDER

Rx	
Hyoscine hydrobromide	$\frac{1}{100}$ gr
Fiat : Pulvis	Mitte : Tales duodecim
Signa : Unus pulvis, mane at nocte sumendum	

Calculation : For (12+3) = 15 powders

Hyoscine hydrobromide for 1 powder = 1/100 gr

$$\frac{1}{100} \times 60 = 0.6 \text{ mg}$$

Hyoscine hydrobromide for 15 powders = 0.6 x 15 = 9 mg

But 9 mg is not a weighable quantity, because Hyoscine hydrobromide is highly potent medicament. Therefore 15 powders containing, 0.6 mg Hyoscine hydrobromide is prepared by triturating with Lactose in two stages, as shown in calculation.

Stage -1

Mix 300 mg of Hyoscine hydrobromide,

With 4700 mg of Lactose

5000 mg of Triturate

i.e 300 mg of Hyoscine hydrobromide is present in 5000 mg of Triturate

$$\therefore 9 \text{ mg of Hyoscine hydrobromide} = \frac{9}{5000} \times 300 = 150 \text{ mg of Triturate}$$

150 mg of triturate consist = 9 mg of Hyoscine hydrobromide.

Stage -2

The minimum weighable quantity on dispensing balance is, 100 mg (or 2 gr = 120 mg)

For 15 powders = 15 x 100 mg = 1500 mg

= 1500 mg lactose – 150 mg triturate

= 1350 mg of lactose is required.

∴ Take 150 mg of Triturate from stage -1, and mix

With 1350 mg of Lactose

Total =1500 mg for 15 powders

$$\therefore \text{Weight for each powder} = \frac{1500}{15} = 100 \text{ mg}$$

$$100 \text{ mg of powder contains} = \frac{9}{1500} \times 100 = 0.6 \text{ mg}$$

Divide the 1500 mg of final mixture, in to 15 parts.

Each powder weighing 100 mg, containing 0.6 mg of Hyoscine hydrobromide.

Type	Ingredients	Quantity in imperial	Quantity in metric
Simple divided powder, containing potent medicament.	Hyoscine hydrobromide	1/100 gr	0.6 mg
	Make: Powder Send: Such 12 powders		
	Direction: One powder to be taken, morning and night.		

Theory:

This is a powder containing single medicament in very small dose, because hyoscine hydrobromide is a potent drug has the maximum dose 0.3 to 0.6 mg, which acts as sedative and parasympatholytic.

The dose of hyoscine hydrobromide is very small, so that it cannot be weighed individually on dispensing balance. Hence it is dispensed in powder form, by diluting with lactose in suitable proportions, in two stages (by double dilution).

Procedure:

Since there will be little wastage (loss) during weighing, mixing and dividing, to manipulate these practical losses, calculate the ingredients for extra powder, than prescribed.

1) Weigh accurately hyoscine hydrobromide and lactose separately (according to calculation for 1st Stage dilution).
2) Mix them uniformly by triturating in a mortar.
3) From this powder mixture, weigh 150 mg and mix with 1350g of lactose, uniformly in geometric dilution method.

Dispensing: Hyoscine hydrobromide is hygroscopic in nature, therefore weigh 100 mg of powder and pack each powder according to pharmaceutical art, in a double wrapper lined with butter paper. Prepare such15 packets and tie with a paper ribbon. Transfer these packets into a suitable cardboard box or tightly closed wide mouthed plastic container and close it tightly, with plastic screw cap..

Direction: One powder to be taken, morning and night.

Storage: Store in a dry place (At temperature not exceeding 25ºC).

Uses: It is used as a sedative or antidepressant. It is also used as, anti parkinsonism agent.

Student's exercise:

1) What is the meaning of potent substance (medicament)? Give examples.
2) How a potent substance is prepared as powder.
3) What type of containers and packing is necessary for powder containing potent medicament?
4) What is the maximum dose of Hyoscine hydrobromide? What is its use?
5) Why lactose is used as diluent?
6) What is codeine phosphate? What are its uses?
7) Briefly explain, how will you dispense the Hyoscine hydrobromide as powder.

EFFLORESCENT SUBSTANCES

Efflorescent substances are some crystalline substances, which liberate water of crystallization wholly or partly after exposure, to humidity or during trituration and hence become wet or liquefy.

Examples for such substances are caffeine, citric acid, codeine, ferrous sulphate. These types of substances are formulated as powders using their anhydrous salts or by mixing such substance with an inert diluent. Before incorporating with other ingredients, these powders should be dispensed in double wrapper lined with wax paper or packed in wide mouthed plastic or glass container sealed with aluminium foil.

Codeine Phosphate	:	60 mg
Caffeine	:	20 mg.

HYGROSCOPIC AND DELIQUESCENT SUBSTANCES

The substances and powders, which absorb moisture from the atmosphere are called as "hygroscopic substances or hygroscopic powders ". But certain substances absorb moisture in a great extent and they liquefies partially or convert into solution form. Such substances (powders) are called as "deliquescent powder".

Eg.
- Ammonium chloride
- Ammonium citrate
- Ammonium bromide
- Potassium citrate
- Ammonium iodide
- Sodium bromide
- Calcium chloride
- Sodium iodide
- Citric acid
- Tartaric acid
- Iron
- Pepsin
- Hyoscine hydrobromide
- Phenobarbitone sodium

Remedy: For dispensing of such substances in the powder form (as powders), following precautions should be taken, to minimize the absorption of moisture from the atmosphere.

1) The hygroscopic substance should not be dispensed in fine state. They should be dispensed in granular form, in order to expose less surface area to the atmosphere.
2) Further, they should be protected by packing in a double wrapper, lined with wax paper. If the substance is very deliquescent in nature, for further wrapping aluminium foil or plastic cover should be used.

Student's exercise:

1) Define efflorescent substances.
2) Give the examples for efflorescent substances.
3) How will you dispense efflorescent substances as powders?
4) Define hygroscopic substances.
5) What is the difference between hygroscopic and deliquescent substances?
6) List out the hygroscopic and deliquescent substances (drugs).
7) Write the dispensing technique for hygroscopic substances.

48 CACHETS

Latin term: Capsula amylacea or Oblatum.

Cachets are unit solid dosage forms of medicament, in which drug is enclosed in a tasteless sheet of rice flour. Cachets are also called as 'Wafer capsules' or 'Capsula amylacea.'

Cachets are mainly used for encloseing of nauseaous or disagreeable drug substances in large doses, from 0.2 to 2 g of medium density. Cachets are prepared by moulding (enclosing) the powdered drug, in a tasteless sheet. This sheet of rice flour (wafer) is prepared by pouring the mixture of rice flour and water, between two hot polished revolving cylinders. When water evaporates, a sheet of wafer is formed, known as cachet.

For filling, the medicament is palced between two sheets of cachets (wafer), which are then sealed either, by wet or dry sealing method.

BPC includes two cachets,

1) Sodium amino salicylate cachet.
2) Sodium amino salicylate with Isoniazid cachet.

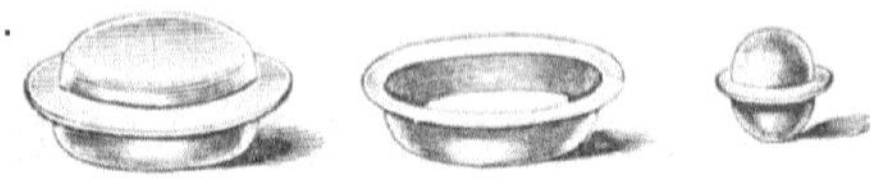

Example for cachets

Sodium amino salicylate is given in a dose of 20 g daily, in the treatment of Tuberculosis. Since dose of drug is high, it is given in the form of cachets of 1.5 to 2 g each (i.e. 10-12 cachets are given per day).

Cachets are very hard to swallow as such, therefore before administration, they should be softened by dipping (immersing) in water for few seconds and placed on the tongue and swallowed with a draught of water. In this way the outer sheet of cachet get softened, but the enclosed drug will remain intact. After swallowing, cachet will disintegrate and powder will be released.

Advantages of cachets:

1) They are easy to prepare, because no complicated machinary is required, compared to tablets.
2) Cachets disintegrate quickly in the stomach.
3) Large doses of drugs can be administered in the form of cachets, compared to tablets and capsules.

Dis-advantages of cachets:

1) They require moistening (softening), before swallowing.
2) They are easily damagable.
3) They can not protect the enclosed drug, from light and moisture.
4) They occupy more space, than the corresponding sizes of capsules or tablets.
5) The contents of cachets can not be greatly compressed, because of the fragile nature of the shells.
6) They are not suitable for filling the drug, by large scale machinary.

Types of Cachets: Cachets are two types,

1 Wet seal cachets

2 Dry seal cachets

(1) Wet seal cachets: These cachets are sealed by moistening the edges with water. A wet seal cachet is made up of two similar convex shaped halves, having flat edges. For sealing, special wet sealing machine is used.

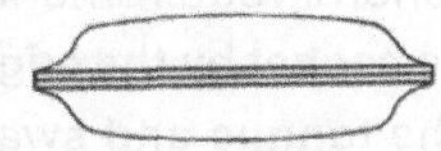

Wet seal cachet

If no machine is available, two wide mouthed bottles may be used for wet sealing. i.e. one half of the cachet is placed on one bottle and a weighed amount of drug is placed in the centre of the cachet. Another half of cachet is placed on the another bottle and its edges is moistened with dump camel's hair brush and superimposed on the first half (first bottle) and pressed the bottles together to get a perfect seal.

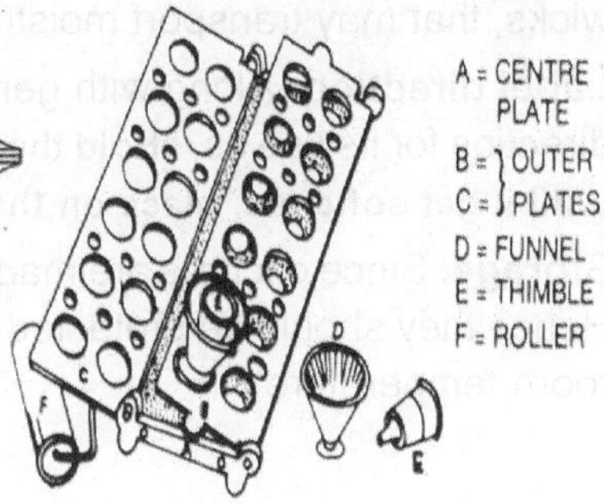

Wet seal cachet machine

After drying for about 15 min at room temperature, cachets should be tested by gently pressing the edges, by rotating between thumb and fore finger.

Example:

- Compound powder of rhubarb and heavy magnesium carbonate.
- Compound mercurous chloride and Sodium bicarbonate, Rhubarb powder are prepared as wet seal cachets.

(2) Dry seal cachets: These cachets are sealed, without using moisture (water). These cachets consists two halves, the upper half and lower half. The diameter of upper half is slightly larger than the lower half.

The powdered drug is filled in the lower half and upper half is fitted over it. The filled cachets are then sealed in a dry sealing machine, by pressing the two halves and removed, as shown in fig.

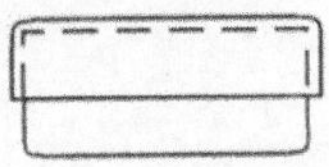

Dry seal cachet

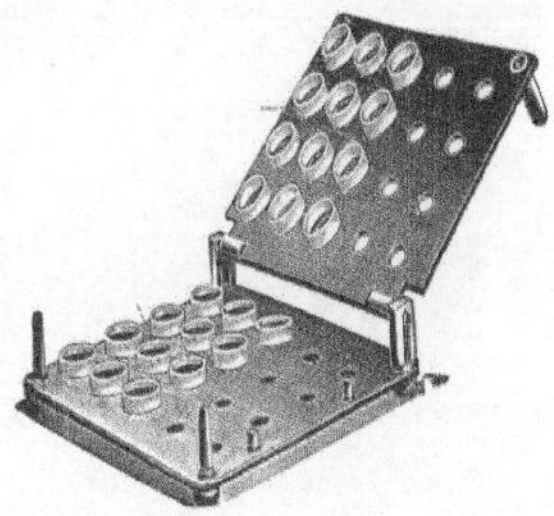

Dry seal cachet machine

Example:

- Sodium amino salicylate and Isoniazid.
- Phenacetin and Caffeine
- Rhubarb powder, Sodium bicarbonate and Eucalyptus oil are prepared as dry seal cachets.

Dispensing (Packing) of cachets: Since cachets are made from sheet of rice flour, they are fragile and hygroscopic in nature. Hence they should be protected from moisture and crushing. Therefore cachets are dispensed in wide mouthed plastic containers or tin containers or vial made up of compartments, in which cachets are packed on their edges or lying flat.

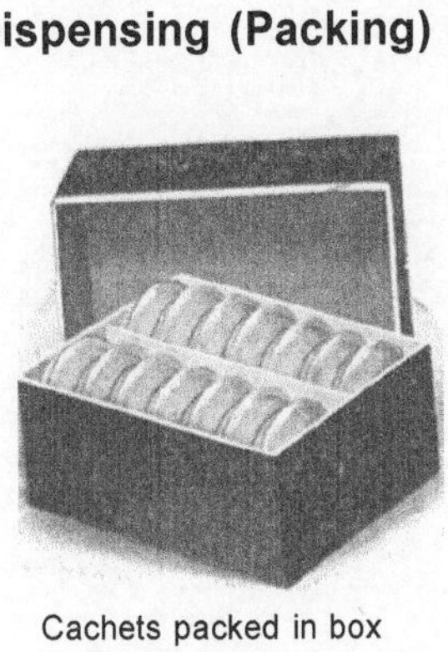

Cachets packed in box

If necessary the compartments may be filled with plastic foam, to prevent the cachets from breaking (movement), due to abrasion during transport. Cotton wool is unsuitable (should not be used) because it adheres to the cachets and fibres may be trapped between the closure and neck of the vial (bottle), these forming minute wicks, that may transport moisture, into the bottle.

Label direction: Along with general requirements of label, cachets should bear a label direction for its use as, **"Hold the cachet by the edge and immerse in water for few seconds until it get softened, place on the tongue and swallow with a draught of water."**

Storage: Since cachets are made from sheet of rice flour, they are hygroscopic in nature. Hence they should be protected from moisture and they should be stored in dry place (at room temperature).

CACHET OF POWDERED RHUBARB

Rx	
Rehi pulverati	gr vii ss
Heavy magnesi carbonatis	gr vii ss
Fiat : Capsula amylacea	Mitte : Tales sex
Signa : Unus capsula amylacea sumendum, post jentaculam.	

Conversion:

gr vii ss → 7.5 grains

15 grains = 1 g

7.5 grains = 0.5 g

Calculation : For 6+2 = 8 Cachets.

Rhubarb powder = 0.5 x 8 = 4 g

Heavy magnesium carbonate = 0.5 x 8 = 4 g.

Type	Ingredients	Quantity in imperial	Quantity in metric	Quantity taken
Cachet, prepared	Powdered rhubarb	7.5 gr.	0.5 g	4 g
by wet sealing	Heavy magnesium carbonate	7.5 gr	0.5 g	4 g
method.	Make: Cachet	Send: Such six.		
	Direction : One cachet to be taken, after break fast.			

Theory:

Rhubarb powder acts as purgative and heavy magnesium carbonate acts as laxative. Hence these are formulated as cachet and used in the evacuation of bowel, during constipation. This cachet is prepared by wet sealing method.

Procedure: If no machine is available for preparation of sheat of rice flour or wafer (cachet) , lozenge board and roller can be used.

A) Preparation of sheat of Rice flour or wafer (cachet)

1) Take a required amount of very fine powder of rice flour in a mortar and add a little amount of water, to make it as a smooth damp mass.
2) Role the mass on a "lozenge board" with the help of roller, for uniform thickness. Before rolling the mass, board and roller should be dusted either with starch, lactose or talc, to prevent the sticking of mass to the board and roller.
3) When the mass is rolled for uniform thickness, a sample cachet is cut with the help of sperical shaped punch, to determine the correct size, shape and thickness of cachet (wafer).
4) If the cachet of suitable thickness, shape and size is obtained, then cut the required number of cachets (wafer) by punch.
5) Spread these cachets (wafer) on a sheat of butter paper or perforated tray and dry at room temperature.

B) Preparation of cachet by wet seal method:

If no machine is available, use two small wide mouthed bottles, for preparation of cachets by wet sealing.

1) Place one of the cachet, on the mouth of one bottle and lightly press at the middle of cachet, to make depression.
2) Accurately weigh rhubarb powder and heavy magnesium carbonate, mix them uniformly in a mortar and place at the centre of the cachet.
3) Place another half of the cachet on another bottle and moisten it's edges with water using dump camel hair brush.
4) Super impose the cachet by inverting the second bottle, press both the bottles together, to get a perfect seal.
5) After preparation of cachets, place them on a white sheet or tile (slab) and allow them for drying, at room temperature for 15 minutes.
6) After drying, cachets should be tested by gently pressing the edges, by rotating between thumb and fore finger.

Dispensing: Select six good cachets which are having perfect seal and pack in wide mouthed plastic or tin container made up of compartments, to prevent the breaking (movement) during transportation. If necessary fill the compartments with plastic foam.

Direction: One cachet to be taken, after breakfast.

Label direction: Hold the cachet by the edge and immerse in water, for few seconds until it get softened and then swallow with a draught of water.

Storage: Store at room temperature

Uses: This cachet is used as laxative (purgative), during constipation.

Similar example for cachet

Rx.

Sodium amino salicylate	1.25 g
Isoniazid	25 mg
Fiat : Capsalama amylacea	Mittee : Tales Decem

Signa : Unus capsula amylacea quartis horis sumendum.

Uses: This cachet is used, in the treatment of tuberculosis.

Question bank:

1) Define cachets.
2) What are the other names for cachets?
3) Which are the cachets official in BPC ?
4) What are the advantages and disadvantages of cachets?
5) Classify the cachets with examples.
6) How will you dispense the cachets?
7) Comments : Cotton wool should not be used, for filling the compartments of cachets container.
8) What direction will you write on the label of cachets?
9) How the cachets are administered ?
10) Briefly explain, how will you prepare cachets by wet sealing.
11) How much dose (quantity) of drug can be incorporated in the cachets?

49 TABLET TRITURATES (T.T.)

Synonym: Moulded tablets or Compressed powders

Latin term: Tabletta

Tablet triturates are powders, moulded into tablets, which are flat, circular disk shaped, prepared by forcing the soft mass into the cavities of the tablet triturate mould. Therefore tablet triturates are also called as "Moulded tablets" or "Compressed powders". Generally potent medicaments and highly toxic drugs, in small doses are prepared in the form of tablet triturates.

Since the medicaments are potent, their dose will be, very less so that, they cannot be compressed into tablets alone. Therefore potent drug is mixed with certain inert diluent like lactose, dextrose or sucrose by trituration and then compressed in to tablets. Hence 'compressed powder' is also called as 'tablet triturates'.

Eg. Potent drugs used in T.T

- Strychnine hydrochloride
- Atropine sulphate
- Morphine
- Calomel (Mercurous chloride)
- Codeine phosphate

Displacement value of medicaments:

For preparation of tablet triturates, "Displacement value" of the medicament should be considered, because the capacity of mould remains same and a particular mould gives a same size of tablet triturates (tablets) but their weight will varies. This variation is due to the differences in the density of the medicament and the diluent.

> Note : For further details of displacement value and its calculation, students are required to see the page no. 393

1) When the proportion (weight) of medicament in a tablet triturate is very small and density difference between medicament and diluent is not so great then, ignore the displacement value of the medicament.
2) If proportion (weight) of medicament is appreciable and density differs considerably than that of diluent (lactose), a suitable correction should be done, using displacement value of the medicament.

Types of Tablet triturates: Tablet triturates are of two types,

1) **Moulded tablets** (Tablet triturates or Dispensing tablets): These tablets are meant for oral administration. They retain their shape, under normal conditions. They are administered by placing them on the tongue and swallowed whole, with a drink of water or they are also administered by crushing into powder.

   Now-a-days, Dispensing tablets are replaced by Compressed tablets or Capsules, to eliminiate the necessity of weighing small quantities of potent substances.

2) **Hypodermic tablets:** These tablets are meant for parenteral administration i.e. tablets will be dissolved in water for injection and resulting solution is injected hypodermically.

   Since the solutions prepared from hypodermic tablets are rarely sterile and now-a-days number of sterile parenteral solutions are available in the market, hypodermic tablets are not used.

Preparation: Tablet triturates are prepared by "Tablet trituration machine". It is made up of stainless steel or plastic. It consists two plates, upper plate and lower plate.

Lower plate consists of 50 to 200 pegs and upper plate consists perforations (holes), exactly the same number of pegs in lower plate. The moulds are available in several sizes, having capacity ranging from 30 to 250 mg. The capacity of mould will be mentioned on their back side.

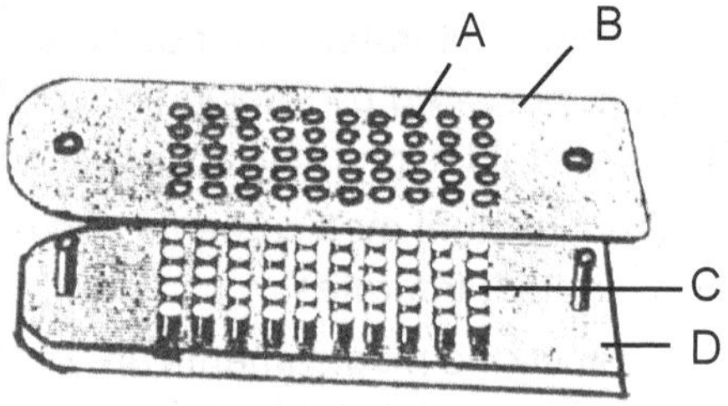

A = Hole B = Upper plate

C = Pegs D = Lower plate

Tablet triturate mould

General method for preparation of tablet triturates:

1) Dilute the potent medicament with a suitable diluent, like lactose, dextrose, sucrose or a mixture of lactose and sucrose by trituration.
2) Using a suitable dilution of alcohol (Usually 60% of alcohol), prepare a soft mass of medicament and diluent.
3) Place the upper plate of the machine on a clean tile or white sheet and press the soft mass into the holes completely, with the help of spatula and remove the excess amount of mass by spatula.
4) After filling, place the upper plate over the lower plate and apply little pressure over the top plate, which will force the plate downward, leaving the moulded tablets on the projected pegs.
5) Spread the ejected tablets as a single layer, on a sheet of paper and dry them by keeping in hot air oven or at room temperature.
6) Generally 50 – 200 tablet triturates can be prepared at a time from a "tablet triturate mould". But now-a days, automatic tablet punching machines (Tablet compressing machines) are available, which can prepare 2500-3000 tablets per minute.

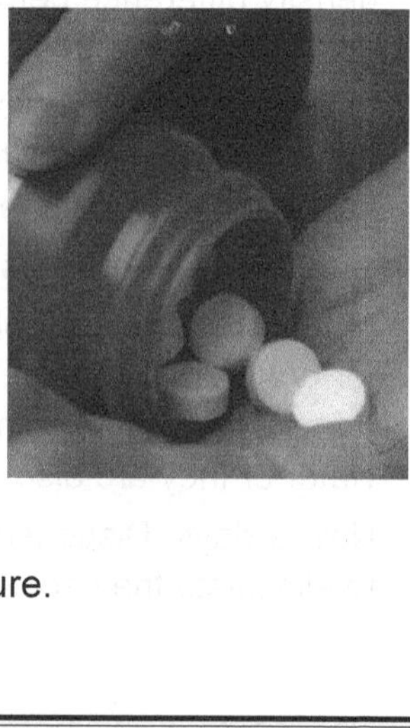

Dispensing (Packing): Since tablet triturates (moulded tablets) are susceptible to crushing and they may deteriorate due to atmospheric moisture, they should be protected by storing in air tight containers. Packing is also done by placing the tablet triturates in a single row, in a narrow tube, sealed with a plug type plastic closure.

Storage: Tablet triturates should be stored at room temperature.

TABLET TRITURATE OF STRYCHNINE HYDROCHLORIDE

Rx	
Strychnine hydrochloride	$\frac{1}{60}$ gr
Fiat: Tabletta	Mitte : Tales quinquaginta
Signa: Unas tabletta, post cibos sumendum.	

Calculation: For (50+10) = 60 tablet triturates.

In this preparation, the weight of Strychnine hydrochloride is very less and density difference is not so great. Therefore ignore the displacement value of strychnine hydrochloride and do not consider for calculation of the quantity of lactose.

The mould capacity is usually 1.5 grains or 100 mg

i.e. For 60 T.T = 60 x 100 mg = 6000 mg (6 g) of total mass

Strychnine hydrochloride for 1 T.T = $\frac{1}{60}$ gr

1 gr = 60 mg so, $\frac{1}{60}$ gr = $\frac{1 \times 60}{60}$ = 1 mg

For 60 T.T = 1 x 60 = 60 mg

Since, Strychnine hydrochloride is a potent drug '60 mg' is not a weighble quantity. Because the minimum weighable quantity for potent drug on dispensing balance is 300 mg.

∴ Tablet triturate is prepared by "Double dilution method" using Lactose as a diluent in two stages as shown below,

Stage- 1 :

Mix 300 mg of Strychnine hydrochloride with 300 mg of Lactose = 600 mg of Triturate.

i.e. 600 mg of triturate contains = 300 mg of Strychnine hydrochloride.

Therefore for 60 mg of strychnine hydrochloride $= \frac{600}{300} \times 60$

= 120 mg of triturate is required

Stage- 2 :

For 60 T.T = 60 X 100 mg = 6000 mg of lactose is required.

∴ 6000 mg of lactose - 120 mg of triturate = 5880 mg of lactose is required.

Mix 120 mg of triturate from stage-1 with 5880 mg of Lactose.

To this triturate add alcohol 60%, sufficient to make soft mass and use for the preparation of T.T.

Revised formula for 60 T.T

Triturate from stage 1 --- 120 mg (≅ 60 mg of Strychnine hydrochloride)

Lactose --- 5880 mg

Alcohol (60%) --- ....q.s...to make mass

Type	Ingredients	Quantity in imperial	Quantity in metric	Quantity taken
Unit solid dosage form - for oral use	Strychnine hydrochloride	1/60 gr	1 mg	60 mg
	Make: Tablet triturate Send: such 50			
	Direction: One tablet triturate to be taken, after meals.			

Theory:

Strychnine hydrochloride is an alkaloidal salt, obtained from the seeds of Strychnus nux-vomica, which acts as central stimulant. Strychnine hydrochloride is a highly potent drug, because it has maximum dose of 1-8 mg. Therefore it cannot be compressed alone as tablets. Hence it is formulated as tablet triturate using lactose as a diluent.

For preparation of 60 tablet triturates, 60 mg of strychnine hydrochloride is required, but 60 mg is not a weighable quantity on dispensing balance. The minimum weighable quantity for potent medicament is 300 mg. Therefore, Tablet triturates of Strychnine hydrochloride is prepared by "double dilution method" with lactose in two stages. Alcohol (60%) is used as a vehicle (Wetting agent) to prepare a soft mass. After preparation of tablet triturate, alcohol evaporates due to its high volatility.

Procedure: Since there will be little wastage during weighing , mixing and preparation, calculate the quantity of ingredients to 5 or 10 extra numbers, than prescribed.

1) Weigh accurately 300 mg of strychnine hydrochloride and 300 mg of lactose. Mix them uniformly by trituration. (Stage-1)
2) From the Stage-1, weigh 120 mg of triturate and triturate with required amount of lactose. (stage-2)
3) To the triturate of stage-2, add alcohol, quantity sufficient to prepare a soft mass.
4) Press this mass into the perforations of the upper plate and press on the pegs of the lower part of the tablet triturate mould.
5) Collect the ejected tablets and arrange in a single row and dry at room temperature, upto complete volatalisation of alcohol (dry at 60 °C in hot air oven.)

Dispensing: After drying, select good 50 tablet triturates and pack in a single row, in a narrow mouthed tube and tightly close with plug type closure or pack in a wide mouthed glass/ plastic container.

Direction: One tablet triturate to be taken, after meals.

Storage: Store in a dry place (At room temperature, not exceeding 25 °C)

Uses: These tablets triturates are used as stimulant.

TABLET TRITURATE OF CALOMEL

Rx	
Calomel	$\frac{1}{30}$ gr
Fiat : Tabletta	Mitte : Vigini quinque
Signa : Unas tabletta, t.i.d post cibos sumendum.	

Calculation : For (25+5) = 30 Tablet triturates

Calomel is very heavy in nature, (has high density), therefore consider the displacement value of Calomel for the determining the quantity of lactose required.

$\frac{1}{30}$ gr = 2 mg (i.e 1 gr = 60 mg so, $\frac{1}{30}$ gr = $\frac{1 \times 60}{30}$ = 2 mg)

For one T.T, Calomel required = 2 mg

For 30 T.T, Calomel required = 2 x 30 = 60 mg

Consider the mould capacity is 1.5 grains or 100 mg.

∴ For 30 T.T : 30 x 100 = 3000 mg of total mass

Displacement value of calomel = 3.74

Therefore 60 mg of Calomel displaces = $\frac{60}{3.74}$ = 16.04 mg of lactose

∴ The quantity of lactose required = 3000-16.04 mg = 2983 mg

Revised formula for 30 T.T:

Calomel --- 60 mg

Lactose --- 2983 mg

Alcohol (60%) --- ..q.s..

Type	Ingredients	Quantity in imperial	Quantity in metric	Quantity taken
Unit solid dosage form, for oral use.	Calomel	1/30 gr	2 mg	60 mg
	Make: Tablet triturate Send: Such 25			
	Direction: One tablet triturate to be taken, after meals.			

Theory:

Calomel is nothing but Mercurous chloride, which acts as cathartic. It is heavy in nature. i.e it has high density. Therefore its displecement value is 3.74 and hence this value should be considered for calculation of lactose.

Procedure: Since there will be little wastage (loss) during weighing, mixing and preparation, to manipulate these practical losses, calculate the quantity of ingredients for at least 5-10 extra than, prescribed.

1) Weigh the required amount of calomel and lactose. Mix them uniformly by trituration.
2) To the triturate, add 60% of alcohol and bind or knead, to get a soft mass.
3) Press this soft mass, into the perforations of the upper plate.

4) Collect the moulded tablets and arrange in a single row and dry at room temperature, upto complete volatalisation of alcohol. (or dry at 60 °C in hot air oven.)

Dispensing: After drying, select good 25 tablet triturates and pack in a single row, in a narrow mouthed tube and tightly close with plug type closure or pack in a wide mouthed glass/ plastic container.

Direction: One tablet triturate to be taken, after meals.

Storage: Store in a dry place (At room temperature, not exceeding 25 °C)

Uses: Calomel tablet triturate is used as cathartic.

Student's exercise:

1) Define Tablet triturates.
2) Comment: Tablets triturates are also called as compressed powders or moulded tablets.
3) Give reason : Why drugs are formulated into tablet triturates?
4) Give the examples for medicaments, which are used in formulation of tablet triturates.
5) What is the capacity of tablet triturate mould?
6) Define displacement value. Why displacement value of medicament should be considered in tablet triturates ?
7) Enlist briefly, the steps involved in the preparation of tablet triturates.
8) Explain how will you dispense the Tablet triturates.
9) Which solvent is used for preparation of Tablet triturates ? Give reason
10) Why lactose is used in preparation of Tablet triturates?
11) Write the uses of Strychnine hydrochloride Tablet triturates.

50 LOZENGES

Latin term : Lozenge- Trochiscus

Lozenges - Troches.

Lozenges are unit solid dosage forms, containing medicament in a sweetened and flavoured base, intended to dissolve slowly in the mouth.

They are mainly used for prolonged action of the medicament, i.e. they are used to give local action on the throat, and to medicate the mouth and throat. Along with medicament they usually consists sugar, flavouring agent and a strong binding agent (gum). Binding agent gives hardness, cohesiveness and ensuring slow release of medicament. Due to the presence of binding agent (gum), lozenges do not disintegrate in the mouth, but dissolves slowly and liberates the active medicament.

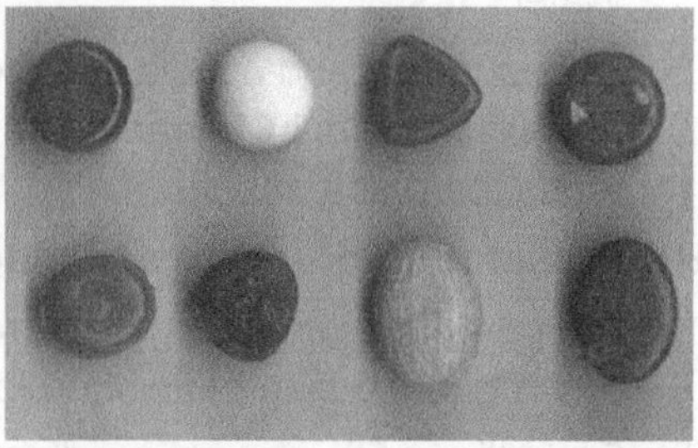

Lozenges

The high contents (concentration) of sugar and gum, produce a sticky solution in the mouth, that causes the medicament to adhere, to the affected surfaces of the throat.

Lozenges are available in various shapes and sizes like round, disc shaped, ablong, oval, rectangle, octagonal, triangle or cylindrical shape as shown in the figure. They usually have weight of 1- 2 g.

Examples: For medicaments used in lozenges.

1)	Antiseptics	Benzalkonium chloride, Formaldehyde
2)	Local anesthetics	Benzocaine
3)	Anti-inflammatory agents	Hydrocortisone
4)	Anti-fungal agents	Amphotericin
5)	Antibiotics	Penicillin
6)	Anti-tussive	Codeine phosphate
7)	Expectorants	Liquorice extract

Preparation of Lozenges: Lozenges are prepared by two methods,

1) By moulding (Moulded lozenges)
2) By compressing (Compressed lozenges).

1) By moulding method: It is a traditional method and most widely used for preparation of lozenges. Lozenges are prepared by moulding method, using 'Lozenge board' and a "roller", as shown in figure.

A) Preparation of mass (base) for lozenges :

The most important stage in the preparation of lozenges is the formation of "lozenge mass". Basically the mass is made up of medicament, powdered sucrose, gum (binding agent), and water. (In certain cases, inert substance like, starch or dextrose is used, to give body or form for lozenges).

Powdered acacia and water are included in the BPC lozenges because, they unite the ingredients to form a mass sufficiently plastic to be rolled and cut without crumbling.

Eg. Simple base

Sucrose (Fine powder) --- 100 g

Acacia (Fine powder) --- 7 g

Water ..q.s... --- to make mass

Take sucrose and acacia in a mortar and add water in small portions, until tough like mass is formed, by kneading and working. Kneading should be continued until mass tends to be soft enough.

B) Preparation of lozenges using base: (Rolling and Cutting)

1) After preparation of soft mass, record the weight of the mass, to determine the size of finished lozenges.
2) For rolling of the mass, use "lozenge board" and "roller". Before rolling and during rolling, board and roller should be dusted either with lactose, starch or talc, to prevent sticking.
3) Roll the mass uniformly on the board by roller.
4) When the mass gets uniform thickness, cut a sample lozenge to determine the correct size, in order to obtain the proper weight.
5) Lozenges can cut from the rolled mass, using punches of specific shape or using "Franciscus lozenge cutter". (Franciscus lozenge cutter is a spring plunges, which ejects the lozenges after cutting.)

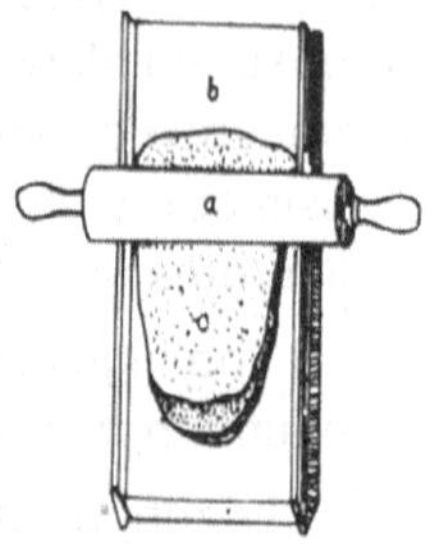

a = Roller
b = Lozenge Board
C = Soft mass(base)

> **Note:** If Franciscus lozenge cutter or punches are not available, students are required to use the caps (closures) of the bottles, to cut the lozenges.

6) After cutting the lozenges, place them on a slab or perforated tray dusted over with starch or talc and dry for 24 hours in a hot air oven at 40 °C to obtain uniform hardness.

Eg. BPC includes two lozenges, prepared by the moulding (traditional) method. Both lozenges are prepared, by using simple base.

A. Compound Bismuth lozenge BPC. consists,
Bismuth carbonate
Calcium carbonate
Heavy Magnesium carbonate
Rose oil
Simple base

B. Liquorice lozenge BPC: (**Synonym**: Brompton cough lozenges) consists,
Liquorice extract
Anise oil
Simple base

2) **By Compression method:** In this method, lozenges are prepared by tabletting technique, using "Tablet compression machine" with the following modifications, to ensure slow disintegration.

a) By applying of very high compression.
b) Without the addition of disintegrant.
c) By incorporating high percentage of binding agent, usually above 50% of sucrose and gum acacia or tragacanth.

Method: In this method, medicament, sucrose and binding agent are mixed together with water, to make a damp mass and this damp mass is passed through the sieve, to obtain granules. These granules are dried and compressed into lozenges, at a high pressure as in tablet compressing machine of specific shape and sizes.

Some medicaments are adversely affected (deteriorate) by the moisture and temperature, which are used for the preparation of granules. In such cases, lozenges are prepared by compressing the mixture of medicament, with previously prepared and dried granules of sucrose or lactose.

Similarly to prevent the volatalization of flavouring agents, they are added after granulation.

Eg. Volatile ingredients like, para-formaldehyde and essential oils are added, after granulation.

Menthol and oils like, lemon oil, anise oil, and eucalyptus oil are dissolved in alcohol and sprayed on to the granules.

Examples for Compressed lozenges

1) **Benzalkonium lozenges:**
Menthol
Thymol
Eucalyptus oil
Lemon oil
Benzalkonium chloride solution
Sucrose or starch

2) **Compound Benzocaine lozenges:**
Benzocaine
Borax
Menthol
Starch or Sucrose

3) **Formaldehyde lozenges** (Formalin throat tablets) :
Para-formaldehyde
Citric acid
Menthol
Lemon oil
Starch or sucrose

4) Hydrocortisone lozenges:

Hydrocortisone sodium succinate

Starch or sucrose

Lemon oil

5) Penicillin lozenges:

Benzyl penicillin

Packing of Lozenges :

Lozenges become mould (soft) in damp conditions, therefore they should packed in air tight containers. Now-a-days, compressed lozenges are packed in strip or blister backings similar to compressed tablets, or packed as individual blister sachets or in a wide mouthed, air tight plastic / glass container.

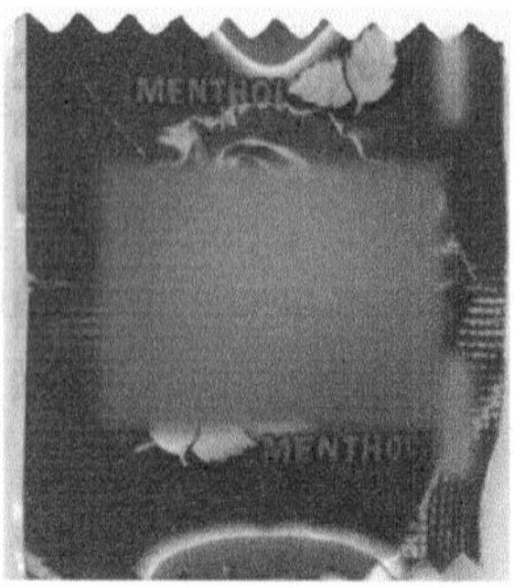

Lozenges packed in sachets

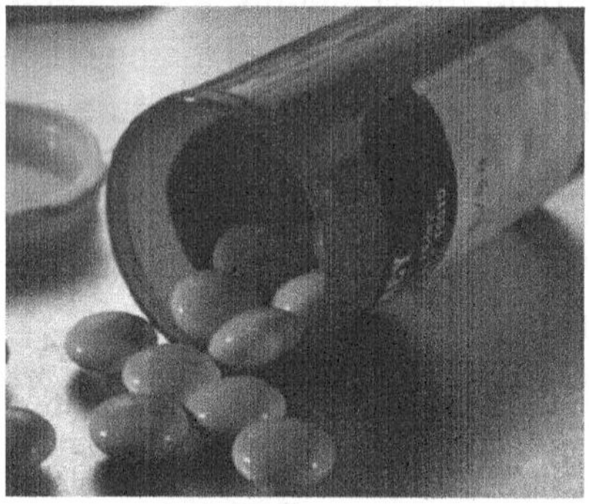

Lozenges packed in wide mouthed container

Storage: Lozenges should be stored in a dry place (at room temperature). In certain cases cool storage is particularly important, when the ingredients or additives are volatile in nature.

COMPOUND BISMUTH LOZENGE B.P.C.

Rx		
Calcii carbonatis	gr ii ss	
Bismuthi carbonatis	gr v	
Heavy magnesii carbonatis	gr ii ss	
Olei rosue	..q.s..	
Simple base….q.s….	gr xv	
Fiat : Trochiscus	Mitte : Tales Quindecim	
Signa : Unus trouchiscus sugendus lente, quatris horis.		

Conversion :

gr v → 5 grains gr ii ss → 2.5 gr = 150 mg

1 gr = 60 mg gr xv → 15 grains = 1 g

5 grains = 300 mg (0.3 g)

Calculation: For (15+5) = 20 lozenges,

Weight of each lozenges is 1 g

For 20 lozenges,

Calcium carbonate = 0.15 x 20 = 3 g

Bismuth carbonate = 0.3 x 20 = 6 g

Heavy magnesium carbonate= 0.15 x 20 = 3 g

Simple base = 8 g

Formula for Simple base for 100 g **Total = 20 g**

Sucrose (Fine powder) = 100 g

Acacia (Fine powder) = 7 g

Water = ..q.s..

But, for 8 g of simple base

$$\text{Sucrose} = \frac{100}{100} \times 8 = 8 \text{ g}$$

$$\text{Acacia} = \frac{7}{100} \times 8 = 0.56 \text{ g}$$

Water …q.s.. = to make mass

Type	Ingredients	Quantity in imperial	Quantity in metric	Quantity taken
Unit solid dosage form	Calcium carbonate	2.5 gr	150 mg	3 g
	Bismuth carbonate	5 gr	300 mg	6 g
	Heavy magnesium carbonate	2.5 gr	150 mg	3 g
Lozenge	Rose oil of commerce	..q.s..	..q.s.	..q.s..
	Simple base….q.s...	15 gr	1 g	20
	Prepare: Lozenge Send: Such 20 Direction: One lozenge to be sucked slowly, every four hours.			

Theory :

Bismuth carbonate acts as anti-diarrhoeal agent. Calcium carbonate and heavy magnesium carbonate acts as antacids. All the ingredients are mixed and prepared as lozenges, using simple base. Simple base is made up of 100 parts of sucrose and 7 parts of acacia gum and water, sufficient to make base. Orange oil is used as flavouring agent.

These lozenges are prepared by moulding method.

Procedure: Since there will be little wastage during the weighing, mixing, punching (preparation), to compensate these practical losses calculate the quantity of ingredients, for at least 15% more, than prescribed.

1) Accurately weigh bismuth carbonate, calcium carbonate and heavy magnesium carbonate and mix uniformly in a mortar.
2) To the powder mixture, add simple base and knead to produce a mass of required consistency at the end, add rose oil and knead the mass, take the weight of the mass (i.e. 'A' g for 20 lozenges.)
3) Dust the lozenge board and roller, either with lactose, starch or talc, to prevent sticking of mass to the board and roller. Roll the mass uniformly on the board, by roller.
4) Cut a sample lozenge with the help of a suitable sized and shaped punch, to determine thickness, shape and consistency. If that lozenge is found to be satisfactory, cut the lozenges of required number and take the weight of them. (It should be A/20 g.)
5) If more or less, adjust the thickness of mass by rolling such that, to get appropriate A/20 by trial and error method.
6) After punching of lozenges, place them on a slab or perforated tray, which is previously dusted with starch or talc and dry for 24 hours in a hot air oven, at 40 °C to obtain uniform hardness.

Dispensing: After complete drying of lozenges, select good 15 lozenges and pack in a tightly closed wide mouthed glass container and label.

Direction: One lozenge to be sucked slowly, every four hours.

Storage: Store in a dry place (or at room temperature not exceeding 25°C)

Uses: Compound bismuth lozenges are used, as anti-diarrhoeal and antacid in the problem of indigestion (dyspepsia).

LIQUORICE LOZENGES B.P.C

Synonym: Brompton cough lozenges

RX	
Liquorice extract	gr iv
Anise oil	M ½
Simple base....q.s...	gr xv
Fiat : Trochiscus	Mitte Tales Vigini quinque
Signa : Unus trochiscus omni hora, sugendus lente.	

Conversion: gr iv → 4 grains   1 Minim = 0.06 ml

1 grain = 60 mg   ½ Minim = 0.03 ml

4 grains = 240 mg

gr xv → 15 grains = 1 g

Calculation for (25+5) = 30 lozenges,

Weight of each lozenges is 1 g

For 30 lozenges,

Liquorice extract	=	240 x 30 = 7.2 g
Anise oil	=	0.03 x 30 = 0.9 ml
Simple base	=	21.9 g ≅ 22 g

		Total = 30 g

Simple base for 100 g:

Sucrose (Fine powder)	100 g
Acacia (Fine powder)	7 g
Water	..q.s..

But for 22 g:

Sucrose = $\frac{100}{100} \times 22 = 22$ g

Acacia = $\frac{7}{100} \times 22 = 1.54$g

Water = …q.s..

Type	Ingredients	Quantity in imperial	Quantity in metric	Quantity taken
Unit solid dosage form	Liquorice extract	4 gr	240 mg	7.2 g
	Anise oil	½ minim	0.03 ml	0.9 ml
	Simple base….q.s...	15 gr	1 g	30 g
	Prepare: Lozenge Send: Such 25 Direction: One lozenge to be sucked slowly, at every one hour.			

Theory:

Extract of Liquorice is prepared by dried root and stolons of Glycyrrhiza glabra. It consists tri-terpenoid saponin, known as glycyrrhizin, which acts as expectorant and demulscent. Therefore extract of liquorice is used for preparation lozenge, for relieving a cough. Anise oil is used as flavouring agent.

These lozenges are prepared by moulding method, using simple base or vehicle (base).

Procedure:

Since there will be little wastage during the weighing, mixing, punching (preparation), to compensate these practical losses, calculate the quantity of ingredients for at least 15%, more than required.

1) Take required amount of liquorice extract and simple base in a mortar and knead them, to get a soft mass of required consistency. At the end, add Anise oil and knead to distribute the oil uniformly. Take the weight of mass (i.e. for 'A' g for 30 lozenges).
2) Dust the lozenge board and roller either with lactose, starch or talc to prevent sticking the mass to board and roller. Roll the mass uniformly, on the board by roller.
3) Cut a sample lozenge with the help of a suitable sized and shaped punch, to determine thickness, shape and consistency. If that lozenge is found to be satisfactory, cut the lozenges of required number and take the weight of them. It should be A/30 g.
4) If more or less, adjust the thickness of mass by rolling, such that to get appropriate A/30, by trial and error method.
5) After punching of lozenges, place them on a slab or perforated tray, which is previously dusted with starch or talc and dry for 24 hours in a hot air oven, at 40°C to obtain uniform hardness.

Dispensing: After complete drying of lozenges, select good 25 lozenges and pack in a tightly closed glass container and label.

Direction: One lozenge to be sucked slowly, at every one hour.

Storage: Store in a dry place (At room temperature, not exceeding 25°C)

Uses: Liquorice lozenges are used, as expectorant and demulscent.

Student's exercise:

1) Define Lozenges. Why they are used ?
2) What is the synonym for lozenges?
3) Comment : Lozenges will disintegrate fastly in the mouth.
4) Why sugar is used in the preparation of Lozenges.
5) Which binding agents are used in Lozenges and why?
6) What are the shapes and sizes of Lozenges?

7) List out the medicaments used in Lozenges and give examples.
8) Classify the Lozenges.
9) What are the basic ingredients of Lozenge base?
10) Comment - Before rolling of the mass, “Lozenge board” and “roller” should be dusted.
11) Which substances are used for dusting of Lozenge board and roller?
12) Give the examples for Lozenges which are available in market.
13) What is “Brompton cough lozenges” ?
14) Comment : Lozenges should be stored in dry place.

51 PASTILLES

Latin term : Pastillus

Pastilles are solid medicated preparations, intended to dissolve slowly in the mouth. Pastilles are similar to lozenges, but they are comparatively softer and transparent, than lozenges and generally contain medicament in gelatin or glycero-gelatin base.

Eg. Only two pastilles are official in BPC

1) Squill pastille
2) Opiate pastille (Synonym: Gee's linctus or Gee's pastille.)

These two pastilles are used, for their mild expectorant activity.

Examples for Pastille's base :

Glycero-gelatin pastille base BPC : This base is used for preparation of squill pastille and Opiate pastille, but it gives soft product, hence quickly dissolves in the mouth. Therefore some modifications are made to make the base hard, by adding agar or sugar in place of some quantity of the gelatin. These bases are less quickly soluble, compare to the glycerol-gelatin base. But this modification has slight disadvantage that, it makes the base opaque.

Examples :

(1) Soft base :

Gelatin	----	1 part
Glycerin	----	2.5 parts
Water	----	2.5 parts

(2) Firm base :

Gelatin	----	30g
Glycerin	----	75g
Acacia	----	8g
Aromatic water	----	60g

(3) More firm base :

Acacia gum	----	18 parts
Sugar	----	6 parts
Water	----	80 parts

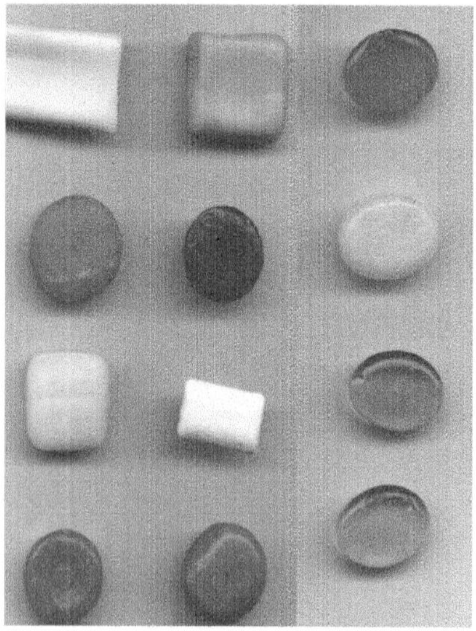

Differents shapes of pastilles

- Since the medicament is intended to have a prolonged local action, the base should be firm enough to ensure that, the pastilles should dissolve very slowly.
- Due to high gelatin content in Glycero-gelatin pastilles, produce a sticky solution in the mouth than lozenges. This property is an advantage, when a local action like antiseptic or anesthetic effect is required in mouth or throat.

- All pastilles are sweetened and flavoured. Some pastilles are dusted with sugar crystallized. Gelatin pastilles usually have weight about – 2 g.

Preparation : Pastilles are prepared by moulding method, using specific shape and sized mould, which is made up of metal. This metal mould consist number of "saucer shaped" cavities.

1) Soften the gelatin in water with the help of heat and add glycerin.
2) Continue the heating, until a clear solution is obtained.
3) Add the medicament to the above glycero-gelatin solution, just before the solution get stiffens, and stir until the mass become firm enough, to remain homogenous.
4) Lubricate the cavities of mould with liquid paraffin. Pour the melted (hot) base in to the cavities of mould up to the brim (surface), to ensure uniformity in size.
5) After preparation, dry the pastilles, by spreading on a sheet of butter paper.

If no machine is available, then Pastilles can also be prepared by the procedure, similar to the lozenges i.e. Roll the mass (base) of pastille on lozenge board for desired thickness. With the help of specific shape and sized punch or sharp knife, cut the base for desired number of pastilles.

- The quantity of medicament in pastilles is usually small. Therefore there is no need to determine the displacement value of the medicament.
- If alkaloidal salts are present in small quantities, they should be dissolved in a small quantity of water, before adding to the base to ensure uniform distribution in the base.

Packing (Dispensing):

Pastilles are packed similar to the lozenges. They are placed in flat boxes with hinged lids, which is made up of metal. The box should be lined with waxed paper and the pastilles are placed in layers, each layer being separated by a piece of waxed paper.

Pastilles are also packed, by wrapping each pastille in a metal foil or waxed paper, to prevent deterioration, when container has been opened (Some times, a vacuum sealed tins are also used, for packing of pastilles).

Storage: Pastilles should be stored in a dry place or at room temperature, not exceeding 25°C.

AMMONIUM CHLORIDE PASTILLE

Rx	
Ammonii chloridi	gr i
Extracti glycyrohiza liquid	M i
Glycero-gelatin...q.s....	gr xxx
Fiat : Pastillus	Mitte : Viginti quinqua
Signa : Unus pastillus, quniquies - sexies in die, lente segendus.	

Conversion:

gr i → 1 grain = 60 mg M i → 1 minim = 0.06 ml

15 grains = 1 g

gr xxx → 30 grains = 2 g

Calculation: For (25+5) = 30 pastilles.

For 1 pastille Ammonium chloride required = 60 mg

For 30 pastilles = 60 mg x 30 = 1.8 g

For 1 pastille, Liquid extract of liquorice required = 0.06 ml

Liquid extract of liquorice = 0.06 x 30 = 1.8 ml

Formula for Glycero-gelatin pastille base (Soft base) for 6 g

Gelatin	---	1 g
Glycerin	---	2.5 ml
Water	---	2.5 ml

But the Mould capacity is 2 g, therefore 30 x 2 = 60 g of base is required.

1) For 6 g of base = 1 g of gelatin is required

For 60 g of base = $\frac{1}{6} \times 60 = 10\ g$

2) For 6 g of base = 2.5 ml of glycerin is required

For 60 g of base = $\frac{2.5}{6} \times 60 = 25\ ml$

3) For 6 g of base = 2.5 ml of water is required

For 60 g of base = $\frac{2.5}{6} \times 60 = 25\ ml$

Revised formula for 30 pastilles:

Ammonium chloride	---	1.8 g
Liquid extract of liquorice	---	1.8 ml
Gelatin	---	10 g
Glycerin	---	25 ml
Water	---	25 ml

Type	Ingredients	Quantity in imperial	Quantity in metric	Quantity taken
Unit solid	Ammonium chloride	1 gr	60 mg	1.8 g
dosage form,	Liquid extract of liquorice	1 minim	0.06 ml	1.8 ml
for oral use.	Glycero-gelatin base...q.s...	30 gr	2 g	60 g
	Make : pastille	Send: Such 25		
Pastille	Direction: One pastille to be sucked slowly, five - six per day.			

Theory:

Ammonium chloride acts as expectorant, Liquid extract of liquorice consists of glycyrrhizin, which acts as expectorant and demulcent. Therefore these drugs are formulated as pastilles, which dissolve slowly in the mouth and gives prolonged effect on the throat.

These pastilles are prepared by using "soft base" – (Glycero-gelatin base). Gelatin dissolves in hot water and forms a solution, which sets as a jelly after cooling. This characteristic of gelatin, is utilized to convert glycerin into solid form, to use as pastilles base.

Glycerin is used as preservative to prevent putrefaction of the gelatin, because it exerts high osmotic pressure, which helps in killing of microorganisms, by withdrawing water from their cells. It also acts as non-volatile hygroscopic emollient. These pastilles are prepared by moulding method, of 2 g capacity mould.

Procedure : To manipulate the practical losses during preparation, calculate the quantity of ingredients, for at least 15% more, than prescribed.

1) The quantity of medicament as compared to the base is very less, therefore do not consider the displacement value of medicament, for the calculation of quantity of base.
2) Heat the glycerin to 100 °C a in closed (covered) china dish, on a water bath.
3) Heat purified water to boiling and add to the weighed quantity of gelatin. Stir gently to dissolve.
4) Add the hot glycerin, to the aqueous solution of gelatin. Stir the mixture gently, to avoid entrapment of air bubbles, until gelatin dissolves completely and gel is formed.
5) Maintain the base at 100 °C for 1 hour, to remove (kill) contaminant microorganisms.
6) To the melted mass, add required quantity of ammonium chloride and liquid extract of Liquorice and mix uniformly
7) Lubricate the mould, with liquid paraffin.
8) Pour the hot mass into the cavities of the lubricated mould and allow it to cool.
9) After cooling, inverse the mould on a sheet of butter paper, to collect the pastilles.

> **Note:** If no machine is available follow the procedure, which is used for preparation of Compound bismuth lozenges.

Dispensing : Select good twenty five pastilles and wrap each pastille in metal foil or waxed (butter) paper. Pack these pastilles in a layer in the metal (Tin) box, which is lined with waxed paper and consist a hinged lid.

Direction : One pastille to be sucked slowly, five - six per day.

Storage : Store in a dry place (or at room temperature not excceding 25 °C)

Uses : These pastilles are used, as expectorant and demulcent in the treatment of cough.

MENTHOL AND EUCALYPTUS OIL PESTILLES

Rx	
Mentholis	gr 1/20
Olei eucalyptus	M ½
Glyco-gelatini…q.s…	gr xxx
Fiat : Pastilles	Mitte : Tales viginti
Signa : Unus pastille quartis horis, lente sumendum.	

Conversion:

1 gr = 60 mg 1 Minim = 0.06ml

1/20 gr = 1/20 x 60 = 3 mg ½ Minim = ½ x 0.06 ml = 0.03 ml

15 grains = 1 g

gr xxx → 30 gr = 2 g

Formula for Glycerogelatin base for 6 g

Gelatin --- 1 g

Glycerin --- 2.5 ml

Water --- 2.5 ml

Calculation: For (20+5) = 25 pastilles, But the mould capacity is 2 g, therefore 25 x 2 = 50 g of base is required.

Gelatin $= \frac{50}{6} \times 1 = 8.35$ g

Glycerin $= \frac{50}{6} \times 2.5 = 20.8$ ml

Water $= \frac{50}{6} \times 2.5 = 20.8$ ml

But mould capacity is 2 g, therefore 25 x 2 g = 50 g of pastille base is required.

Menthol = 3 mg x 50 = 150 mg

Eucalyptus oil = 0.03 ml x 50 = 1.5 ml

Type	Ingredients	Quantity in imperial	Quantity in metric	Quantity taken
Unit solid	Menthol	1/20 grains	3 mg	150 mg
dosage form,	Eucalyptus oil	½ minim	0.03 ml	1.5 ml
for oral use.	Glycero-gelatin base…q.s..	30 grains	2 g	50 g
	Make: Pastille	Send: such twenty		
Pastille.	Direction : One pastille to be sucked slowly every four hours			

Theory :

Menthol is main constituent of peppermint oil, which is obtained by steam distillation of the fresh flowering tops of the plant, Mentha-piperita. Menthol acts as antiseptic, stimulant, counter irritant and flavouring agent.

Eucalyptus oil is a volatile oil, obtained by the distillation of fresh leaves of Eucalyptus globulus. It consists mainly ciniole, known as eucalyptol which acts as antiseptic, expectorant and counter irritant.

Because of antiseptic, expectorant action and their flavouring properties, menthol and eucalyptus oil are formulated as pastilles, to relieve the cough and to treat the throat infections, because pastilles dissolves slowly and gives effect of medicaments for prolonged time, on the mucous membrane of the throat.

Procedure : To manipulate the practical losses during preparation, calculate the quantity of ingredients for at least 15% more, than prescribed.

1) The quantity of medicament as compared to the base is very less. Therefore do not consider the displacement value of medicament, for calculation of the quantity of base.
2) Heat the glycerin to 100 °C, in a closed (covered) china dish, on a water bath.
3) Heat purified water, to boiling and add to the weighed quantity of gelatin. Stir gently to dissolve
4) Add the hot glycerin to the aqueous solution of gelatin. Stir the mixture gently to avoid entrapment of air bubbles until gelatin dissolves completely and gel is formed.
5) Maintain the base at 100 °C for 1 hour to remove (kill) contaminant microorganisms.
6) Cool the melted mass to room temperature. Dissolve menthol in eucalyptus oil and add to Glycero-gelatin base and mix uniformly.
7) Lubricate the mould with liquid paraffin.
8) Pour the hot mass into the cavities of the lubricated mould and allow it to cool.
9) After cooling, inverse the mould on a sheet of butter paper to collect the pastilles.

Dispensing : Select good twenty pastilles and wrap each pastille in metal foil or waxed (butter) paper. Pack these pastilles in a layer in the metal (Tin) box which is lined with waxed paper and consist a hinged lid.

Direction : One pastille to be sucked slowly, every four hours.

Storage : Store in a cool place to prevent the volatalization of menthol and eucalyptus oil and to prevent softening of the pastille, at higher temperature.

Uses : These pastilles are used as antiseptic and expectorant, in the relieving of cough and throat infections.

Student's exercise:

1) Define pastilles. How they differ from lozenges?
2) Give the examples for official lozenges.
3) What is pastilles base. How it can be modified to dissolve slowly ?
4) Write ingredients of Simple pastilles base, Firm base and More firm base.
5) What is the advantage of Glycero-gelatin base to be used in preparation of lozenges?
6) Briefly explain the preparation of pastilles.
7) How will you pack the pastilles?
8) Which are the ingredients used in ammonium chloride pastilles and write its uses.
9) What is soft base? How it is prepared?
10) Comment : Glycerin prevents the putrifaction of gelatin.
11) Comment : Gelatin should be heated at 100 ºC for preparation of Glycero-gelatin base.
12) What direction will you write on the label of pastilles?
13) Define demulscent and expectorant.

52 INCOMPATIBILITIES

Incompatibility is defined as, "a change resulting from mixing of two or more antagonistic substances and an undesirable product is formed, which may affect the safety, efficacy, appearance and stability of the pharmaceutical preparation."

Incompatibility may occur during compounding, formulation, manufacturing, packing, dispensing, storage or administration of drugs.

Types of incompatibilities: The incompatibilities are mainly of three types,

1) Physical incompatibility
2) Chemical incompatibility
3) Therapeutic incompatibility.

1) Physical incompatibility:

Physical incompatibility is obtained, when two or more than two substances are combined together, a physical change takes place and an unacceptable product is formed.

Physical incompatibility occurs, due to the some of the physical properties of drugs and additives such as,

- Immiscibility
- Insolubility
- Precipitate formation and
- Liquefaction of solid materials.

The physical changes are visible and can be easily corrected by applying the pharmaceutical skill, to obtain a product of uniform dosage, an attractive appearance and therapeutic activity.

The physical incompatibilities may be corrected, by using the following methods,

1) By changing the order of mixing of ingredients of the prescription.
2) By emulsification.
3) By the addition of suspending agent.
4) By changing the form of ingredients.
5) By the addition or substitution of therapeutically inactive substance (excipients).

Precipitate yielding interactions:

Depending upon the types of precipitates, different methods are adopted for dispensing of such prescriptions, They are :

Method – A : This method is suitable for diffusible precipitates.

1) Divide the vehicle into two equal portions.
2) Dissolve one of the reacting substances in one of the portion and the other substance in the another portion.
3) Mix the two portions, by slowly adding one portion to the other with rapid and constant stirring.

Method – B : This method is suitable for indiffusible precipitates,

1) Divide the vehicle in to two portions.
2) Dissolve one of the reacting substance in one portion.

3) Place second portion of vehicle in a mortar and incorporate suitable amount of compound tragacanth powder (2 g/100 ml of preparation) with constant trituration, until a smooth mucilage is produced.

4) Add and dissolve the other reacting substance to the mucilage. Add the solution of first reactant to the mucilage slowly with rapid stirring.

2) Chemical incompatibility:

Chemical incompatibility is obtained (formed) as a result of chemical interaction between ingredients of the prescription, due to that a toxic or inactive product may be formed.

Chemical incompatibilities occur, due to the chemical properties (reaction) of drugs and additives like,

- pH change.
- Oxidation – reduction.
- Acid – base hydrolysis.
- Double decomposition.
- Complex formation.

These reactions may be noticed by,

- Precipitation.
- Effervescence.
- Decomposition.
- Colour change or Explosion.

Therefore, during dispensing of such prescriptions, precautions should be taken, either to prevent the formation of harmful product or to correct them.

The prescription having chemical incompatibility should be dispensed only after its correction, by the prescriber.

Types of chemical incompatibilities : There are two types of chemical incompatability.

1) Tolerated incompatibility.
2) Adjusted incompatibility.

1) Tolerated incompatibility:

In tolerated incompatibility, the chemical interactions can be minimized by changing the order of mixing or mixing the solutions in dilute forms, without any alteration in the active ingredients (formulation) of the prescription.

2) Adjusted incompatibility:

In adjusted incompatibility, the chemical interaction can be prevented by the addition or substitution of any of the ingredient of the prescription with another substance, which is having equal (similar) therapeutic value.

Examples for chemical incompatibility:

1) Alkaloidal incompatibility :
   a) Alkaloidal salts with alkaline substances.
   b) Alkaloidal salts with soluble iodides.
   c) Alkaloidal salts with tannins.
   d) Alkaloidal salts with salicylate.
   e) Alkaloidal salts with soluble iodides and bromides.
2) Soluble salicylate incompatibility :
   a) Soluble salicylate with ferric salt.
   b) Soluble salicylate with alkali bicarbonates.
   c) Soluble salicylate and benzoates with acids.
3) Chemical incompatibilities causing evaluation of CO_2:
   a) Sodium bicarbonate with soluble calcium or magnesium salts.
   b) Bismuth sub nitrate and sodium bicarbonate.
   c) Borax with sodium bicarbonate and glycerin.
4) Miscellaneous chemical incompatibilities :
   a) Soluble barbiturates with ammonium bromide.
   b) Potassium chlorate with oxidisable substances.
   c) Incompatibility of emulsifying agents.
   d) Colour stability of dye.
   e) Quinine sulphate with iodides.

3) Therapeutic incompatibility:

Therapeutic incompability occurs as a result of prescribing certain drugs to the patients, with the intension to produce a specific degree of action, but the nature or intensity of the action produced by the drug will be different from the intension of the prescriber. The therapeutic incompability occurs due to prescribing,

- Error in dosage.
- Over dose or improper dose.
- Contraindicated drugs.
- Synergic and antagonistic drugs.
- Drug interactions.

PHYSICAL INCOMPATIBILITY : MIXTURE OF CHALK POWDER WITH TINCTURE OF CATECHU

Rx	
Cretae pulverati	gr xxx
Tincturae of catechu	M xxx
Aquam cinnamoni... q.s. ...	fl.oz i
Fiat : Mistura	Mitte : fl.oz i
Signa : Cochleare magnum, b.i.d sumendum.	

Conversion :

gr xxx → 30 grains　　M xxx → 30 minims

15 grains = 1 g　　15 minims = 1 ml

30 grains = 2 g　　30 minims = 2 ml

Calculation : For fl.oz i → 30 ml

Chalk powder $= \frac{2}{30} \times 30 = 2$ g

Tincture of catechu $= \frac{2}{30} \times 30 = 2$ ml

Cinnamon water ...q.s...... = 30 ml

Compound powder of tragacanth = 2 g /100 ml

But, for 30 ml $= \frac{2}{100} \times 30 = 0.6$ g

Revised Formula:

Chalk powder	---	2 g
Tincture of catechu	---	2 ml
Compound powder of tragacanth	---	0.6 g
Cinnemon water... q.s. ...	---	30 ml

Type	Ingredients	Quantity in imperial	Quantity in metric	Quantity taken
Physical incompatibility, showing insolubility	Chalk powder	30 gr	2 g	2 g
	Tincture of catechu	30 minims	2 ml	2 ml
	Cinnamon water....q.s....	1 fl.oz	30 ml	30 ml
	Make : Mixture　Send : 30 ml Direction: One tablespoonful to be taken, two times a day.			

Uses: In this preparation, chalk powder acts as an adsorbent and produces its action by covering the intestinal mucous membrane. It also acts as antacid. Tincture of catechu contains tannic acid, which acts as an astringent. Therefore this preparation is used in the treatment of diarrhoea.

Incompatibility: This prescription shows physical incompatibility, because chalk powder is indiffusible in nature, which gets precipitate, when added to the aqueous system.

Remedy :

- This incompatibility can be prevented by following method 'B' for precipitate yielding combination i.e, using a suspending agent, which makes the indiffusible precipitate of prepared chalk into diffusible, evenly in the vehicle for longer time, so as to ensure that accurate amount of dose can be measured.
- In this preparation, cinnamon water is used as vehicle, which is medicinally active. Therefore compound powder of tragacanth is used as a suspending agent, in the concentration of 2 g / 100 ml.

Procedure:

1) Weigh accurately, chalk powder and transfer to a mortar.
2) To this powder, add calculated quantity of compound tragacanth powder and mix thoroughly.
3) Measure $\frac{3}{4}^{th}$ of final volume of cinnamon water, and add a small portion to mortar and triturate, to form smooth cream.
4) Add tincture of catechu in to the center of the cream, with continuous trituration and transfer to a measure and adjust the final volume, with cinnamon water.

Dispensing: Transfer this mixture to a narrow mouthed glass bottle, close it thoroughly with metallic screw cap, polish and label.

Direction: One tablespoonful to be taken, two times a day.

Storage: Store in a cool place.

Auxilliary label: SHAKE WELL BEFORE USE.

PHYSICAL INCOMPATIBILITY: MIXTURE OF MAGNESIUM CARBONATE, SODIUM BICARBONATE AND CITRIC ACID

Rx	
Magnessi carbonatis	3 i
Sodii bicarbonatis	3 i
Acidi citratis	3 i
Aquam...q.s.....	fl.oz viii
Fiat : Mistura	Mitte : fl.oz ii
Signa : Cochleare magnum, post singular cibos sumendum.	

Conversion :

3 i → 1 drachm   fl.oz i → 1 fl.oz = 30 ml

1 drachm = 4 g   fl.oz viii → 8 fl.oz= 240 ml

Calculation : For fl.oz ii → 60 ml

Magnessium carbonate $= \frac{4}{240} \times 60 = 1$ g

Sodium bicarbonate $= \frac{4}{240} \times 60 = 1$ g

Citric acid $= \frac{4}{240} \times 60 = 1$ g

Water ....q.s....... = 60 ml

Type	Ingredients	Quantity in imperial	Quantity in metric	Quantity taken
Physical incompatibility, showing insolubility	Magnesium carbonate	1 dr	4 g	1 g
	Sodium bicarbonate	1 dr	4 g	1 g
	Citric acid	1 dr	4 g	1 g
	Purified water .....q.s...	8 fl. oz	240 ml	60 ml
	Make : Mixture	Send : 60 ml		
	Direction: One tablespoonful to be taken, after each meal.			

Uses: In this preparation, magnesium carbonate and sodium bicarbonate acts as antacids. Hence this mixture is used as an antacid preparation.

Incompatibility: This prescription shows physical incompatibility, if any changes in the order of mixing, because

a) If citric acid is reacted first with sodium bicarbonate, some amount of magnesium carbonate will be remaing insoluble and a suspension will be formed.

b) If citric acid reacts with magnesium carbonate first, both magnesium carbonate and sodium bicarbonate are soluble and a clear solution will be obtained.

This preparation also involves the incompatibility of causing evaluation of carbon dioxide, due to acid-base reaction between citric acid, sodium bicarbonate and magnesium carbonate. Therefore the reaction should be allowed to complete evaluation of $CO_{2,}$ before transferring the mixture to a dispensing bottle and then closed. Otherwise, it may lead to the explosion with the bursting of bottle, due to excessively increased pressure of the gas, inside the bottle.

Remedy: This physical incompatibility can be prevented by changing the order of mixing like,

- Initially prepare a suspension of magnesium carbonate, with half quantity of water. To this suspension, add citric acid in small amounts and allow the effervescence (Co_2) to cease completely.
- Dissolve sodium bicarbonate in remaining amount of water and add to the above solution and allow the effervescence, to cease completely and then dispensed.

Procedure:

1) Weigh separately magnesium carbonate, sodium bicarbonate and citric acid.
2) Take magnesium carbonate in a mortar and add half the quantity of water with trituration, until a smooth suspension is formed.
3) Dissolve the citric acid in a small portion of water and add to the above suspension and let the effervescence ceases completely. Filter the solution, if any foreign particles present.
4) Dissolve sodium bicarbonate in a small portion of water by stirring.
5) Mix the above two solutions and let the effervescence ceases completely.
6) Transfer the solution to a measure and make up the final volume with water.

Dispensing: Transfer the mixture to a narrow mouthed glass bottle, close it thoroughly with metallic screw cap, polish and label.

Direction: One tablespoonful to be taken, after each meal.

Storage: Store in a cool place.

Other examples for physical incompatibility, which are already discussed in the other categories. Students are required to be refer in the concern category:

S.n.	Example		Category	Page no.
1)	Rx. Castor oil Cinnamon water…q.s..	 - 10 ml - 25 ml	Emulsion	329
2)	Rx. Menthol Camphor Ammonium chloride Light magnesium carbonate	 - 5 g - 5 g - 30 g - 60 g	Insufflation Eutectic powder for external use	492
3)	Rx. Phenacetin Caffeine Orange syrup Water … q.s.…	 - 3 g - 1 g - 12 g - 90 ml	Mixture containing indiffusible solid	47
4)	Rx. Sulphadimidine Orange syrup Benzoic acid solution Amaranth solution Chloroform water… q.s.…	 - 1 g - 2 ml - 0.2 ml - 0.1 ml - 10 ml	Mixture containing indiffusible solid	51
5)	Rx. Bismuth carbonate Prepared chalk Light kaolin Tincture of catechu Purified water q.s.	 - 1 g - 1 g - 4 g - 2 ml - 30 ml	Mixture containing indiffusible solid.	53
6)	Rx. Ethereal tincture of lobelia Potassium iodide Purified water q.s.	 - 2 g - 8 ml - 180 ml	Mixture containing precipitate forming liquid.	56
7)	Rx. Camphor Menthol Light kaolin	 - 1.33 g - 0.66 g - 2 g	Eutectic powder, meant for internal use	507

CHEMICAL INCOMPATIBILITY : ALKALOIDAL SALT WITH ALKALINE SUBSTANCE

Rx	
Strychnine hydrochloride solution	M XC
Spiritus ammoniae aromatici	M LX
Aquam..... q.s. ...	fl.oz iv
Fiat : Mistura	Mitte : fl.oz ii
Signa : Cochleare magnum post singular cibos sumendum.	

Conversion :

M XC → 90 minims　　M LX → 60 minims = 4 ml

15 minims = 1 ml

90 minims = 6 ml　　fl.oz iv → 4 fl. oz = 120 ml

Calculation : For fl.oz ii → 2 fl.oz = 60 ml

Strychnine hydrochloride solution = $\frac{6}{120} \times 60 = 3\text{ ml}$

Aromatic spirit of ammonia = $\frac{4}{120} \times 60 = 2\text{ ml}$

Water .....q.s..... = 60 ml

Type	Ingredients	Quantity in imperial	Quantity in metric	Quantity taken
Chemical incompatibility.	Strychnine HCl solution	90 minims	6 ml	3 ml
	Aromatic spirit of ammonia	60 mminims	4 ml	2 ml
	Water ..q.s...	4 fl.oz	120 ml	60 ml
	Make : Mixture　　Send : 60 ml Direction: One tablespoonful to be taken, after each meal.			

Uses: Strychnine hydrochloride is an alkaloidal salt, obtained from the tincture of Nux-vomica. Strychnine hydrochloride acts as CNS stimulant and aromatic spirit of ammonia acts as stimulant. Therefore this preparation is used as stimulant, in nervous disorder like epilepsy.

Incompatibility: This prescription shows tolerated type chemical incompatibility, because strychnine hydrochloride is an alkaloidal salt, but aromatic spirit of ammonia is an alkaline substance. When they react together, precipitate of strychnine will be formed because,

a) The quantity of strychnine hydrochloride prescribed is much more than its solubility.

b) Even though aromatic spirit of ammonia contains alcohol, which is in negligible quantity, to dissolve the precipitated strychnine.

Remedy:

- The precipitate of strychnine, so formed is diffusible in nature. Therefore the precipitate formation is prevented or minimised by mixing the reacting substances in dilute forms to a maximum extent, without altering the active ingredients of the preparation.
- Strychnine hydrochloride solution is dissolved in half of the portion of water and aromatic spirit of ammonia is dissolved in remaining portion of water and these solutions should be mixed slowly with continuous stirring, which avoids the formation of diffusible precipitate.

Procedure:

1) Divide the purified water into two equal portions.
2) Mix strychnine hydrochloride solution in one portion of the water.
3) Mix aromatic spirit of ammonia with little quantity of water.
4) Mix both the solutions slowly by continuous stirring.
5) Transfer the solution to a measure and make up the final volume with water.

Dispensing: Strychnine hydrochloride is sensitive to the light, therefore transfer the mixture to a ambered colored, narrow mouthed glass bottle, and close it thoroughly with metallic screw cap, polish and label.

Direction: One tablespoonful to be taken, after each meal.

Storage: Store in a cool place.

Auxilliary label: SHAKE WELL BEFORE USE.

CHEMICAL INCOMPATIBILITY : ALKALOIDAL SALT WITH SALICYLATE

Rx	
Quinine hydrochloride	gr i sss
Sodii salicylatis	gr LX
Aquam...... q.s. ...	fl.oz iii
Fiat : Mistura	Mitte : fl.oz i
Signa : Cochleare magnum, post cibos sumendum	

Conversion :

gr i sss → 1.75 grains	gr LX → 60 grains
15 grains = 1 g	15 grains = 1 g
1.75 grains = 0.12 g	60 grains = 4 g

Calculation : For fl.oz i → 1 fl.oz = 30 ml

Quinine hydrochloride = $\frac{0.12}{90} \times 30 = 0.04$ g (40 mg)

Sodium salicylate = $\frac{4}{90} \times 30 = 1.2$ g

Water ....q.s...... = 30 ml

For 30 ml,

40 mg of Quinine hydrochloride is required. But it is not a weighable quantity on dispensing balance. 100 mg is minimum weighble quantity on dispensing balance..

Therefore, dissolve 100 mg Quinine hydrochloride in 10 ml water.

i.e.10 ml solution contains = 100 mg Quinine hydrochloride

for 40 mg of Quinine hydrochloride = $\frac{40}{100} \times 10 = 4$ ml

Compound powder of tragacanth = 2 g / 100 ml

For 30 ml = $\frac{2}{100} \times 30 = 0.6$ g

Revised Formula :

Quinine hydrochloride solution (1%)	---	4 ml
Sodium salicylate	---	1.2 g
Compound powder of tragacanth	---	0.6 g
Water ....q.s... ...	---	30 ml

Type	Ingredients	Quantity in imperial	Quantity in metric	Quantity taken
Chemical incompatibility.	Quinine hydrochloride	1.75 gr	1.20 g	40 mg
	Sodium salicylate	60 gr	4 g	1.2 g
	Water.....q.s...	3 fl.oz	90 ml	30 ml
	Make : Mixture Send : 30 ml Direction: One tablespoonful to be taken, after meals.			

Uses: Quinine hydrochloride is an alkaloidal salt, which reduces the malarial fever and sodium salicylate acts as analgesic. Therefore these drugs are combinedly used in the treatment of malarial fever (associated with body pain).

Incompatibility: This prescription shows chemical incompatibility, because quinine hydrochloride is an alkaloidal salt, which when reacts with sodium salicylate, it will be precipitate out as quinine salicylate. This precipitate is indiffusible in nature.

Remedy: The indiffusible precipitate of quinine salicylate is made into diffusible by following the method B, for precipitate yielding combination i.e. by using a suspending agent like compound powder of tragacanth in the concentration of 2 gm / 100 ml of the total mixture.

$$\underset{\text{Indiffusible ppt}}{Quinine\ Salicylate} \xrightarrow[\text{(Suspending agent)}]{\text{Compound powder of tragacanth}} \underset{\text{Ppt}}{Quinine\ Salicylate\ (Diffusible)}$$

Procedure:

1) Weigh separately sodium salicylate and compound powder of tragacanth and transfer into mortar. Triturate them to mix properly.
2) Weigh accurately quinine hydrochloride and dissolve in little quantity of water. Add this solution into the mortar. Mix well by trituration.
3) Transfer the above mixture into measuring cylinder.
4) Rinse the pestle and mortar with water and then transfer to the measuring cylinder.
5) Adjust the final volume with water, mix well.

Dispensing: Quinine hydrochloride is sensitive to the light, therefore transfer the mixture to an amber colored, narrow mouthed glass bottle, close it thoroughly with metallic screw cap, polish and label.

Direction: One tablespoonful to be taken, after meals.

Storage: Store in a cool place.

Auxilliary label: SHAKE WELL BEFORE USE.

CHEMICAL INCOMPATIBILITY- SOLUBLE SALICYLATES WITH ALKALI BICARBONATE

Rx	
Sodium salicylatis	3 ii
Sodium bicarbonate	3 ii
Sodium metabisulphite	gr i s
Aqua chloroformi...q.s....	fl.oz iv
Fiat : Mistura	Mitte : fl.oz i
Signa : Cochleare magnum mane et nocte sumendum.	

Conversion :

3 ii → 2 drachms	gr i s → 1.25 grains	fl.oz iv → 4 fl. oz
1 drachm = 4 g	15 grains = 1 g	1 fl.oz = 30 ml
2 drachms = 8 g	1.25 grains = 0.08 g	4 fl.oz = 120 ml

Calculation : For fl.oz i → 1 fl.oz = 30 ml

Sodium salicylate = $\frac{8}{120} \times 30 = 2\text{ g}$

Sodium bicarbonate = $\frac{8}{120} \times 30 = 2\text{ g}$

Sodium metabisulphite = $\frac{0.08}{120} \times 30 = 0.02\text{ g}$

Chloform water ...q.s...... = 30 ml

Type	Ingredients	Quantity in imperial	Quantity in metric	Quantity taken
Chemical incompatibility.	Sodium salicylate	2 dr	8 g	2 g
	Sodium bicarbonate	2 dr	8 g	2 g
	Sodium metabisulphite	1.25 gr	0.08 g	0.02 g
	Chloroform water...q.s....	4 fl.oz	120 ml	30 ml
	Make : Mixture	Send : 30 ml		
	Direction: One tablespoonful to be taken, morning and night.			

Uses: Sodium salicylate acts as analgesic. Hence this mixture is used for relieving of pain.

Incompatibility:

- This prescription shows chemical incompatibility, involving reaction between sodium salicylate and sodium bicarbonate i.e. when sodium salicylate alone is administered orally it reacts with hydrochloric acid of the stomach and leads to the formation of precipitate of salicylic acid.

- The liberated salicylic acid causes irritation to the gastric mucosa and pain in the stomach. Therefore whenever sodium salicylate is prescribed, it is usually given along with equal the quantity of sodium bicarbonate, as that of sodium salicylate. Since sodium bicarbonate is alkaline in nature, neutralizes the gastric secretion and also minimizes the formation of precipitate of salicylic acid.
- But when sodium salicylate is in the solution form, with an alkali like sodium bicarbonate, the mixture absorbs oxygen from the atmosphere and becomes reddish brown in colour.
- This change of colour does not effect the therapeutic efficacy of the preparation, but it may leads to confusion in the mind of patients that, the medicament has spoiled and they may not wish to use the preparation (mixture).

Remedy: To prevent the oxidation and hence the colour change, antioxidant like, sodium meta bisulphite (0.1%) is used.

> **Note:** To avoid (mask) the colour change, a colouring agent like liquid extract of liquorice or caramel may be used, which darkens the colour of the mixture or patient may be warned, about the colour change before dispensing.

Procedure:

1) Accurately weigh sodium salicylate, sodium bicarbonate and sodium metabisulphite.
2) Dissolve sodium salicylate and sodium bicarbonate in ¾ th quantity of chloroform water by stirring.
3) To the above solution, add sodium metabisulphite and dissolve by stirring and filter the solution through muslin cloth, to remove if any foreign particles present.
4) Transfer the content to a measure and adjust the final volume with chloroform water

Dispensing: Transfer the mixture to a narrow mouthed glass bottle, close it thoroughly with metallic screw cap, polish and label.

Direction: One tablespoonful to be taken, morning and night.

Storage: Store in a cool place.

CHEMICAL INCOMPATIBILITY - SOLUBLE SALICYLATES WITH ACID

Rx	
Sodii salicylatis	gr VL
Syrupi lemolis	fl. 3 iii sss
Aqum... q.s. ...	fl.oz ii
Fiat : Mistura	Mitte : fl.oz i
Signa : Cochleare magnum, b.i.d sumendum.	

Conversion :

gr VL → 45 grains
15 grains = 1 g
45 grains = 3 g

fl. 3 iii sss → 3.75 fl. drachms
1 fl. drachm = 4 ml
3.75 fl. drachms = 15 ml
fl.oz ii → 2 fl. oz = 60 ml

Calculation : For fl.oz i → 1 fl.oz = 30 ml

Sodium salicylate = $\frac{3}{60} \times 30 = 1.5\,\text{g}$

Lemon syrup = $\frac{15}{60} \times 30 = 7.5\,\text{ml}$

Water... ...q.s.... = 30 ml

Type	Ingredients	Quantity in imperial	Quantity in metric	Quantity Taken
Chemical incompatibility	Sodium salicylate	45 gr	3 g	1.5 g
	Lemon syrup	3.75 fl. dr	15 ml	7.5 ml
	Water....q.s....	2 fl.oz	60 ml	30 ml
	Make : Mixture	Send : 30 ml		
	Direction: One tablespoonful to be taken, two times a day.			

Uses: In this preparation, Sodium salicylate acts as analgesic. Therefore this mixture is used in the relief of pain. Lemon syrup is used as flavouring and sweetening agent.

Incompatibility: This prescription shows adjusted type chemical incompatibility, because of acid-base reaction between lemon syrup and sodium salicylate i.e. lemon syrup contains citric acid, due to its strong acidic nature, it decomposes sodium salicylate into salicylic acid.

Remedy:

- In this prescription, lemon syrup is used for its flavouring and sweetening taste. Therefore to prevent the above problem, instead of using lemon syrup, use simple syrup as sweetening agent and tincture of lemon as flavouring agent, without altering the therapeutic action of the preparation.
- The ratio of simple syrup and tincture of lemon for 10 ml is,

  Simple syrup - 9.5 ml

  Tincture of lemon - 0.6 ml

  Even though tincture of lemon contains citric acid, it is in a lesser quantity so that, it cannot decompose the sodium salicylate in to salicylic acid.

According to the ratio (Formula)

For 10 ml lemon syrup, 9.5 ml of simple syrup and 0.6 ml of tincture of lemon are required.

But for 7.5 ml of lemon syrup,

a) Simple syrup $= \frac{9.5}{10} \times 7.5 = 7.125$ ml

b) Tincture of lemon $= \frac{0.6}{10} \times 7.5 = 0.45$ ml

Revised Formula :

Sodium salicylate	---	1.5 g
Simple syrup	---	7.125 ml
Tincture of lemon	---	0.45 ml
Water... q.s. ...	---	30 ml

Procedure:

1) Accurately weigh required quantity of sodium salicylate and dissolve in ¾ th quantity of water in a beaker.
2) Filter the solution through a muslin cloth, directly to a previously tared amber coloured (calibrated) bottle.
3) To the filtrate, add measured quantity of simple syrup and tincture of lemon and mix well and adjust the final volume with remaining amount of water.

Dispensing: Transfer the mixture to a narrow mouthed glass bottle, close it thoroughly with metallic screw cap, polish and label.

Direction: One tablespoonful to be taken, two times a day.

Storage: Store in a cool place.

CHEMICAL INCOMPATIBILITY : SOLUBLE SALICYLATES WITH FERRIC SALTS

Rx	
Sodii salicylatis	3 i
Ferric chloride solution	M xv
Sodii bicarbonatis	3 ii
Aquam... q.s. ...	fl.oz vi
Fiat : Mistura	Mitte : fl.oz ii
Signa : Cochleare amplum omni nocte, sumendum	

Conversion :

3 i → 1 drachm — M XV → 15 minims = 1 ml

1 drachm = 4 g

2 drachms = 8 g — fl.oz vi → 6 fl.oz = 180 ml

Calculation : For fl.oz ii → 2 fl.oz = 60 ml

Sodium salicylate = $\frac{4}{180} \times 60 = 1.33$ g

Ferric chloride solution = $\frac{1}{180} \times 60 = 0.33$ ml

Sodium bicarbonate = $\frac{8}{180} \times 60 = 2.66$ g

Water...q.s...... = 60 ml

Type	Ingredients	Quantity in imperial	Quantity in metric	Quantity taken
Chemical incompatibility.	Sodium salicylate	1 dr	4 g	1.33 g
	Ferric chloride solution	15 minims	1 ml	0.33 ml
	Sodium bicarbonate	2 dr	8 g	2.66 g
	Water....q.s....	6 fl.oz	180 ml	60 ml
	Make : Mixture	Send : 60 ml		
	Direction: One tablespoonful to be taken, at every night.			

Uses: Sodium salicylate acts as analgesic and ferric chloride acts as powerful astringent and also used in anemia. Therefore this preparation is used as iron supplement, during haemorrhage associated with pain.

Incompatibility: This prescription shows the (adjusted type) chemical incompatibility, involving reaction between sodium salicylate with ferric salts. i.e when ferric chloride reacts with sodium salicylate, ferric salicylate will be precipitated out, which is violet in colour and also insoluble and indiffusible in water. This prescription also associated with incompatibility of evolution of carbon dioxide gas.

Remedy:

- The precipitate of ferric salicylate is freely soluble in presence of alkali like sodium bicarbonate or potassium bicarbonate and hence a clear (solution) mixture will be formed.
- After the addition of ferric chloride solution to the mixture of sodium salicylate and sodium bicarbonate, effervescence will be produced due to evolution of CO_2, because of acid-base reaction.
- Therefore, allow the reaction mixture to complete, until effervescence ceases completely (complete evolution of CO_2), before adjusting the final volume with water (before transferring the mixture in to the dispensing bottle and then corked).

Procedure:

1) Accurately weigh the required quantity of sodium salicylate, sodium bicarbonate and measure ferric chloride solution separately and dissolve in the ¾th quantity of purified water by stirring.
2) To the above solution, add ferric chloride solution with continuous stirring and allow the effervescence (CO_2), to cease completely.
3) Filter the solution through muslin cloth and transfer the filtrate to a measure. Adjust the final volume with purified water.

Dispensing: Transfer the solution to a narrow mouthed, amber coloured bottle, close it thoroughly with metallic screw cap, lined with polyethylene wad (liner), polish and label.

Direction: One tablespoonful to be taken, at every night.

Storage: Store in a cool place.

CHEMICAL INCOMPATIBILITY – SOLUBLE SALICYLATE WITH ALKALOIDAL SALT

Rx	
Sodii salicylatis	gr xv
Caffeine citratis	gr ix
Aquam... q.s. ...	fl.oz i
Fiat : Hastus (Draught)	Mitte : fl.oz i
Signa : Statim sumat.	

Conversion :

3 XV → 15 grains — gr ix → 9 grains

15 grains = 1 g — 15 grains = 1 g

9 grains = 0.6 g

Calculation : For fl.oz i → 1 fl.oz = 30 ml

Sodium salicylate = $\frac{1}{30} \times 30 = 1$ g

Caffeine citrate = $\frac{0.6}{30} \times 30 = 0.6$ g

Water... q.s... = 30 ml

Type	Ingredients	Quantity in imperial	Quantity in metric	Quantity taken
Chemical incompatibility.	Sodium salicylate	15 gr	1.0 g	1 g
	Caffeine	9 gr	0.6 g	0.3 g
	Water.....q.s......	1 fl.oz	30 ml	30 ml
	Make : Draught Send : 30 ml Direction: Take at once (To be taken, as a single dose).			

Uses: This is a mixture used as a draught. Caffeine citrate acts as CNS stimulant and caffeine also acts as CNS stimulant, which is specially used for headache and migraine. Sodium salicylate acts as analgesic. Therefore this preparation is used, in the treatment of migraine, associated with headache.

Incompatibility: This prescription shows adjusted type of chemical incompatibility i.e. caffeine citrate is a mixture of equal weights of caffeine and citric acid. Citric acid is acidic in nature (reaction) and present in excess quantity, than required but caffeine is a weak base.

Due to the acidic nature of Caffeine citrate, it decomposes sodium salicylate into salicylic acid, which is indiffusible in nature and hence it does not remain evenly distributed in the vehicle for longer time.

Remedy:

- Caffeine is basic in nature, and has similar therapeutic effect of caffeine citrate. Therefore decomposition of salicylic acid is prevented by substituting (replacing) caffeine citrate by half of its quantity of caffeine.
- Even though caffeine is insoluble in water, but in presence of sodium salicylate it forms a readily soluble compound. Therefore half quantity of caffeine is required, to solublize with the sodium salicylate.

Caffeine citrate is substituted by Caffeine, half of its quantity.

$$\therefore \text{ Caffeine required is } = \frac{0.6}{2} = 0.3 \text{ g}$$

Revised Formula :

Sodium salicylate	=	1 g
Caffeine	=	0.3 g
Water... q.s. ...	=	30 ml

Procedure:

1) Accurately weigh sodium salicylate and caffeine and dissolve in half of the portion of water.
2) Strain the solution through a plug of cotton wool, to remove foreign particles or any undissolved substance, if present.
3) Transfer the content to a measure and adjust the final volume with water.

Dispensing: Transfer the solution to a narrow mouthed, amber coloured bottle, close it thoroughly with metallic screw cap, lined with polyethylene wad (liner), polish and label.

Direction: Take at once (To be taken, as a single dose).

Storage: Store in a cool place.

CHEMICAL INCOMPATIBILITY – SOLUBLE BARBITURATE WITH AMMONIUM BROMIDE

Rx	
Phenobarbitone sodium	gr ix
Ammonium bromide	3 ii
Aquam... q.s. ...	fl.oz iv
Fiat : Mistura	Mitte : fl.oz i
Signa : Cochleare amplum omni nocte capiendus.	

Conversion :

gr ix $\rightarrow$ 9 grains
15 grains = 1 g
9 grains = 0.6 g

3 ii $\rightarrow$ 2 drachms
1 drachm = 4 g
2 drachms = 8 g
fl.oz iv $\rightarrow$ 4 fl.oz = 120 ml

Calculation : For fl.oz i $\rightarrow$ 1 fl.oz = 30 ml

Phenobarbitone sodium = $\frac{0.6}{120} \times 30 = 0.15$ g

Ammonium bromide = $\frac{8}{120} \times 30 = 2$ g

Water... q.s. ... = 30 ml

Type	Ingredients	Quantity in imperial	Quantity in metric	Quantity taken
Chemical incompatibility	Phenobarbitone sodium	9 gr	0.6 g	0.15 g
	Ammonium bromide	2 dr	8 g	2 g
	Water.....q.s......	4 fl.oz	120 ml	30 ml
	Make : Mixture Send : 30 ml Direction: One tablespoonful to be taken, at every night.			

Uses: Phenobarbitone sodium acts as hypnotic and anticonvulsant. Ammonium bromide acts as sedative. Therefore these drugs are used in combination, to give sedative / hypnotic and anticonvulsant effect in epileptic patients.

Incompatibility : This prescription shows adjusted type chemical incompatibility i.e. Phenobarbitone sodium is a soluble barbiturate, when it reacts with ammonium bromide, ammonium ion decomposes phenobarbitone sodium, into indiffusible and poorly soluble phenobarbitone.

Phenobarbitone sodium + Ammonium bromide $\xrightarrow{\text{ammonium ion}}$ Sodium bromide + Ammonia + Phenobarbitone

(Indiffusible and poorly soluble)

Remedy:

- Salts like ammonium bromide, sodium bromide and potassium bromide are having similar therapeutic (sedative) action. Their sedative action is due to the "bromide ions".
- Therefore the decomposition of phenobarbitone sodium can be prevented by, without altering the therapeutic effect of the preparation by replacing ammonium bromide with equivalent amount of other bromide like sodium bromide, where sodium ions does not reacts with soluble phenobarbitone sodium.
- The pharmacological (therapeutic) action of sodium bromide and ammonium bromide is similar, but the intensity of sedative action, depends on the amount of bromide radicals present (used). Therefore equivalent amount of sodium bromide should be calculated, by considering the molecular weights of both ammonium bromide and sodium bromide.

Ammonium bromide is replaced by Sodium bromide

$\therefore$ Consider their molecular weight, for the calculation.

Molecular weight of Ammonium bromide = Molecular weight of Sodium bromide

$(NH_4Br) \rightarrow (14 + 4 + 80) = (NaBr) \rightarrow (23 + 80)$

$98 = 103$

i.e. for 98 g of (Ammonium bromide), 103 g of (Sodium bromide) is required.

$\therefore$ for 1 g NH_4Br, the amount of NaBr required = $\frac{103}{98} \times 1 = 1.05$ g

But, for preparation of 30 ml of preparation, 2 g NH_4Br is required.

Therefore, for 2 g of NH_4Br, the amount of NaBr required = $\frac{103}{98} \times 2 = 2.1$ g

Hence replace 2 g of NH_4Br with 2.1 g of NaBr to prepare a clear mixture.

Revised Formula :

Phenobarbitone sodium	---	0.15 g
Sodium bromide	---	2.1 g
Water... q.s. ...	---	30 ml

Procedure:

1. Accurately measure $\frac{3}{4}^{th}$ quantity of purified water and divide into two equal portions.
2. Dissolve the required amount of phenobarbitone sodium, in one portion of water with stirring.
3. Separately dissolve sodium bromide, in another portion of water by stirring.
4. Mix both the solutions uniformly, with continuous stirring. Filter the solution through a muslin cloth, to remove if any foreign particles present.
5. Transfer the filtrate to a measure and adjust the final volume with water.

Dispensing: Phenobarbitone sodium is sensitive to the light. Therefore transfer the solution to a amber coloured, narrow mouthed glass bottle, close thoroughly with metallic screw cap, polish and label.

Direction: One tablespoonful to be taken, at every night.

Storage: Store in a cool place.

CHEMICAL INCOMPATIBILITY - CAUSING EVOLUTION OF CARBON DIOXIDE GAS

(BORAX WITH SODIUM BICARBONATE AND GLYCERIN)

Rx	
Sodii bicarbonatis	gr xxii ss
Boracis	gr xxii ss
Liquidi phenolis	M xi s
Glyerini	fl. 3 vi s
Aquam... q.s. ...	fl. 3 xxv
Fiat : Mistura	Mitte : fl.oz i
Signa : Utendus more dicto.	

Conversion :

gr xxii ss → 22.5 grains
15 grains = 1 g
22.5 grains = 1.5 g

fl. 3 vi s → 6.25 fl. drachms
1 fl. drachm = 4 ml
6.25 fl. drachms = 25 ml
fl. 3 xxv → 25 fl. drachms = 100 ml

M xi s → 11.25 minims
15 minims = 1 ml
11.25 minims = 0.75 ml

Calculation : For fl.oz i → 1 fl.oz = 30 ml

Sodium bicarbonate = $\frac{1.5}{100} \times 30 = 0.45$ g

Borax = $\frac{1.5}{100} \times 30 = 0.45$ g

Liquified phenol = $\frac{0.75}{100} \times 30 = 0.225$ ml

Glycerin = $\frac{25}{100} \times 30 = 7.5$ ml

Water... q.s. ... = 30 ml

Type	Ingredients	Quantity in imperial	Quantity in metric	Quantity taken
Chemical incompatibility.	Sodium bicarbonate	22.5 gr	1.5 g	0.45 g
	Borax	22.5 gr	1.5 g	0.45 g
	Liquified phenol	11.25 minims	0.75 ml	0.225 ml
	Glycerin	6.25 fl. dr	25 ml	7.5 ml
	Water.....q.s......	25 fl. dr	100 ml	30 ml
	Make : Mixture	Send : 30 ml		
	Direction: To be used, as directed.			

Uses: This mixture is used as spray solution (Nasal spray), for the treatment of nasal congestion as a nasal decongestant, because sodium bicarbonate dissolves the mucous. Borax and liquid phenol acts as bacteriostatic and glycerin increases the viscosity of the preparation, to adhere the droplets of the spray on the mucous membrane of the nose, for longer time.

Incompatibility:

This prescription shows chemical incompatibility, causing evolution of carbon dioxide gas due to acid-base reaction i.e. when borax glycerin and sodium bicarbonate are mixed together in presence of water, borax hydrolyses into boric acid and sodium meta per borate.

The liberated boric acid reacts with glycerin and coverts into monobasic glycerol boric acid which is strong acidic in nature.

When glyceryl-boric acid reacts with base like, sodium bicarbonate, it causes effervescence due to the liberation of carbon dioxide gas.

$$\underset{\text{Borax}}{Na_2B_4O_7} + 3H_2O \longrightarrow \underset{\text{Sodium meta borate}}{2NaBO_2} + \underset{\text{Boric acid}}{2H_3BO_3}$$

$$\underset{\text{Glycerin}}{2C_3H_5(OH)_3} + \underset{\text{Boric acid}}{2H_3BO_3} \longrightarrow \underset{\text{Glyceryl boric acid}}{(C_3H_5OH)_2 \cdot HBO_4} + 2H_2O$$

If this reaction mixture is dispensed as such, without complete evolution of carbon dioxide and mixture is transferred immediately to the bottle and closed, there are chances of explosion with bursting of the bottle, due to excessively increased pressure of gas, inside the bottle.

Remedy:

- For dispensing of this type of prescription mix borax, sodium bicarbonate and glycerin with water in a open vessel (mortar) and allow the reaction to complete, so that effervescence ceases completely (or complete evolution of CO_2).
- Transfer the solution to a dispensing bottle, to this solution incorporate phenol. Close thoroughly with metallic screw cap and mix the content uniformly by shaking the bottle.
- In certain cases, if the reaction proceeds very slowly, then hot vehicle (water) would be used to hasten (increase) the reaction.

Procedure:

1) Heat the water, up to 60°C.
2) In an open vessel (mortar), dissolve borax in ¾th quantity of hot water. To this solution, add glycerin and mix well.
3) To the above reaction mixture, add required quantity of sodium bicarbonate and mix well. Allow the reaction mixture, for complete evolution of effervescence (CO_2).

Dispensing: After complete evolution of CO_2, transfer the content to a previously calibrated, narrow mouthed, amber coloured glass bottle and add liquid phenol. Close thoroughly with metallic screw cap and mix well by shaking. Polish and label.

Direction: To be used as directed.

Storage: Store in a cool place.

CHEMICAL INCOMPATIBILITY – CAUSING EVOLUTION OF CARBON DIOXIDE

(MAGNESIUM SULPHATE AND SODIUM BICARBONATE MIXTURE)

Rx	
Magnesii sulphatis	3 iv
Sodii bicarbonatis	3 ii
Aquam pipermente... q.s. ...	fl.oz iv
Fiat : Mistura	Mitte : fl.oz ii
Signa : Cochleare maximum, b.i.d. capiendus.	

Conversion:

3 iv → 4 drachms — fl.oz iv → 4 fl.oz

1 drachm = 4 g — 1 fl.oz = 30 ml

4 drachms = 16 g — 4 fl.oz = 120 ml

2 drachms = 8 g

Calculation : For fl.oz ii → 2 fl.oz = 60 ml

Magnesium sulphate = $\frac{16}{120} \times 60 = 8$ g

Sodium bicarbonate = $\frac{8}{120} \times 60 = 4$ g

Peppermint water... q.s. ... = 60 ml

Type	Ingredients	Quantity in imperial	Quantity in metric	Quantity taken
Chemical incompatibility.	Magnesium sulphate	4 dr	16 g	8 g
	Sodium bicarbonate	2 dr	8 g	4 g
	Peppermint water ...q.s...	4 fl.oz	120 ml	60 ml
	Make : Mixture	Send : 60 ml		
	Direction: One tablespoonful to be taken, two times a day.			

Uses: Sodium bicarbonate acts as antacid and magnesium sulphate acts as a purgative. Therefore this mixture is used in the treatment of dyspepsia. Peppermint water is used as a flavoured vehicle, to mask the saline taste of sodium bicarbonate.

Incompatibility: This prescription shows the chemical incompatibility, causing evolution of carbon dioxide gas i.e. when alkali like sodium bicarbonate reacts with soluble magnesium sulphate, double decomposition reaction occurs. This reaction leads to the formation of insoluble magnesium carbonate and evolution of carbon dioxide.

$$MgSO_4 + 2NaHCO_3 \longrightarrow Mg(HCO_3)_2 + Na_2SO_4$$

Magnesium sulphate, Sodium bicarbonate

$$4Mg(HCO_3)_2 \longrightarrow 3MgCO_3 + Mg(OH)_2 + 5CO_2\uparrow + 3H_2O$$

Insoluble magnesium carbonate, Carbon dioxide

Remedy:

- The liberated magnesium carbonate is diffusible in nature, therefore no suspending agent is required.
- The reaction mixture should be allowed to react completely so that effervescence (CO_2) should cease completely, before transferring into the bottle.
- The reaction between sodium bicarbonate and magnesium sulphate is very slow, at room temperature. Therefore to accelerate the reaction, preparation should be heated (or use the hot vehicle). But in this preparation, peppermint water is used as a vehicle. If the peppermint water is heated, it losses its flavour due to its volatility at higher temperature.
- Therefore replace the peppermint water by large portion of hot water and a small portion of concentrated peppermint water in the ratio of 3:1 respectively.

Procedure:

1) Heat the water, up to 60 °C (do not boil). Take this hot water in a mortar.
2) To the hot water, add accurately weighed, sodium bicarbonate and magnesium sulphate, slowly with continuous stirring.
3) Allow the reaction mixture, until effervescence ceases completely (complete evolution of CO_2) and allow to cool, to the room temperature.
4) Filter the solution through muslin cloth to remove, if any foreign particles present.
5) Transfer the filtrate to a measure, add required quantity of concentrated peppermint water and mix well.

Dispensing: Transfer the mixture to a narrow mouthed clear or amber coloured glass bottle, close it thoroughly with metallic screw cap, polish and label.

Direction: One tablespoonful to be taken, two times a day.

Auxillary label: SHAKE WELL BEFORE USE.

Storage: Store in a cool place.

CHEMICAL INCOMPATIBILITY – QUININE SULPHATE WITH IODIDES

Rx	
Quininae sulphatis	gr xx iv
Acidi sulphuric diluti	fl. 3 i
Potassi iodidi	3 ii
Aquam... q.s....	fl.oz vi
Fiat : Mistura	Mitte : fl.oz ii
Signa : Cochleare amplum, t.i.d. capiendus.	

Conversion :

gr xx iv → 24 grains | 3 i → 1 drachm
15 grains = 1 g | 1 drachm = 4 g
24 grains = 1.6 g | 2 drachms = 8 g
fl. 3 i → 1 fl. drachm | fl.oz vi → 6 fl.oz
1 fl. drachm = 4 ml | 1 fl.oz = 30 ml
 | 6 fl.oz = 180 ml

Calculation : For fl.oz ii → 2 fl.oz = 60 ml

Quinine sulphate = $\frac{1.6}{180} \times 60 = 0.53$ g

Dilute sulphuric acid = $\frac{4}{180} \times 60 = 1.33$ ml

Potassium iodide = $\frac{8}{180} \times 60 = 2.66$ g

Water... q.s. = 60 ml

Type	Ingredients	Quantity in imperial	Quantity in metric	Quantity taken
Chemical incompatibility.	Quinine sulphate	24 gr	1.6 g	0.53 g
	Dilute sulphuric acid	1 fl. dr	4 ml	1.33 ml
	Potassium iodide	2 dr	8 g	2.66 g
	Water......q.s.......	6 fl.oz	180 ml	60 ml
	Make : Mixture Send : 60 ml			
	Direction: One tablespoonful to be taken, three times a day.			

Uses: Quinine sulphate is an alkaloidal salt, which acts as anti-malarial. Potassium iodide acts as expectorant and also used as source of iodine. Dilute sulphuric acid is used to dissolve quinine sulphate.

Incompatibility: This prescription shows chemical incompatibility i.e. in this prescription, dilute sulphuric acid is used to dissolve quinine sulphate because, it is not freely soluble in water. When this preparation is freshly prepared, a clear solution will be formed. But after keeping more than three days the following reaction takes place,

$$H_2SO_4 + KI_2 \xrightarrow{oxidation} Hydroiodic\ Acid$$

$$Hydroiodic\ Acid \xrightarrow{Partially\ oxidised\ by\ Dil\ Sulphuric\ Acid} Free\ Iodine$$

In the mixture Quinine sulphate

+ Iodine → Herapathite / Iodo sulphite of quinine

+ Hydroiodic acid (Bronze or Olive green scales)

a) Dilute sulphuric acid reacts with the potassium iodide and liberates hydro-iodic acid.
b) This hydro-iodic acid is partially oxidized by remaining amount of dilute sulphuric acid and free iodine will be liberated.
c) In this mixture, when quinine sulphate, hydro-iodic acid and free iodine are combined together, a new compound will be formed, which is called as "Herapathite" or "Iodo-sulphite of quinine". This reaction is called as "Herapath reaction".
d) This formed herapathite deposits as bronze or olive green scales, inside the bottle. It is undesirable and preparation looks non-elegant.

Remedy: There are two methods to avoid incompability,

- To avoid the incompatibility, mixture should be dispensed to the patients in such a way that, all the doses of preparation should be finished with in three days. Then dispense this preparation as it is, without any alterations.
- If the preparation is to be dispensed for more than 3 days, then supply potassium iodide solution in one bottle and quinine sulphate and dilute sulphuric acid solution in another bottle. The patient should be advised, to mix both solutions for necessary dose, before use.

Procedure:

Method-A: For the mixture that should be used with in 3 days.		**Method-B: For the mixture, that is to be used for more than 3 days.**
1)	Dissolve Quinine sulphate in half portion of purified water.	Dissolve Potassium iodide in water and dispensed in a narrow mouthed amber coloured glass bottle.
2)	To the above solution, add dilute sulphuric acid with continuous stirring.	Dissolve Quinine sulphate in dilute sulphuric acid and dispense separately, in a narrow mouthed clear glass bottle.
3)	Dissolve potassium iodide in little portion of water and add to the above solution and mix uniformly.	**Direction:** The label on the the container should bear suitable direction to the patients that, "Mix the specific amount (dose) of the solutions before use".

4)	Transfer the content to a measure and adjust the final volume with water and mix well.	
5)	Transfer the solution to a narrow mouthed amber coloured glass bottle, close thoroughly with metallic screw cap,polish and label.	

Auxilliary label : SHAKE WELL BEFORE USE.

Direction: One tablespoonful to be taken, three times a day.

Storage: Store in a cool place.

Student's exercise:

1) Define incompatibility and classify.
2) How a Physical incompatibility is identified?
3) Explain the methods used for prescription, showing precipitate formation.
4) What are the reasons for physical incompatibility?
5) How a chemical incompatibility occurs ?
6) How a chemical incompatibility is noticed?
7) Explain the different types of chemical incompatibility.
8) Give the example for Tolerated type of incompatibility.
9) Give the best example for adjusted type of chemical incompatibility.
10) What is therapeutic incompatibility? How it occurs?
11) Give examples for prescriptions showing physical incompatibility, due to immiscibility and insolubility.
12) Give the examples for prescriptions showing physical incompatibility due to liquification.
13) Which prescription shows the incompatibility of evaluation of carbon dioxide?
14) What is the remedy for following prescription :

    Rx

Magnesium carbonate	4 g
Sodium bicarbonate	8 g
Citric acid	8 g
Purified water	240 ml

15) What is strychnine hydrochloride? What is its use?
16) Rx

Quinine hydrochloride	1.2 g
Sodium salicylate	4 g
Water... q.s.	90 ml

    Which type of incompatibility is observed in the above prescription and why?. What is the remedy for that?
17) Write short note on the following prescription :

    Rx

Quinine Salicylate	8 g
Sodium Bicarbonate	8 g
Sodium metabisulphite	0.08 g
Chloroform water ..q.s.	120 ml

18) Give the examples for chemical incompatibility associated with soluble salicylates.
19) Explain about the following prescription and give the solution (remedy) for that :

Rx

Phenobarbitone sodium	0.6 g
Ammonium bromide	8 g
Water q.s.	120 ml

20) What is Herapath reaction? How it occurs?
21) How can you solve the prescription showing Herapath reaction?
22) Which are the different methods used to correct the physical incompatibilities ?
23) What is the difference between tolerated and adjusted type of incompatibilities?
24) Explain the various reasons, which are responsible for therapeutic incompatibilities.

:SYNONYMS:

Sr.no	Name of the Experiments	Synonym
1.	Phenobarbitone elixir U.S.P	Elixir of Luminal
2.	Tolu syrup	Balsam of tolu syrup
3.	Lemon syrup	Citric acid syrup
4.	Compound ferrous sulphate syrup B.P.C	Parrish's food
5.	Compound Iodine throat paint	Mandl's paint
6.	Aluminium acetate ear drops	Barow's solution
7.	Zinc sulphate – Sulphurated potash lotion	White lotion N.F
8.	Crystal violet and Brilliant green paint	Corn solvent
9.	Aqueous iodine solution I.P.	Lugol's solution
10.	Weak iodine solution I.P.	Iodine tincture
11.	Cresol with soap solution	Lysol
12.	Chlorxylenol solution B.P.C	Roxenol
13.	Magnesium hydroxide mixture B.P	Milk of Magnesia **or** Cream of magnesia **or** Magnesium hydroxide oral suspension
14.	Arachis oil emulsion	Ground nut oil emulsion **or** Peanut oil emulsion
15.	Liquid paraffin emulsion B.P	Liquid paraffin oral emulsion
16.	Calcium soap emulsion	Lime cream **or** Calamine zinc oxide lime cream
17.	Oily calamine lotion B.P	Calamine soap emulsion **or** Lime cream
18.	Hydrocarbon ointment base	Paraffin ointment **or** Oleogenous base **or** Fatty base
19.	Emulsifying ointment B.P	Emulsion base
20.	Compound benzoic acid ointment	Whitfield's ointment
21.	Compound iodine ointment	Non-staining iodine ointment
22.	Vanishing cream	Foundation cream
23.	Zinc gelatin paste	Unna's paste
24.	Zinc salicylic acid paste	Lassar's paste
25.	Compound aluminium paste B.P.C	Baltimore paste
26.	Compound Rhubarb powder B.P.C	Gregory's powder
27.	Effervescent compound powder B.P.C	Seidlitz powder
28.	Formaldehyde Lozenges	Formalin throat tablets
29.	Liquorice Lozenges B.P.C	Brompton cough lozenges

DEFINITIONS

1) **Abrasion :** Rubbing of the surface of the skin or mucous membrane due to some mechanical injury (or removal of epidermis of skin or mucous membrane).
2) **Abscess :** A localized collection of pus, formed by tissue disintegration and surrounded by inflammation.
3) **Acne :** An inflammatory disease of the skin, with the formation of an eruption of pimples or pastules.
4) **Acrid taste :** Sharp or biting to the taste.
5) **Anaesthetic :** Drugs producing insensibility to the (external impressions) touch or pain OR An agent that produce loss of sensation of pain. It may be a local or general.
6) **Analgesics:** Agents that relieve the pain by depressing sensory nerve centers or reducing conductivity of nerve fibers. (Drugs that relieve the pain without loss of consciousness.)
7) **Anemia :** A condition of inadequate RBC's or hemoglobin in the blood.
8) **Anodyne:** An agent which relieves the pain, but it is milder than analgesic.
9) **Antacid :** An agent that neutralizes hyper-acid conditions of stomach OR An agent which counter act acidity.
10) **Antacid :** An agent that reduces or neutralizes the activity of the gastric juice.
11) **Anthelmintic :** Substance used to expel the worms, out of intestine like threadworms, tapeworms, round worms.
12) **Antibacterial :** An agent which destroys or suppress the growth or reproduction of bacteria.
13) **Anticonvulsant :** An agent (drug) which checks (stops) convulsions.
14) **Anti-depressant :** A drug that alleviates the symptoms of depression.
15) **Anti-diarrhoeals :** Agents which stops, rapid passage of feacal matter through gastrointestinal tract and frequent passage of liquid faeces.
16) **Antidote :** An agent which acts against poison by physical, chemical or physiological means or An agent, which counteract the poison.
17) **Antiemetic :** The drug which prevents or reduces nausea and vomiting.
18) **Antifungal :** An agent, antagonizing the fungal growth.
19) **Antihistamines :** Drugs having an histamine antagonistic action. These are used in the treatment of allergy.
20) **Anti-histaminic :** Relating to drugs, which antagonize the action of histamine.
21) **Anti-Infective :** Drug which counteract the infection
22) **Anti-Inflammatory :** Agents which counteracts or suppress inflammation.
23) **Antiprotozal :** An agent which destroys the protozoa.
24) **Anti-pruretic :** An agent which relieves or prevents itching.
25) **Antipyretic :** A drug which reduces body temperature (fever).
26) **Anti-rheumatic :** An agent which prevents or relieves the rheumatism symptoms like stiffness or swelling of muscles and joints with pain.
27) **Antiseptic** : An agent used to check (inhibit) the growth or development of microorganisms on living tissue.

28) **Antispasmodic :** The drug which prevent or relieve spasm of voluntary or involuntary muscles.

29) **Antitussive :** The drug which is effective against cough (Agents that prevents or relieves the cough.)

30) **Appetizer :** Drug or substance, which stimulates appetite (desire of food).

31) **Arthralgia :** Pain in joints.

32) **Arthritis :** A chronic systemic disease, primarily of the joints.

33) **Arthritis :** Inflammation of the joints (Rheumatoid arthritis).

34) **Asthma :** Breathing problem accompanied by wheezing caused, by a spasm of the bronchial tube or by swelling of mucous membrane.

35) **Astringent :** An agent, which precipitates the proteins and causes contraction of tissues, thereby checking or diminishing the bleeding or excessive discharge.

36) **Bactericide :** A chemical substance (agent) used to kill bacteria OR Agent which is capable of killing bacteria.

37) **Bacteriostatic :** Agent which inhibits the bacterial growth, without killing the bacteria.

38) **Bitter tonics :** Drugs which have bitter taste and used as appetizer.

39) **Bowel :** The Intestine

40) **Bronchial asthma :** A chronic syndrome characterized by breathlessness, resulting from bronchial spasm and wheezing.

41) **Bronchitis :** Inflammation of bronchi (bronchial mucous membrane)

42) **Bronchodilator :** Agents which dilates the bronchi OR Agent causing an increase in lumen of the bronchial tube.

43) **Calluses :** Localized hyperplasia of the horny layer of the epidermis due to friction.

44) **Calomel :** Mercurous chloride.

45) **Carminative :** A substance which removes excessive gas from the G.I.T. (agents used to relief of fluctulance).

46) **Cathartic :** An active purgative, usually producing severe evacuation, which may or may not be accompanied with pain. or An agent causing active movement of bowels (powerful purgative to hasten emptying) (Drugs used to promote defaecation).

47) **Cold :** A virus infection, involving the upper respiratory tract, characterized by watery nasal discharge and sneezing.

48) **Colitis :** Inflammation of the colon.

49) **Colon :** The division of the large intestine extending from the caecum to the rectum.

50) **Conjunctiva :** The delicate, transparent membrane, which covers the front of the eye and lines the inner surface of eyelids.

51) **Conjunctivitis :** Inflammation of the conjunctiva OR Inflammation of the delicate membrane lining of eyelids and cover the eye bases.

52) **Conspicious :** Clearly seen.

53) **Constipation :** It is a condition, in which defecation is delayed and hard stool is formed for various reasons.

54) **Cornea :** Anterior external surface of eye ball.

55) **Counter irritant :** A substance which produce superficial irritation, intended to relieve some other irritation.

56) **Crystalluria :** The excretion of crystalline material in the urine.

57) **Cycloplegic :** Eliminates the power of optical accommodation by paralyzing ciliary muscles of the eye ball (Paralysis of ciliary muscles).
58) **Dandruff :** White scales cast off from the scalp.
59) **Decant :** To pour off gently the upper clear solution, leaving the sediment in the vessel.
60) **Decongestant :** Agent which relieves the congestion.
61) **Demulcent :** A substance which exerts a soothing or protective influence on the surface of the alimentary canal.
62) **Deodorant :** An agent that destroys (removes) odour, especially disagreeable odour.
63) **Depressant :** An agent which lowers the nervous or functional activity.
64) **Diagnosis :** The determination of nature of disease (Art of distinguishing one disease from another).
65) **Diagnostic agents :** Agents (substances) used for diagnosis.
66) **Diaphoretic :** An agent which produce perspiration or sweating.
67) **Diarrhoea :** Frequent discharge of more or less fluid fecal matter from bowel.
68) **Diuretic :** Substance which produce diuresis or Increases the excretion of urine by the kidneys.
69) **Dyspepsia :** Impairment of function of digestion. (i.e. a condition of pain or disorder of abdomen or chest, which may be associated with other disturbances like nausea, or impairment of digestion after meals.
70) **Eczema :** A skin disease, involving inflammation, redness, itching, weeping, oozing etc.
71) **Effervescence :** To bubble and to froth up (or excessive bubbles rising to the surface of liquid) due to production of carbon dioxide or some other gas.
72) **Effervescent :** Bubbling tending to effervesce when freed from pressure or an effective solution.
73) **Emetic :** An agent which induce or produce vomiting.
74) **Emollient :** A substance which softens and soothen the skin when applied locally.
75) **Euphoria :** Feeling of well being, optimism, cheerfulness.
76) **Evacuation :** A substance which helps in excretion of faeces.
77) **Expectorant :** Promotes the expulsion of mucous or cough from the respiratory tract.
78) **Fibrositis :** Inflammation of fibrous connective tissue.
79) **Fistula :** An unnatural narrow channel, leading from an abscess cavity such as duct of gland, anus.
80) **Germicide :** An agent which destroys germs or pathogenic microbes.
81) **Haemorrhoids (piles) :** Dilation of veins near anus (A disease has inflamed condition of the veins of the lower inflamed condition of the veins by the lower end of the bowel). It is also called as "Piles".
82) **Haemorrhoids :** Swelling at the anal region (Piles).
83) **Haemostatic :** Arresting the flow of blood within the vessels.
84) **Halitosis:** Bad breath.
85) **Healing :** A process of cure (a closing of a wound).
86) **Humectant :** A substance that is used for moistening (a moistening substance and gives cooling sensation).

87) **Hypnotics :** Drugs that induce sleep, without cerebral excitement.

88) **Ichthamol :** Synthetic, syrupy liquid used as a local skin anti-infective.

89) **Indigestion :** Lack or failure of digestion.

90) **Infection :** A process by which a disease is communicated, from the person to another person.

91) **Inflammation :** Reaction of tissues to any injury yielding redness, heat, pain and swelling.

92) **Insomnia :** Inability of sleep (sleepless ness).

93) **Intestinal colitis :** Inflammation of the colon.

94) **Intoxication :** State of poisoning.

95) **Intraocular pressure :** Pressure exerted within the eye ball due to humors.

96) **irrigation :** Washing by a stream of water (washing out of cavity or wounded surface, with a stream of fluid.)

97) **Irritant :** An agent which when used locally, produces more or less inflammation or Any material (substance) that causes irritation of a tissue.

98) **Isotonic :** Denoting solutions having the same osmotic pressure.

99) **Isotonic solution :** Denoting a solution having the same tonicity as another solution, with which it is compared (a solution which has the same osmotic pressure as that of body cells.)

100) **Isotonicity :** (1) The duality (quality) of maintaining a uniform tone or tension.
(2) The property of a solution, having same osmotic pressure as that of another solution.

101) **Itching :** Irritation of the skin (An unpleasant condition of the skin which causes irritation).

102) **Keratin :** A fibrous protein, that forms the body's horny tissues.

103) **Keratolytic:** Agent separating or loosening the horny layer of the epidermis.

104) **Kidney stones :** Granular mass composed of oxalates, phosphates and carbonates. Kidney stones are the crystalline masses, found in the pelvis of the kidney.

105) **Lachryma :** Tears.

106) **Lachrymal :** Arrangement attached to the eyes for moistening and cleaning.

107) **Lachrymal secretion :** Secretion of eye (tear secretion).

108) **Laevulose :** Fructose or fruit sugar.

109) **Lard :** Purified fat detained from hog. The sole nutrient fat.

110) **Laryngitis :** Inflammation of the Larynx.

111) **Larynx :** The organ of Voice.

112) **Laxative :** Mild purgative or an agent that acts to promote evacuation of the bowel.

113) **Lesion :** (1) Single infected patch of a skin disease (2) a circumscribed area of pathologically altered tissue (3) Any pathological or traumatic discontinuity of tissue.

114) **Lint :** Cotton fiber soft and wooly for dressing wounds.

115) **Lubricant :** Agent which reduces friction between substances or parts.

116) **Malaria:** Periodic fever, caused by the presence of certain protozoa of the genus plasmodium in the blood. An infectious disease transmitted by mosquitoes.

117) **Migraine :** A familiar symptom complex of periodic attacks of vascular headache associated with irritability, nausea, vomiting (A common condition of re-occuring intense headache).

118) **Miotic (Myotic) :** An agent that decrease the pupil size by contraction.

119) **Mucosa :** A Mucous membrane.

120) **Mucus (Mucous):** A slimy secretion derived from mucous membrane.

121) **Mydriatic :** An agent (drug) that dilates the pupil of eye.

122) **Myolgia :** Pain in the spinal cord.

123) **Narcotic :** Drug which produces sleepines or A habit forming agent.

124) **Nasopharynx :** A part of pharynx which lies above the level of the soft palate.

125) **Nausea :** Vomiting sensation (feeling that vomiting is about to take place).

126) **Neuralgia :** Severe sharp pain along the course of a nerve (Nerve pain).

127) **Ophthalmia :** Inflammation of the eye.

128) **Ophthalmic :** Relation to eye.

129) **Otalgia :** Pain in the ear – ear ache.

130) **Otitis :** Inflammation of the ear.

131) **Otorrhoea :** A discharge from the ear.

132) **Pain :** A localized sensation of discomfort, distress or agony, resulting from the stimulation of specialized nerve ending.

133) **Palatable :** Pleasant to taste.

134) **Pediatric :** Children.

135) **Pediatrics :** Medicinal science relating to care of children and treatment of their diseases.

136) **Peristaltic movement : (Peristalsis) :** Wave of concentration passing along the alimentary canal for visible distance.

137) **Pharyngitis :** Inflammation of pharynx.

138) **Pharynx :** Passage (way) for air from nasal cavity to larynx and food from mouth to esophagus.

139) **Piles :** Dilated blood vessels in the rectal mucosa forming a vascular tumour.

140) **Placenta :** The oval or discoid spongy structure in the uterus of mammals through which the fetus derives the nourishment.

141) **Plaster :** External medicinal preparation in which the constituents are formed into an ointment and spread upon muslin skin or paper.

142) **Pliable (Pliability) :** The capacity of bend or twisted easily.

143) **Poison :** Any substance taken into the body by ingestion, inhalation, injection or absorption that interferes with normal physiological functions.

144) **Poisonous :** The toxic state produced by introduction of a poison into the body.

145) **Porous :** A pore or a small opening.

146) **Potable :** Water suitable for drinking.

147) **Potency :** Strength of medicine.

148) **Potent :** Highly effective medicine at lower doses.

149) **Pouch :** A pocket like space or sac of the peritoneum.

150) Preservative : A substance or preparation added to product for destroying or inhibiting the multiplication of microorganisms.

151) Prickly heat : An itchy rash of small raised red spots.

152) Prophylaxes : The prevention of disease

153) Protective : (1) Affording defense or immunity (2) An agent that affords defense against a detertorious influence.

154) Pruritus : Sever itching.

155) Psoriasis : A dermatitis consists a dull red lesions surrounded by characteristics salivary sealing OR A common chronic disease of the skin in which raised rough red dense areas appear covered with fine silvery scales.

156) Pupil : The contractile opening at the centre of the iris of the eye.

157) Purgative : An agent that causes evacuation of the intestinal contents.

158) Pus: Liquid product of inflammation composed of albuminous substances thin fluid and leucocytes or their remains generally yellow in colour.

159) Pyrogen : A toxin that causes fever.

160) Rancid : Having a disagreeable smell or taste from partial decomposition or a fat due to oxidation.

161) Rashes : General term applied to any eruption of the skin (Temporary eruption of the skin).

162) Reducing agent : A substance that stops oxidation or loses electrons easily.

163) Remedy : Any thing that cures, palliation or prevents diseases.

164) Rheumatism : A term used for acute/chronic conditions characterized by inflammation, stiffness of muscles, soreness and pain in joints and associated structures.

165) Rheumatoid : Resembling rheumatism, associated with rheumatoid arthritis.

166) Rheumatoid arthritis : A disease characterized by pain, swelling and redness of the affected joints (is one of the rheumatic disorder).

167) Rhinitis : inflammation of the mucous membrane of the nose.

168) Rickets : A condition in infants and childhood caused by deficiency of Vitamin'D' with disturbance of normal ossification, marked by bending and distoration of the bones.

169) Rubificient : Agent causes redness to the skin. (An agent that reddens the skin by producing a local congestion, the vessel becoming dilated and the supply of blood increased.).

170) Sailogogue : An agent that promotes the copious flow of saliva.

171) Saline : A solution of salt and water having the same osmotic pressure as that of blood.

172) Saline purgative : A salt such as Epsom salt used to produce evacuation of the bowel, due to osmotic action on intestinal lining.

173) Saliva : The clear, alkaline viscid secretion of salivary glands. It serves to moisten and soften the food and contains amylase a digestive enzyme.

174) Salivation : The process of action of salivating or an excessive flow of saliva.

175) Scabicide : An agent used to treat scabies.

176) Scabies : A contagious skin disease, caused by itch mite (causing intense itching).

177) **Scalp :** The skin covering the cranium (The skin part of the head covered with hair).

178) **Scar :** A mark left by the natural separation of the organ or a mark remaining after the healing of a wound.

179) **Scurvy :** A condition due to deficiency of ascorbic acid (Vitamin-C) in the diet and marked by weakness, anemia, spongy gums, a tendency to mucocutaneous haemorrhages (OR a deficiency disease characterized by haemorrhagic. manifestations and abnormal formation of bones and teeth which is and abnormal formation of bones and teeth which is due to deficiency of Vitamin'C').

180) **Sedative :** (1) A drug that reduces excitement (2) Agent which lowers the functional activities or substances which quiet the nervous system substances, which induces sleep.

181) **Sinusitis :** Inflammation of sinus.

182) **Sore throat :** Inflammation of the tonsils, pharynx or larynx.

183) **Sprain :** A joint injury in which, some of the fibers of a supporting ligament are ruptured but the continuity of the ligament remains intact.

184) **Stain :** Any dye or compound used for colouration.

185) **Stimulant :** An agent that improves normal functions of the system.

186) **Stomachic :** A medicine which promotes the functional activity of the stomach.

187) **Sunburns :** Injury to the skin with erythemia, tenderness and blistering following excessive exposure to sunlight and produced by ultraviolet rays.

188) **Surgical dressings :** A sterile protective covering of gauge or other substances applied to an operative wound.

189) **Synonym :** A word which has the same meaning.

190) **Tonsillitis :** Inflammation of the tonsils.

191) **Ulcer :** An open sore or lesion of the skin mucous membrane accompanied by sloughing of inflamed necrotic tissue which does not tend to heal quickly.

192) **Vasoconstrictor :** Agent causing constriction of the blood vessels (Any agent which causes a narrowing of the lumen of blood vessels).

193) **Verrucas :** A common wart, a hyperplastic epidermal lesion with a horny surface and usually occurring on the dorsa of the hands and fingers.

MARKETED PREPARATIONS OF DOSAGE FORM

1. Mixtures:

Sr.no	Brand name	Active Ingredients	Manufacturer
1.	Wokadine	Providone-Iodine	Wockhardt
2.	Cetavlon.conc	Certimide 20% w/v	ICI
3.	Perinorm	Metoclopramide	Ipca
4.	Duphalac	Lactulose	Duphar-Interfran
5.	Cizoran	Haloperidol	Stadmed
6.	Fepanil	Paracetcmol	Citadel
7.	Tinavate	Tolnaftate	Dabur

2. Elixirs:

Sr.no	Brand name	Active Ingredients	Manufacturer
1.	Piperazine	Piperazine citrate	Burroughs Wellcome
2.	Betonin elixir	Vitamin B-Complex	Boots Pharma
3.	Etophylate elixir	Etophylline	Walter Bushnell
4.	Caliphylate elixir	Theophyline	Cadila Pharma
5.	Asmotone elixir	Ephedrine	East India

3. Linctuses:

Sr.no	Brand name	Active Ingredients	Manufacturer
1.	Ascoril	Bromhexine	Glenmark
2.	Asthalin	Salbutamol	Cipla
3.	Avil expectorant	Pheniramine maleate	Hoechst Roussel
4.	Bronchosolvin	Guiaphenesin	Ipca.
5.	Mucosol	Turbutalin	Strazeneca
6.	Piriton expectorent	Chlorpheniramine maleate	Glaxo
7.	Codine linctus	Codeine sulphate	Infone

4. Syrups:

Sr.no.	Brand name	Active Ingredients	Manufacturer
1.	Corex	Chlorpheniramine maleate	Pfizer
2.	Crocin	Paracetamol	Duphar-Interfran
3.	Polybion	Multivitamin	E-Merck
4.	Althrocin	Erythromycin	Alembic
5	Minicycline dry syrup	Doxycyclin	Plethico
6.	Medler	Pseudoephedrine	Comed
7.	Salmodil Plus	Terbutaline	FDC

5. Mouthwashes:

Sr.no	Brand name	Active Ingredients	Manufacturer
1.	Tantum	Benzydamine Solution	Elder Pharma Ltd.
2.	Dettolin	Chloroxylenol	Reckitt & Colman
3.	Listrine liquid	Thymol & Eucalyptol	Warner
4	Providine	Providone	Stadmed
5.	Flohex	Flohexidine	Dr.Reddy
6.	Clohex	Chlorhexidine	

6. Gargles:

Sr.no	Brand name	Active Ingredients	Manufacturer
1.	Wokadine gargle	Providone - Iodine	Wockhardt
2.	Iodolan	Providone - Iodine	East India
3.	Thymoral	Methyl salicylate	Rays lab.
4.	Kemicetine	Chloramphemicol	Mac
5.	Senquel-AD	Potassium nitrate	Group

7. Throat paints:

Sr.no	Brand name	Active Ingredients	Manufacturer
1.	Candid throat paint	Clotrimazole	Glenmark
2.	Dentex gum paint	Tannic acid	Dermocare
3.	Paint of Iodine compound (Mandl's Paint)	Iodine	Alpine Pvt. Ltd.
4.	Paintex Paint	Clove Oil	Mendine

8. Throat sprays:

Sr.no	Brand name	Active Ingredients	Manufacturer
1.	Budenase AQ	Budesonide	Protec
2.	Asthalin	Salbutamol	Cipla

9. Eye drops :

Sr. no	Brand name	Active Ingredients	Manufacturer
1.	Acivir	Acyclovir	Cipla
2.	Chlormet	Chloramphenicol	Milmet
3.	Ciplox	Ciprofloxacin	Cipla
4.	Zoxan	Ciprofloxacin	FDC
5.	Oflox	Ofloxacin	Protec
6.	Milbeta	Betamethasone	Milmet
7.	Dicloran	Diclofenac	Unique
8.	Allercrom	Sodium Cromoglycate	FDC

10. Eye lotions:

Sr.no	Brand name	Active Ingredients	Manufacturer
1.	Ocupres	Timolol	Cadila Pharma.
2.	Timolet GFS	Timolol	Milmet
3.	Ciplox	Ciprofloxacin	Cipla
4.	Norflox	Norfloxacin	Cipla
5.	Flurisone	Flurometholone	Micro vision

11. Eardrops:

Sr.no	Brand name	Active Ingredients	Manufacturer
1.	Candibootic	Clotrimazole	Glenmark
2.	Betnesol	Betamethasone	Glaxo Smithkline
3.	Confiox ear drops	Ciprofloxacin	Concept
4.	Garamycin	Gentamicin	Fulford
5.	Phytoral	Ketoconazole	Brown & Burk
6.	Biomycetin	Chloramphenicol	Juggat

12. Eardrops:

Sr.no	Brand name	Active Ingredients	Manufacturer
1.	Candibootic	Clotrimazole	Glenmark

13. Nasal drops:

Sr.no	Brand name	Active Ingredients	Manufacturer
1.	Chromotop	Sodium Cromoglycate	Astra Zeneca
2.	Nasivion	Oxymetazoline	E-Merck
3.	Nasomet	Xylometazoline	Milmet
4.	Decon	Xylometazoline	Cadila Pharma.
5.	Fenox nasul drop	Phenylephrine HCL	Knoll Pharma.

14. Nasal spray:

Sr.no	Brand name	Active Ingredients	Manufacturer
1.	Beclate nasal spray	Beclomethasone	Cipla
2.	Budenase AQ	Budesonide	Protec
3.	Fintal nasal spray	Sodiumm Chromoglycate	Rhone-Poulenc
4.	Healex	Polyvinyl Polymer	Rhone-Poulenc

15. Nasal wash

Sr.no	Brand name	Active Ingredients	Manufacturer
1.	Nasivion	Oxymetazoline	E-Merck
2.	Rhinocort Aqua	Budesonide	Astra zeneca

16. Inhalations:

Sr.no	Brand name	Active Ingredients	Manufacturer
1.	Chromotop	Sodium Chromoglycate	Astra zeneca
2.	Ifiral	Sodium Chromoglycate	Unique
3.	Beclate inhaler	Beclomethazone	Cipla
4.	Flomist	Fluticazone Propionate	Cipla
5.	Vicks inhaler		Procter & Gamble
6.	Amrutanjan maha inhaler		Amrutanjan

17. Douches:

Sr. no	Brand name	Active Ingredients	Manufacturer
1.	Betadine	Providone - Iodine	Win-Medicine

18. Enemas:

Sr.no	Brand name	Active Ingredients	Manufacturer
1.	Laxicion enema (0.25% Solution)	Dioctyl sodium sulphosuccinate	Stadmed
2.	Practo-Clyss	Sodium dihydrogen phosphate	Comteck Lab.
3.	Mesacol (5-Amino salicylic acid)	Mesalazine	Sun Pharma.
4.	Neotomic enema	Glycerine	USV

19. Lotions:

Sr.no	Brand name	Active Ingredients	Manufacturer
1.	Candid	Clotrimazole	Glenmark
2.	Lotril	Clotrimazole	Gufic
3.	Zole	Miconazole	Rexcel
4.	Crotorax	Crotamiton	SPPL
5.	Acnederm	Clindamycin	Abbott
6.	Betnovate scalp	Betamethasone	Glaxo Smithkline
7.	Fluticate	Fluticazone Propionate	TTK Pharma
8.	Caladrya lotion	Calamine	Pfizer

20. Liniments:

Sr.no	Brand name	Active Ingredients	Manufacturer
1.	Turpentine liniment	Turpentine oil	Grima Healthcare
2.	Turpentine liniment	Turpentin oil	Arora Pharma.
3.	Methyl salicylate liniment	Methyl salicylate	Alpine Industries

21. Paints:

Sr.no	Brand name	Active Ingredients	Manufacturer
1.	Toss Gum paint	Iodine & Potassium iodine	Ind-Swif.
2.	Candid mouth paint	Clotrimazole	Glenmark
3.	Nifugal	Clotrimazole	Biddle Sawyer

22. Official Solutions:

Sr.no	Brand name	Active Ingredients	Manufacturer
1.	Soludine	Providone - Iodine	Lincoln
2.	Wockadine	Providone - Iodine	Wockhardt

23. Emulsions:

Sr.no	Brand name	Active Ingredients	Manufacturer
1.	Agrol emulsion	Liquid Paraffin	Warner Hindustan
2.	Cremaffin pink	Milk of magnesia	Knoll Pharma
3.	Laxol-P	Liquid Paraffin	Medochem Lab.
4.	Magafin emulsion	Milk of magnesia	Reliable Lab.
5.	Phenolax	Liquid Paraffin	Rays Lab.

24. Ointments:

Sr.no	Brand name	Active Ingredients	Manufacturer
1.	Painstop	Wintergreen oil	Welable
2.	Wokadin	Providone - Iodine	Wockhardt
3.	Fusiderm	Sodium fusidate	Indipharma
4.	Supri cort	Fluconazole	Glenmark
5.	Kargan	Gentamycin	Karlin
6.	Micodol	Miconazole	Dolphin
7.	Mupirax	Mupirocin	Micro Lab.
8.	Betadine ointment	Providone - Iodine	Win Medicare
9.	Ring cutter ointment	Salicylic acid	Jagsonpal

25. Medicated Creams:

Sr.no	Brand name	Active Ingredients	Manufacturer
1.	Betnovate-N cream	Betamethasone valerate	Glaxo
2.	Savlon cream	Cetrimide	ICI Ltd.
3.	Sofradex	Dexamethasone acetate	Roussel
4.	Soframycin	Framycetin sulphate	Roussel
5.	Lobate	Clobetasole propionate	Nicholas paramal
6.	Dermatop	Prednicarbate	Hoechst marion
7.	Fluticare	Fluticasone propionate	Lyka
8.	Candid-B	Beclomethasone and Clotrimazole	Glenmark

26. Pastes:

Sr.no	Brand name	Active Ingredients	Manufacturer
1.	Emoform	Potassium nitrate	JL Morison
2.	Senquel	Potassium nitrate	Group
3.	Stolin tooth paste	Tannic acid	Group
4.	Toss tooth paste	Strontium chloride	Ind-Swift
5.	Zinc and salicylic acid paste (Lesar's paste)	Zinc and salicylic acid	Agrawal pharma
6.	Desent tooth paste	Strontium chloride	Indico Ltd.

27. Jellies:

Sr.no	Brand name	Active ingredients	Manufacturer
1.	Clomax vaginal gel	Clotrimazole	Bombay tablet
2.	Candid-V gel	Clotrimazole	Glenmark
3.	VG-Gel	Metronidazole	Lekar pharma.
4.	Gyno-Daktarin	Miconazole	Ethnor pharma.
5.	Rejois vaginal gel	Polycarbophil	Astra Zeneca
6.	Acneclin gel	Clindamycin	Themis Chemicals
7.	Lynx gel	Lincomycin	Wallace
8.	Xylocaine gel	Lignocain	Astra Zeneca

28. Suppositories:

Sr.no	Brand name	Active Ingredients	Manufacturer
1.	Dulcolax Suppositories	Bisacodyl	German Remedies
2.	Lanolax Suppositories	Bisacodyl	Bliss Pharma
3.	Cisapro Suppositories	Cisapride	Cadila health care
4.	Ciza Suppositories	Cisapride	Intas
5.	Cifomed-TZ	Ciprofloxacin & Tinidazole	Aglomed
6.	Anomex	Hydrocortisone acetate	Bliss

29. Pessaries:

Sr.no	Brand name	Active Ingredients	Manufacturer
1.	Betadine vaginal pessaries	Providone - Iodine	Win Medicare
2.	Candid-V pessaries	Clotrimazole	Glenmark
3.	Provid pessaries	Providone - Iodine	Bliss Pharma
4.	Wokadine	Providone - Iodine	Wockhardt
5.	Kemicetine vaginal	Chloramphenicol	Mac Pharma
6.	Myconip	Lactic acid	Uni-Sankyo

30. Powders:

Sr.no	Brand name	Active Ingredients	Manufacturer
1.	Candid	Clotrimazole	Glenmark
2.	Zole	Miconazole	Rexcel
3.	Wokadine	Providone – Iodine	Wockhardt
4.	Steradent	Sodium perborate	Reckitt & Colman
5.	Bismag powder	Sodium bicarbonate and Light magnesium carbonate	Geoffrey manners
6.	Prequest powder	Sodium chloride	Parke-Davis Ltd.
7.	Novamox dry syrup	Amoxycillin	Cipla
8.	Ampark dry syrup	Ampicillin	Parke-Davis Ltd.
9.	Ceff dry syrup	Cephalexin	Lupin lab Ltd.

31. Dusting powders:

Sr.no	Brand name	Active Ingredients	Manufacturer
1.	Nebasulf dusting powder	Neomycin sulphate	Pfizer Ltd.
2.	Cibazole dusting powder	Sulphathiazole	Ciba-Geigy Ltd.

32. Effervescent powder / granules :

Sr.no	Brand name	Active Ingredients	Manufacturer
1.	Eno fruit salt effervescent powder	------	Glaxo Smithkline
2.	Cetri- soda effervescent powder	Sodium bicarbonate	Abbott

33. Lozenges:

Sr.no	Brand name	Active Ingredients	Manufacturer
1.	Alex cough lozenges	Dextromethorphan HBr	Gracewell
2.	Cherana cough lozenges	Noscapine	Knoll Pharma.
3.	Dequadin lozenges	Dequalinium chloride	Wellcome
4.	Cofsits	Ginger lemon	Cipla
5.	Strepsils	-------	Boots Ltd.